Document Smart

The A-to-Z Guide to Better Nursing Documentation

Fourth Edition

Clinical Editor

Teri Capriotti, DO, MSN, CRNP, RN

Clinical Professor
Villanova University
M. Louise Fitzpatrick College of Nursing
Villanova, Pennsylvania

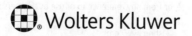

Philadelphia • Baltimore • New York • London
Buenos Aires • Hong Kong • Sydney • Tokyo

Executive Editor: Nicole Dernoski
Development Editor: Maria M. McAvey
Editorial Coordinator: Mary Woodman
Senior Production Project Manager: Alicia Jackson
Design Coordinator: Elaine Kasmer
Manufacturing Coordinator: Kathleen Brown
Marketing Manager: Linda Wetmore
Prepress Vendor: S4Carlisle Publishing Services

Fourth edition

9 8 7 6 5 4 3 2 1

Printed in China

Library of Congress Cataloging-in-Publication Data

ISBN-13: 978-1-975120-73-3
ISBN-10: 1-975120-73-6

Library of Congress Control Number: 2019943395

---

shop.lww.com

DEDICATION

I would like to dedicate this book to my grandsons, Ethan and Caleb Wolinsky.

Teri

Contributors

Jeanette M. Anderson, MSN, RN
JMA Nursing Consultant
Fort Worth, Texas

Cheryl Brady, MSN, RN, CNE
Senior Lecturer, Nursing Faculty
Kent State University
Salem, Ohio

Teri Capriotti, DO, MSN, CRNP, RN
Clinical Professor
Villanova University
M. Louise Fitzpatrick College of Nursing
Villanova, Pennsylvania

Misty B. Conlan, MSN, RN, CPN
Adjunct Clinical Assistant Professor
Villanova University
M. Louise Fitzpatrick College of Nursing
Villanova, Pennsylvania

Kim Cooper, RN, MSN
Nursing Department Chair
Ivy Tech Community College
Terre Haute, Indiana

Linda C. Copel, PhD, RN, PMHCNS, BC, CNE, ANEF, NCC, FAPA
Professor
Villanova University
M. Louise Fitzpatrick College of Nursing
Villanova, Pennsylvania

Carol A. Devlin, MSN, BSN, RNFA, CNOR
PhD Student
Robert Wood Johnson Foundation Future of Nursing Scholar, Adjunct Clinical Faculty
Villanova University
M. Louise Fitzpatrick College of Nursing
Villanova, Pennsylvania

Susan B. Dickey, PhD, RN
Associate Professor
Secretary of the Temple University Faculty Senate, 2016-18
Department of Nursing, Temple University
College of Public Health
Philadelphia, Pennsylvania

Meredith M. Greenle, PhD, RN, CRNP, CNE
Assistant Professor
Villanova University
M. Louise Fitzpatrick College of Nursing
Villanova, Pennsylvania

Gwendolyn M. Hamid, BA, MSN, RN
Adjunct Clinical Instructor
Villanova University
Villanova, Pennsylvania

Melissa O'Connor, PhD, MBA, RN
Associate Professor
Distinguished Educator in Gerontological Nursing
Villanova University,
M. Louise Fitzpatrick College of Nursing
Claire M. Fagin Fellow /Patricia G. Archbold Scholar / National Hartford Center of Gerontological Nursing Excellence
Villanova, Pennsylvania

Alanna Owens, BSN, RN
Graduate Assistant
Villanova University
M. Louise Fitzpatrick College of Nursing
Villanova, Pennsylvania

Noel C. Piano, RN, MS
Instructor/Coordinator
Lafayette School of Practical Nursing
Lafayette, Louisiana

Monica N. Ramirez, PhD, RN
Associate Professor
University of the Incarnate Word
San Antonio, Texas

PREVIOUS EDITION ADVISORY BOARD

Deborah Hutchins Allen, RN, MSN, FNP, APRN-BC, AOCNP

Jeanette M. Anderson, RN, MSN

Sharon Baranoski, MSN, RN, CWCN, APN-CCNS, FAAN

Valerie A. Barron, RN, BC, MS, CCRN

Marissa U. Camanga-Reyes, RN, MN, CNS

Kim Cooper, RN, MSN

Kim R. Davis, RN, MSN

Laurie Donaghy, ADN, RN, CEN

Christine Greenidge, APRN, BC, MSN, DHA

Kathleen M. Hill, RN, MSN, CCNS-CSC

Julia Anne Isen, RN, MS, FNP-C

Susan M. Kilroy, RN, MS

Linda Laskowski-Jones, RN, APRN, BC, MS, CCRN, CEN

Cyndie Miculan, RN, MSN, ONC, CE-BC

Nicolette C. Mininni, RN, MED, CCRN

Monica Narvaez Ramirez, RN, MSN

Lauren R. Roach, LPN, HCSD

Amanda Stefancyk, RN, MSN, MBA

Allison Terry, RN, MSN, PhD

Genevieve M. Thul, RN, BSN

Suzanne P. Weaver, RN, BSN, RHIT, CPHQ

PREVIOUS EDITION CONTRIBUTORS

Jeanette M. Anderson, RN, MSN

Marissa U. Camanga-Reyes, RN, MN, CNS

Kim Cooper, RN, MSN

Kim R. Davis, RN, MSN

Laurie Donaghy, ADN, RN, CEN

Julia Anne Isen, RN, MS, FNP-C

Susan M. Kilroy, RN, MS

Cyndie Miculan, RN, MSN, ONC, CE-BC

Monica Narvaez Ramirez, RN, MSN

Lauren R. Roach, LPN, HCSD

Allison Terry, RN, MSN, PhD

Genevieve M. Thul, RN, BSN

Suzanne P. Weaver, RN, BSN, RHIT, CPHQ

Foreword

In all areas of health care practice, complete and timely documentation of a patient's care remains a key factor in achieving positive treatment outcomes. As the number of people and disciplines involved in patient care expands, comprehensive and accurate communication among health care providers is essential. Time to document is becoming a scarce commodity. With increases in workload, the nurse needs to know how to be concise in charting while making sure crucial information is entered into the patient's record.

Document Smart: The A-to-Z Guide to Better Nursing Documentation is an easy-to-use reference covering all aspects of documentation about patient care, from the assessment of patient data to the formulation of effective patient goals and optimal nursing interventions, evaluation of treatment, and patient teaching and education.

There is specific content regarding the Health Insurance Portability and Accountability Act (HIPAA) regulations, which are essential to follow when documenting and communicating about patient care.

The text also contains information about charting in the electronic health record (EHR). Electronic health records are used across most health care settings at this time; however, individual institutions use different EHR software programs. These different EHR software programs pose a challenge for the presentation of electronic charting in this book. It is up to the nurse and other health care providers to obtain training in their individual facility to understand how to chart within the institution's EHR. This book offers examples of essential information to document; however, it is not able to demonstrate how to use specific forms of EHRs.

Document Smart has synthesized information from many sources to recommend how to deliver safe and high-quality nursing care. Recommendations for safe nursing interventions from The Joint Commission are included. Measures needed for safe administration of medications from the Institute of Safe Medication Practices (ISMP) are included. The Quality and Safety Education (QSEN) Institute competencies have also been used to teach how to perform safe and high-quality nursing documentation and interventions.

A new list of current nursing diagnoses from NANDA International (NANDA-I) is included in this book. Health care institutions vary in their recommendations for using the approved NANDA-I nursing diagnoses in charting about patient care. It is up to the nurse to review individual facility policies regarding the use of NANDA-I terminology.

No matter where the nurse practices, from hospital to outpatient to home health care settings, the nurse will find that *Document Smart* is a valuable resource for performing safe and high-quality patient care documentation.

Teri Capriotti, DO, MSN, CRNP, RN
Clinical Professor
Villanova University
M. Louise Fitzpatrick College of Nursing
Villanova, PA

Contents

INTRODUCTION

DOCUMENTATION (in alphabetical order)

Computerized and Electronic Health Records

THE ELECTRONIC HEALTH RECORD

Throughout this book there will be references to the electronic health record (EHR), sometimes called the electronic medical record (EMR) or computerized medical records. Health information technology (HIT) has emerged as a key tool for making necessary improvements in health care quality and cost. EHRs are a major component of HIT that have been advocated to enhance patient safety and efficiency of patient care. As a part of the American Recovery and Reinvestment Act of 2009, all public and private health care providers were required to adopt and demonstrate the use of EMRs by January 1, 2014 in order to maintain their existing Medicaid and Medicare reimbursement levels. Since that date, the use of electronic medical and health records has spread worldwide and shown its many benefits to health organizations everywhere. Given the current mandate requiring the use of EHRs, automated nursing documentation will affect the work of every nurse.

EHRs are real-time, patient-centered records. They make information available instantly, at the time of patient care. EHRs bring patient information from different sources together into one digital record. An EHR can bring information from current and past health care providers, emergency visits, school and workplace clinics, pharmacies, laboratories, and medical imaging facilities.

In 2003, the Institute of Medicine identified basic health care delivery functions that EHR systems should be capable of performing in order to promote greater safety, quality, and efficiency in health care delivery.

- contain information about a patient's medical history, diagnoses, medications, immunization dates, allergies, images, consultations, and lab and procedure results
- offer access to evidence-based tools that providers can use in making decisions about a patient's care
- streamline providers' workflow to provide seamless interprofessional communication

- increase organization and accuracy of patient information
- support institutional administrative processes
- assist providers provide patient education and report population health data; to accelerate the use of HIT, in 2009, Congress passed and President Obama signed into law the Health Information Technology for Economic and Clinical Health (HITECH) Act, which is part of the American Recovery and Reinvestment Act

HITECH makes incentive payments available to hospitals and health care professionals who adopt EHRs certified by the Office of the National Coordinator for Health Information Technology and use them effectively in the course of care. EHRs have been associated with reductions in medication administration errors and improved nursing documentation; nursing communication and workflow are enhanced as well. As of May 2015, more than $20.5 billion in Medicare EHR incentive program payments and $9.7 billion in Medicaid EHR incentive program payments have been made.

There are many different EHR software systems, and different types of health care settings use individualized designs that suit the needs of their providers and patient population.

The process of nursing documentation within EHRs is primarily data entry into discrete fields in rows and columns similar to a spreadsheet. Flow sheets are commonly used by nurses within the EHR. Documentation of nursing care in the EHR occurs in real time at the point of care. Patient physiologic monitors, lab results, and imaging studies are commonly linked to EHR documentation systems. This reduces the need of recording some patient care data as was done in the past in handwritten nurse notes. However, patient physiologic monitors are rarely fully integrated with the EHR, requiring nurses to manually enter some data into the EHR. Many EHR systems are still evolving to capture all the details of nursing care. It is recognized that standardized terminologies used in EHRs may not contain all concepts reflecting nursing care. Therefore, some handwritten nursing notes may still be a needed component in EHRs.

POSITIVE AND NEGATIVE EFFECTS OF EHR ON PATIENT CARE

A literature review by Waneka and Spetz (2010) on the impact of EHR systems on nursing care was found to be generally positive. Overall, EHRs are associated with reductions in medication administration errors and time spent on documentation, as well as improved quality of nursing documentation. Nurse communication and workflow seem to be positively influenced by technology as studies have identified nurse satisfaction with improved integration of technology systems into workflow processes, such as documentation, medication, and patient discharges and transfers.

One of the greatest disadvantages of EHRs is the difficulty in maintaining privacy and addressing security risks. More specifically, viable EHR systems must constantly work to prevent unauthorized patient information access that may originate from internal and external pathways. Internal threats to private patient information may result from such things as poor password management, irresponsible employees, and transparent physical security measures. External threats include unauthorized access to protected health information by hackers and theft of electronic devices containing health information (Amatayabul, 2011).

In a research survey, 7,000 nurses responded negatively to questioning about the nurses' experience with documentation requirements in the EHR (Stokowski, 2013). Some of the nurse's comments in the study included:

- I feel like a data entry clerk.
- We're "nursing" the medical record rather than the patient.
- I need a stenographer to follow me around during my work and record everything I see, discover, think, evaluate, and do.
- I "nurse" a computer instead of a patient, and it's made very clear that the computer input is more important than the patient.
- I rest easy at night knowing I didn't sacrifice bedside care to click boxes on a screen.
- In reality, we don't need to do anything at all for the patient, as long as we document that we did.
- I never thought I would see the day when a machine would need to be cared for more than my patient.

To remedy any problems that are discovered in the course of electronic documentation, nurses are encouraged to keep a list of EHR functions that they believe need to be improved. This list should be shared with hospital leadership and the information technology (IT) team responsible for upgrading, revising, and maintaining the system (Burns, Gassert, & Cipriano, 2008).

Researchers in patient safety assert that problems can occur when clinical staff automatically trust that EHR systems are working properly.

Health care providers need to be constantly vigilant regarding their documentation in the EHR. Data mistakes via copy–paste transactions often occur. Use of templates with automatic data population can be inaccurate. Recurring errors should trigger investigation by health IT specialists within the organization. The EHR is a tool that is still evolving. Mistakes and errors provide valuable lessons that both clinicians and health IT developers could use to reduce the risk of harm in the future (Rouleau et al., 2017).

BENEFITS OF EHR FOR PATIENTS

EHRs affect not only providers and health care agencies, but also patients. EHRs can enhance the patients' ability to follow their own health care plans. EHRs facilitate a patient's ability to review and re-review information contained in the record, to absorb medical information at their own pace, to question what is not understandable, to provide additional information that has not been solicited, and to report additional information. A recent study was conducted by Reed and colleagues to determine whether utilization of an EHR system could positively impact health outcomes among over 169,000 patients with diabetes. Study participants who had access to their health care information demonstrated significant improvements in their hemoglobin A1C values, lipid levels, and frequency of monitoring, particularly among those whose diabetes was not previously well controlled (Reed et al. 2012).

WHEN USING EHRS (ALSO CALLED COMPUTERIZED HEALTH RECORDS), THE NURSE NEEDS TO BE SURE TO MAINTAIN CONFIDENTIALITY

- Never share

Never give your password or computer code to anyone—including another nurse in the unit, a nurse serving temporarily in the unit, or a health care provider. Your health care facility can issue a short-term password that allows infrequent users to access certain records.

- Log off

After you log into a computer terminal, don't leave the terminal unattended. Although some computer systems have a timing device that automatically shuts off the user after an idle period, you should get into the habit of logging off the system before leaving the terminal.

- Don't display

Don't leave information about a patient displayed on a monitor where others can see it. Also, don't leave print versions or excerpts of the medical record unattended.

- Never use the organization or facility computer for personal use.
- Never document another health care provider's notes.

REFERENCES

Amatayabul, M. K. (2011). *Electronic health records: A practical guide for professionals & organizations* (5th ed.). Chicago, IL: American Health Information Association.

Burns, L. B., Gassert, A. C., & Cipriano, P. F. (2008). Smart technology, enduring solutions. *Journal of Healthcare Information Management, 22*(4), 24–30.

Reed, M., Huang, J., Graetz, I., Brand R., Hsu, J., Fireman, B., & Jaffe, M. (2012). Outpatient electronic health records and the clinical care and outcomes of patients with diabetes mellitus. *Annals of Internal Medicine, 157*(7), 482–489.

Rouleau, G., Gagnon, M. P., Cote, J., Payne-Gagnon, J., Hudson, E., & Dubois, C. H. (2017). Impact of information and communication technologies on nursing care: Results of an overview of systematic reviews. *Journal of Medical Internet Research, 19*(4), e122.

Stokowski, L. A. (2013). Electronic nursing documentation: charting new territory. *Medscape.*

Waneka, R., & Spetz, J. (2010). Hospital information technology systems' impact on nurses and nursing care. *Journal of Nursing Administration, 40*(12), 509–514.

SAFE MEDICATION ADMINISTRATION AND USE OF BAR CODES ON MEDICATIONS

Nurses must follow a series of steps for safe and accurate medication administration. Within the curriculum of nursing education, medication administration is taught in a step-by-step manner. The "rights of medication administration" are a commonly taught system for safe and accurate administration of medication. There are a few different sets of "rights of medication" administration in the literature: 5, 9, 10, and 12 rights of medication administration (Bourbonnais & Caswell, 2014; Chu, 2016; Elliot & Liu, 2010; Jones & Trieber, 2018).

The following are the 12 rights of medication administration:

1. right patient
2. right medication
3. right dosage of medication
4. right route of medication
5. right time for medication
6. right assessment of patient prior to administration of medication
7. right medication preparation
8. right expiration date on medication
9. right of patient to refuse medication
10. right of patient to understand reason for medication
11. right documentation of medication administration
12. right evaluation of medication effect

The following rules to follow are of particular importance:

- Check the patient identification bracelet.
- Have the patient state his/her name.
- Address the patient by name prior to drug administration.
- Always double-check medication order if patient questions the medication.
- Check the drug label three times before administration.

With each step in the process there is potential for error, because of interruptions, complexity of tasks, and not following the "rights" of medication administration. Medication errors in hospitals can lead to patient harm. It is estimated that one in three hospital adverse events are related to a medication. This can be a medication error, adverse effect, overdose, or allergic reaction (Office of Disease Prevention and Health Promotion, 2018). In the past, researchers found that medication errors were responsible for approximately 7,000 deaths each year, with a national cost annually of $2 billion (Institute of Medicine, 1999). Studies also estimated that there were approximately 6.5 adverse events related to medication use per 100 inpatient admissions. The majority of these adverse events were preventable (Bates et al., 1995).

Prior to institution of bar code medication administration (BCMA), studies found that the majority of medication errors that affected a hospitalized patient occurred when the medication was incorrectly administered at the patient's bedside (Bates et al., 1995).

A study by Wideman and colleagues (2010) found that the incidence of adverse drug events was highest in the medical ICU, followed by the general medical units and the general surgical units. More than one-fourth of these events were due to preventable errors.

To help prevent such errors, technology has been developed to verify medications with an electronic medication administration system using bar codes. Bar code verification technology has been used as a strategy for reducing medication errors (Macias, Bernabeu-Andreu, Arribas, Navarro, & Baldominos, 2018; Poon, et al., 2010; Wideman, Whittler, & Anderson, 2010). It does so by guiding users through the appropriate medication verification process, recording medication administration data correctly, and alerting the users to potential errors, all at the patient's bedside (DeYoung, VanderKooi, & Barletta, 2009). Paoletti and colleagues (2007) found that the BCMA system reduced medication errors by 54% and significantly improved pharmacy–nursing communication interactions. DeYoung et al. (2009) found that BCMA reduced medication errors in the adult ICU by 56%. Many investigators have found that the bar code system helps to ensure that the "rights of medication administration" in nursing are implemented (Agrawal & Glasser, 2009; Macias et al., 2018; Wideman et al., 2010).

Nurses retrieve medications from an automatic medication dispensing system in a medication room. Nurses then commonly use a mobile workstation that is brought to the patient's bedside. At this workstation at the patient's bedside, the documentation of medication administration occurs at the point of care in real time (Bowers et al., 2015).

When a nurse scans a patient's wristband using a handheld scanning device (see Figures 1 to 3), the electronic record opens to the patient's medication administration record (MAR). The BCMA software guides the nurse in reviewing the MAR and determining which medications are due for patient administration. After selecting and preparing the medications for administration, the nurse scans the bar code on the unit dose medication package. If the scanned medication matches

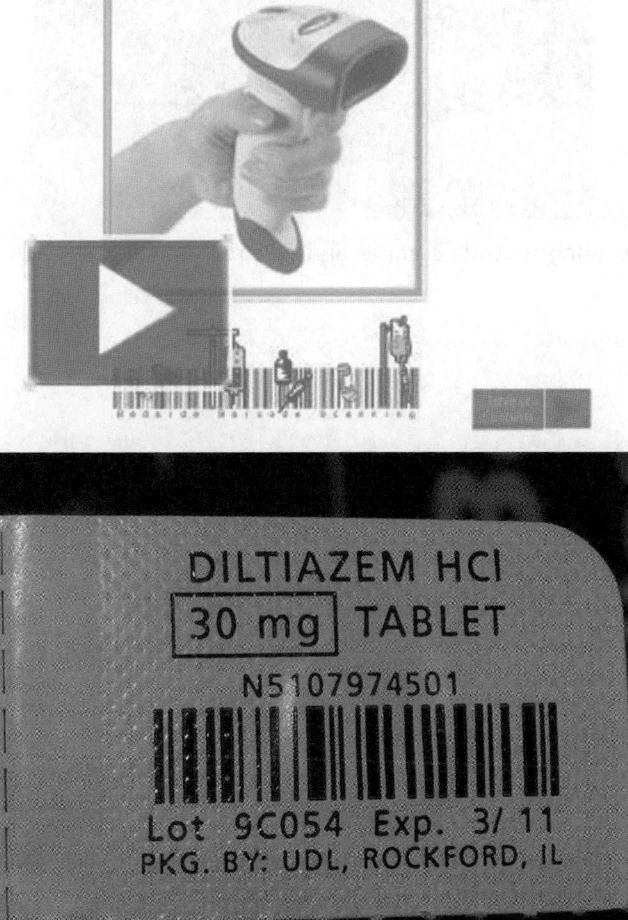

FIG 1: Barcode scanner and medication barcode.

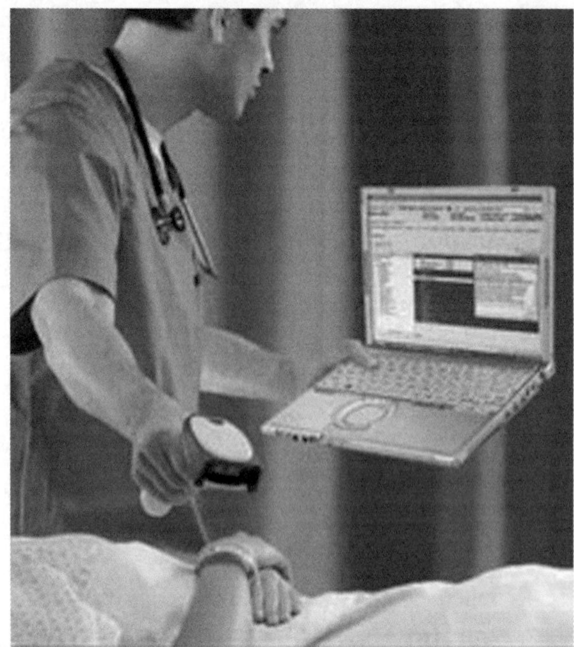

FIG 2: Nurse using barcode scanner and electronic medication administration record.

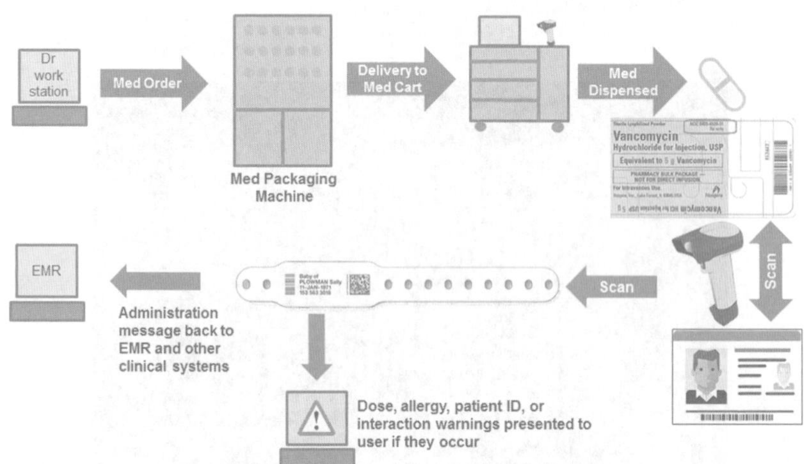

FIG 3: Barcode medication administration workflow from health care provider entry of medication order to pharmacy medication packaging to med cart on unit that contains medication to nurse who dispenses medication and uses barcode scanner on the patient to electronic medication administration record.

the medication on the profile, including dose, route, and time, the nurse completes the verification process and administers the medication. However, if the drug is not on the patient's medication profile, the dose is too high or too low, the dosage form is incorrect for the intended route of administration, or the administration time is too early or too late, an alert is generated to warn the nurse of a potential medication error (Bowers et al., 2015).

Despite increasing usage of BCMA, evidence of the effectiveness of the bar code technology has been limited and mixed. Several studies have highlighted certain unintended consequences of its implementation, with some users either bypassing this technology or relying on the technology without using nursing judgment, increasing the risk of errors (Rack, Dudjak, & Wolf, 2012).According to a study by Bowers et al. (2015), medication safety is paramount to patient care. The data retrieved during this study indicate that BCMA has the potential to be a valuable tool when used at the bedside to ensure that the "rights of medication administration" are conducted. Medication information displayed on the mobile workstation at the bedside ensures that the most current orders are being implemented. Technology does not, however, replace the keen observation of the nurse when determining the advisability of any medication or treatment. This technology is a tool that when used appropriately can enhance the ability to provide safe care (McNulty, Donnelly, & Lorio, 2009).

REFERENCES

Agrawal, A., & Glasser, A. R. (2009). Barcode medication administration implementation in an acute care hospital and lessons learned. *Journal of Healthcare Information Management, 23*(4), 24–29.

Bates, D. W., Cullen, D. J., Laird, N., Petersen, L. A., Small, S. D., Servi, D., . . . Hallisey, R. (1995). Incidence of adverse drug events and potential adverse drug events: Implications for prevention. *JAMA, 274,* 29–34.

Bourbonnais, F. F., & Caswell, W. (2014). Teaching successful medication administration today: More than just knowing your 'rights'. Nurse Education in Practice, *14*(4), 391–395.

Bowers, A. M., Goda, K., Bene, V., Sibila, K., Piccin, R., Golla, S., . . . Zell, K. (2015). Impact of bar code medication administration. *Computers, Informatics, & Nursing, 33*(11), 502–508.

Chu, R. Z. (2016). Simple steps to reduce medication errors. Nursing, *46*(8), 63–65.

DeYoung, J. L., VanderKooi, M. E., & Barletta, J. F. (2009). Effect of bar-code-assisted medication administration on medication error rates in an adult medical intensive care unit. *American Journal of Health System Pharmacy, 66*(12), 1110–1115.

Elliott, M., & Liu, Y. (2010). The nine rights of medication administration: An overview. *British Journal of Nursing, 19*(5), 300–305.

Institute of Medicine. (1999). *To err is human: Building a safer health system.* Washington, DC: National Academy Press.

Jones, J. H., & Treiber, L. A. (2018). Nurses' rights of medication administration: Including authority with accountability and responsibility. *Nursing Forum, 53*(3), 299–303.

Macias, M., Bernabeu-Andreu, F. A., Arribas, I., Navarro, F., & Baldominos, G. (2018). Impact of a barcode medication administration system on patient safety. Oncology Nursing Forum, *45*(1), E1–E13.

McNulty, J., Donnelly, E., & Iorio, K. (2009). Methodologies for sustaining Barcode medication administration compliance. *Journal of Healthcare Information Management, 23*(4), 30–33.

Office of Disease Prevention and Health Promotion. (2018, October 11). *Adverse drug events.* Retrieved from https://health.gov/hcq/ade.aspPaoletti, R. D., Suess, T. M., Lesko, M. G., Feroli, A. A., Kennel, J. A., Mahler, J. M., & Sauders, T. (2007). Using bar-code technology and medication observation methodology for safer medication administration. *American Journal of Health-System Pharmacy, 64*(5), 536–543.

Poon, E. G., Keohane, C. A., Yoon, C. S., Ditmore, M., Bane, A., Levtzion-Korach, O., . . . Gandhi, T. K. (2010). Effect of bar-code technology on the safety of medication administration. *New England Journal of Medicine, 362*(18), 1698–1707.

Rack, L. L., Dudjak, L. A., & Wolf, G. A. (2012). Study of nurse workarounds in a hospital using barcode medication administration system. *Journal of Nursing Care Quality, 27*(3), 232–239.

Wideman, M. V., Whittler, M. E., & Anderson, T. M. (2010). Barcode medication administration: Lessons learned from an intensive care unit implementation. *Advances in Patient Safety, 3,* 437–451.

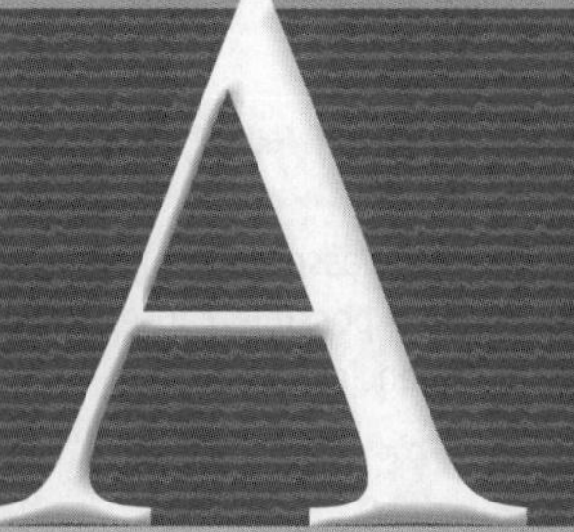

ABUSE, SUSPECTED

Abuse may be suspected in any age group, cultural setting, or environment. The patient may readily report being abused or may fear reporting the abuser. Types of suspected abuse include neglect and physical, sexual, emotional, and psychological abuse.

In most states, nurses are required by law to report signs of abuse in children, older adults, and individuals with disabilities. (See *Common signs of neglect and abuse,* page 2.) The nurse should use the appropriate channels for the facility and report his or her suspicions to the appropriate administrator and agency. Document suspicions on the appropriate form for the facility or in the nurse's notes. If the patient is a child, interview the child alone, and try to interview caregivers separately to note inconsistencies with histories. An injunction can be obtained to separate the abuser and the abused, ensuring the patient's safety until the circumstances can be investigated.

Remember, certain cultural practices that produce bruises or burns, such as coin rubbing in Vietnamese groups, may be mistaken for child maltreatment. Regardless of cultural practices, the judgment of child maltreatment is decided by the department of social services and the health care team. (See *The nurse's role in reporting abuse,* page 3.)

Essential Documentation

When documenting, the nurse should record only the facts and be sure to leave out personal opinions and judgments. Record the time and date of the entry. Provide a comprehensive history, noting inconsistencies in histories, evasive answers, delays in treatment, medical attention

COMMON SIGNS OF NEGLECT AND ABUSE

If the assessment reveals any of the following signs, the nurse should consider neglect or abuse as a possible cause and document the findings. Be sure to notify the appropriate people and agencies.

Neglect

- Failure to thrive in infants
- Malnutrition
- Dehydration
- Poor personal hygiene
- Inadequate clothing
- Severe diaper rash
- Injuries from falls
- Failure of wounds to heal
- Periodontal disease
- Infestations, such as scabies, lice, or maggots in a wound

Abuse

- Recurrent injuries
- Multiple injuries or fractures in various stages of healing
- Unexplained bruises, abrasions, burns, bites, damaged or missing teeth, strap or rope marks
- Head injuries or bald spots from pulling out hair
- Bleeding from body orifices
- Genital trauma
- Sexually transmitted diseases in children
- Pregnancy in young girls or women with physical or mental handicaps
- Verbalized accounts of being beaten, slapped, kicked, or involved in sexual activities
- Precocious sexual behaviors
- Exposure to inappropriately harsh discipline
- Exposure to verbal abuse and belittlement
- Extreme fear or anxiety

Additional Signs

- Mistrust of others
- Blunted or flat affect
- Depression or mood changes
- Social withdrawal
- Lack of appropriate peer relationships
- Sudden school difficulties, such as poor grades, truancy, or fighting with peers
- Nonspecific headaches, stomachaches, or eating and sleeping problems
- Clinging behavior directed toward health care providers
- Aggressive speech or behavior toward adults
- Abusive behavior toward younger children and pets
- Runaway behavior

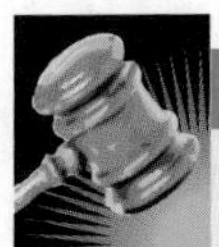

LEGAL CASEBOOK

THE NURSE'S ROLE IN REPORTING ABUSE

Nurses play a crucial role in recognizing and reporting incidents of suspected abuse. While caring for patients, the nurse may note evidence of apparent abuse. If such evidence is found, the nurse must pass the information along to the appropriate authorities. In many states, failure to report actual or suspected abuse constitutes a crime.

Because nurses may hesitate to file an abuse report because of the fear of repercussions, it is important to remember that the Child Abuse Prevention and Treatment Act protects against liability. If the nursing report is bona fide (i.e., filed in good faith), the law protects from any suit filed by an alleged abuser.

sought at other hospitals, and the person caring for the individual during the incident. Document the physical assessment findings using illustrations and photographs as necessary (per police department and social service guidelines). Describe the patient's response to treatments given. Record the names and departments of people notified within the facility. Provide the names of people notified outside the facility, such as social services, the police department, and welfare agencies. Record any visits by these agencies. Include any teaching or support given.

Nursing Documentation of Abuse

06/08/2019	1700	**NURSING ASSESSMENT:** Circular burns 2 cm in diameter noted on lower right and left scapulae in various stages of healing while auscultating breath sounds. Pt. states these injuries occurred while playing with cigarettes he found at his babysitter's home. When parents were questioned separately as to the cause of injuries on child's back, mother stated the child told her he fell off a swing and received a rope burn. Father stated he had no idea of the child's injuries. Parents stated the child is being watched after school until they get home by the teenager next door, Sally Johnson. Parents stated that their son doesn't like being watched by her anymore, but they don't know why. Parents state they're looking into alternative care suggestions. ________
		NURSING INTERVENTION: Dr. M. Gordon notified of injuries and examined pt. at 1645. Social worker, Nancy Stiller, and nursing supervisor, Nancy Taylor, RN, notified at 1650. ________
		________ **Joanne M. Allen, RN**

ACTIVITIES OF DAILY LIVING

Activities of daily living (ADLs) checklists are standard forms completed on each shift by the nursing staff and, in some cases, the patient performing the activities. After completion, the nurse reviews and signs them. These forms tell the members of the health care team about the patient's abilities, degree of independence, and special needs so that they can determine the type of assistance each patient requires. Tools that are useful in assessing and documenting ADLs include the Katz index, the Lawton Instrumental Activities of Daily Living Scale, and the Barthel index and scale.

Essential Documentation

The nurse should be sure to include the patient's name, the date and time of the evaluation, and the nurse's name and credentials.

On the Katz index, the nurse ranks the patient's ability in six areas:

- bathing
- dressing
- toileting
- transferring
- continence
- feeding

For each ADL, check whether the patient can perform the task independently, needs some help to perform the task, or cannot perform the task without significant help. (See *Katz index*, page 5.)

The Lawton scale evaluates the patient's ability to perform complex personal care activities necessary for independent living, such as:

- using the telephone
- cooking or preparing meals
- shopping
- doing laundry
- managing finances
- handling medications
- using transportation
- doing housework

Rate the patient's ability to perform these activities using a three-point scale: (1) completely unable to perform task, (2) needs some help, or (3) performs activity independently. (See *Lawton Instrumental Activities of Daily Living Scale*, page 6.)

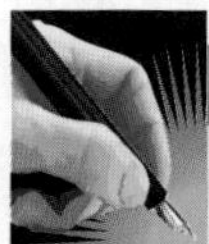

AccuChart

KATZ INDEX

Below you'll find a sample of the Katz index, which is used to assess six basic activities of daily living.

Evaluation Form **Name** Harold Kaufmann **Date** 6/1/19

For each area of functioning listed below, check the description that applies.

Indicates independence (1 point)	Indicates dependence (0 points)
Bathing: Sponge bath, tub bath, or shower. ☑ Receives no assistance; or only needs help with one area; gets into and out of tub, if tub is usual means of bathing.	❑ Receives assistance in bathing more than one part of the body or getting into or out of the tub or shower. Cannot bathe self.
Dressing: Gets outer garments and underwear from closets and drawers and uses fasteners, including suspenders, if worn. ☑ Gets clothes and gets completely dressed without assistance.	❑ Receives assistance in getting clothes or in getting dressed or stays partly or completely undressed.
Toileting: Goes to the room termed "toilet" for bowel movement and urination, cleans self afterward, and arranges clothes. ☑ Goes to toilet room, cleans self, and arranges clothes without assistance. May use object for support, such as cane, walker, or wheelchair, and may manage night bedpan or commode, emptying it in the morning.	❑ Doesn't go to toilet room for the elimination process or needs help in cleaning self or arranging clothes after elimination.
Transfer ☑ Moves into and out of bed and chair without assistance. May use object, such as cane or walker, for support.	❑ Doesn't get out of bed on own or needs assistance.
Continence ☑ Controls urination and bowel movement completely by self.	❑ Supervision helps keep control of urination or bowel movement, or catheter is used, or is incontinent.
Feeding ☑ Feeds self without assistance. Food may be prepared by someone else.	❑ Receives assistance in feeding or is fed partly or completely through tubes or by I.V. fluids.

Evaluator: Holly Sebastian, RN

Overall points: 6

6 points = Independence
0 points = Very Dependent

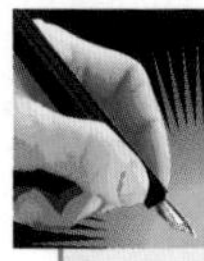

AccuChart

LAWTON INSTRUMENTAL ACTIVITIES OF DAILY LIVING SCALE

The Lawton Instrumental Activities of Daily Living Scale evaluates more sophisticated functions—known as instrumental ADLs—than the Katz index. Patients or caregivers can complete the form in 10 to 15 minutes. For each category, circle the item description that most closely resembles the client's highest functional level (either 0 or 1).

Name Martha Lutz **Rated by** Nancy Kline, RN **Date** February 13, 2019

Ability to Use Telephone
1. Operates telephone on own initiative; looks up and dials numbers 1
2. Dials a few well-known numbers .... (1)
3. Answers telephone, but does not dial 1
4. Does not use telephone at all 0

Shopping
1. Takes care of all shopping needs independently 1
2. Shops independently for small purchases .... (0)
3. Needs to be accompanied on any shopping trip 0
4. Completely unable to shop 0

Food Preparation
1. Plans, prepares, and serves adequate meals independently 1
2. Prepares adequate meals if supplied with ingredients .... (0)
3. Heats and serves prepared meals or prepares meals but does not maintain adequate diet 0
4. Needs to have meals prepared and served 0

Housekeeping
1. Maintains house alone with occasional assistance (heavy work) 1
2. Performs light daily tasks such as dishwashing, bed making .... (1)
3. Performs light daily tasks, but cannot maintain acceptable level of cleanliness 1
4. Needs help with all home maintenance tasks1
5. Does not participate in any housekeeping tasks 0

Laundry
1. Does personal laundry completely 1
2. Launders small items, rinses socks, stockings, etc .... (1)
3. All laundry must be done by others 0

Mode of Transportation
1. Travels independently on public transportation or drives own car 1
2. Arranges own travel via taxi, but does not otherwise use public transportation .... (1)
3. Travels on public transportation when assisted or accompanied by another 1
4. Travel limited to taxi or automobile with assistance of another 0
5. Does not travel at all 0

Responsibility for Own Medications
1. Is responsible for taking medication in correct dosages at correct time .... (1)
2. Takes responsibility if medication is prepared in advance in separate dosages 0
3. Is not capable of dispensing own medication0

Ability to Handle Finances
1. Manages financial matters independently (budgets, writes checks, pays rent and bills, goes to bank); collects and keeps track of income 1
2. Manages day-to-day purchases, but needs help with banking, major purchases, etc .... (1)
3. Incapable of handling money 0

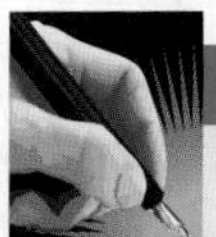

ACCUCHART

Barthel Index

The Barthel index, shown here, is used to assess the patient's ability to perform 10 ADLs, document findings for other health care team members, and reveal improvement or decline.

Date December 14, 2019
Patient's name Joseph Amity
Evaluator John Kaiser, RN

Action	Unable	With help	Independent
Feeding (if food needs to be cut = help)	0	5	(10)
Moving from wheelchair to bed and return (includes sitting up in bed)	0	5 to (10)	15
Personal toilet (wash face, comb hair, shave, clean teeth)	0	0	(5)
Getting on and off toilet (handling clothes, wipe, flush)	0	(5)	10
Bathing self	0	0	(5)
Walking on level surface (or, if unable to walk, propelling wheelchair)	0	0	(5) or 15
Ascending and descending stairs	0	(5)	10
Dressing (includes tying shoes, fastening fasteners)	0	(5)	10
Controlling bowels	0	5	(10)
Controlling bladder	0	(5)	10

Definition and Discussion of Scoring

A person scoring 100 is continent, feeds himself, dresses himself, gets up out of bed and chairs, bathes himself, walks at least a block, and can ascend and descend stairs. This doesn't mean that he's able to live alone; he may not be able to cook, keep house, or meet the public, but he's able to get along without attendant care.

Feeding

10 = Independent. The person can feed himself a meal from a tray or table when someone puts the food within his reach. He must be able to put on an assistive device, if needed, cut the food, use salt and pepper, spread butter, and so forth. Also, he must accomplish these tasks in a reasonable time.

5 = The person needs some help with cutting food and other tasks, as listed above.

0 = Unable

Moving from wheelchair to bed and return

15 = The person operates independently in all phases of this activity. He can safely approach the bed in his wheelchair, lock brakes, lift footrests, move safely from bed, lie down, come to a sitting position on the side of the bed, change the position of the wheelchair, if necessary, to transfer back into it safely, and return to the wheelchair.

10 = Either the person needs some minimal help in some step of this activity, or needs to be reminded or supervised for safety in one or more parts of this activity.

5 = The person can come to a sitting position without the help of a second person but needs to be lifted out of bed, or needs a great deal of help with transfers.

0 = Unable to sit with balance

Handling personal toilet

5 = The person can wash hands and face, comb hair, clean teeth, and shave. He may use any kind of razor but he must be able to get it from the drawer or cabinet and plug it in or put in a blade without help. A woman must put on her own makeup, if she uses any, but need not braid or style her hair.

0 = Needs assistance with grooming

(continued)

BARTHEL INDEX *(continued)*

Getting on and off toilet

10 = The person is able to get on and off the toilet, unfasten and refasten clothes, prevent soiling of clothes, and use toilet paper without help. He may use a wall bar or other stable object for support, if needed. If he needs to use a bed pan instead of toilet, he must be able to place it on a chair, use it competently, and empty and clean it.

5 = The person needs help to overcome imbalance, handle clothes, or use toilet paper.

0 = Dependent

Bathing self

5 = The person may use a bath tub or shower or give himself a complete sponge bath. Regardless of method, he must be able to complete all the steps involved without another person's presence.

0 = Dependent

Walking on a level surface

15 = The person can walk at least 50 yards without help or supervision. He may wear braces or prostheses and use crutches, canes, or a walkerette, but not a rolling walker. He must be able to lock and unlock braces, if used, get the necessary mechanical aids into position for use, stand up and sit down, and dispose of the aids when he sits. (Putting on, fastening, and taking off braces is scored under Dressing).

10 = Walks with assistance of one person more than 50 yards.

5 = If the person can't ambulate but can propel a wheelchair independently, he must be able to go around corners, turn around, maneuver the chair to table, bed, toilet, and other locations. He must be able to push a chair at least 1508 (45.7 m). Don't score this item if the person receives a score for walking.

0 = Unable to walk.

Ascending and descending stairs

10 = The person can go up and down a flight of stairs safely without help or supervision. He may and should use handrails, canes, or crutches when needed, and he must be able to carry canes or crutches as he ascends or descends.

5 = The person needs help with or supervision of any one of the above items.

0 = Unable

Dressing and undressing

10 = The person can put on, fasten, and remove all clothing (including any prescribed corset or braces) and tie shoe laces (unless he requires adaptations for this). Such special clothing as suspenders, loafers, and dresses that open down the front may be used when necessary.

5 = The person needs help in putting on, fastening, or removing any clothing. He must do at least half the work himself and must accomplish the task in a reasonable time. Women need not be scored on use of a brassiere or girdle unless these are prescribed garments.

0 = Dependent

Controlling bowels

10 = The person can control his bowels without accidents. He can use a suppository or take an enema when necessary (as in spinal cord injury patients who have had bowel training).

5 = The person needs help in using a suppository or taking an enema or has occasional accidents.

0 = Incontinent

Controlling bladder

10 = The person can control his bladder day and night. Spinal cord injury patients who wear an external device and leg bag must put them on independently, clean and empty the bag, and stay dry, day and night.

5 = The person has occasional accidents, can't wait for the bed pan or get to the toilet in time, or needs help with an external device.

0 = Incontinent or catheterized

The total score is less significant or meaningful than the individual items because these indicate where the deficiencies lie. Any applicant to a long-term care facility who scores 100 should be evaluated carefully before admission to see whether admission is indicated. Discharged patients with scores of 100 shouldn't require further physical therapy but may benefit from a home visit to see whether any environmental adjustments are needed.

The Barthel index and scale is used to evaluate:

- feeding
- moving from wheelchair to bed and returning
- performing personal hygiene
- getting on and off the toilet
- bathing
- walking on a level surface or propelling a wheelchair
- going up and down stairs
- dressing and undressing
- maintaining bowel continence
- controlling the bladder

Score each ADL according to the amount of assistance the patient needs. Over time, results reveal improvement or decline. Another scale, the Barthel self-care rating scale, evaluates function in more detail. (See *Barthel index*, pages 7 and 8.)

ADVANCE DIRECTIVE

An advance directive is a legal document used as a guideline for the medical care of a patient with an advanced disease or disability who is no longer able to indicate his or her own wishes. Advance directives also include living wills (which instruct the health care provider regarding life-sustaining treatment) and durable powers of attorney for health care (which name another person to act on the patient's behalf for medical decisions in the event that the patient cannot act for him- or herself).

Because laws vary from state to state, the nurse must be sure to find out how his or her state's laws apply to nursing practice and to the medical record.

If a patient has previously executed an advance directive, the nurse should request a copy for the chart and make sure the health care provider is aware of it. Many health care facilities routinely make this request a part of admission procedures. (See *Advance directive checklist*, page 10.)

Essential Documentation

The nurse should document the presence of an advance directive and notify the health care provider. Include the name, address, and telephone number of the person entrusted with decision-making power. The nurse should indicate that he or she has read the advance directive

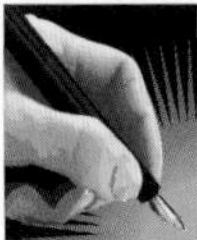

AccuChart

ADVANCE DIRECTIVE CHECKLIST

The Joint Commission requires that information on advance directives be charted on the admission assessment form. However, some facilities also use checklists like the one shown here.

ADVANCE DIRECTIVE CHECKLIST

I. DISTRIBUTION OF ADVANCE DIRECTIVE INFORMATION

- A. Advance directive information was presented to the patient: .... ☑
  1. At the time of preadmission testing .... ☑
  2. Upon inpatient admission .... ☐
  3. Interpretive services contacted.......... ☐
  4. Information was read to the patient .... ☐
- B. Advance directive information was presented to the next of kin as the patient is incapacitated.......... ☐
- C. Advance directive information wasn't distributed as the patient is incapacitated and no relative or next of kin was available.......... ☐

Susan Long, RN	7/01/19
RN	Date

II. ASSESSMENT OF ADVANCE DIRECTIVE UPON ADMISSION

	Upon admission		Upon transfer to Critical Care Unit	
	YES	NO	YES	NO
A. Does the patient have an advance directive?	☑	☐	☐	☐
If yes, was the attending physician notified?	☑		☐	
B. If he has no advance directive, does the patient want to execute an advance directive?	☐	☐	☐	☐
If yes, was the attending physician notified?	☐		☐	
Was the patient referred to resources?	☐		☐	
	Susan Long, RN			
	RN		RN	
	7/01/19			
	Date		Date	

III. RECEIPT OF AN ADVANCE DIRECTIVE AFTER ADMISSION

- A. The patient has presented an advance directive after admission and the attending physician has been notified.

RN	Date

and has placed a copy in the chart. If the patient's wishes differ from those of his or her family or health care provider, make sure that the discrepancies are thoroughly documented in the chart.

If a patient does not have an advance directive, the nurse should document that the patient was given written information concerning his or her rights under state law to make decisions regarding his or her health care. If the patient refuses information on an advance directive, document this refusal using the patient's own words, in quotes, if possible. Document any conversations with the patient regarding his or her decision making. Document that proof of competence was obtained (usually the responsibility of the medical, legal, social services, or risk management department).

Nursing Documentation Regarding Patient Advanced Directive		
7/28/2019	1000	**NURSING INTERVENTION:** Pt. admitted with an advance directive. Dr. Wellington notified at 0950 about advance directive in chart. Copy of advance directive read and placed in medical record, and copy forwarded to Melissa Edwards in Risk Management. Mary Gordon, pt.'s daughter, has durable power of attorney for health care (123 Livingston Drive, Newton, VT, phone: 123-456-7890). ________ **Carol Edwards, RN**

ADVICE TO PATIENT BY TELEPHONE

Nurses, especially those working in hospital emergency departments (EDs), frequently get requests to give advice to patients by telephone. A hospital has no legal duty to provide a telephone advice service, and the nurse has no legal duty to give advice to anyone who calls. The nurse should check the facility's policy and procedure manual to determine whether nurses are allowed to give telephone advice.

The best response to a telephone request for medical advice is to tell the caller to come to the hospital because the nurse or other health care provider cannot assess the caller's condition or treat him or her over the phone. One exception is a life-threatening situation, in which someone needs immediate care, treatment, or referral.

If nurses do dispense advice over the phone, they should keep in mind that a legal duty arises the minute the nurse says, "OK, let me tell you what to do." This creates a nurse–patient relationship, and the nurse is responsible for any advice given. The nurse who starts to give advice by telephone cannot decide midway through that the situation is too difficult to handle and simply hang up; that could be considered abandonment. The nurse must give appropriate advice or a referral.

Essential Documentation

If the nurse's facility allows telephone advice or has a triage service, there should be a system of documenting such calls—for example, by using a telephone log. The log should include:

- date and time of the call
- caller's name, if he or she will give it
- caller's address
- caller's request or reason for seeking care
- disposition of the call, such as giving the caller a poison-control number or suggesting that the caller come to the ED for evaluation
- name of the person who made that disposition

The nurse should document the information given to the patient. (See *Logging calls for telephone advice* below.)

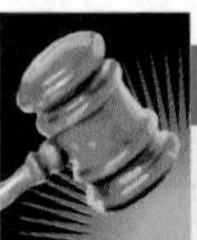

LEGAL CASEBOOK

LOGGING CALLS FOR TELEPHONE ADVICE

Some nurses hesitate to use a log to record advice given by telephone because they assume that if they do not document, they will not be responsible for the advice they give. This assumption is faulty. A patient may make only one call to the hospital, usually about something important to him or her. The patient will remember that; the nurse may not.

The telephone log can provide evidence and refresh the nurse's recollection of the event. For example, it may remind the nurse that he or she did not tell the patient to take two acetaminophen tablets to lower a fever of 105°F (40.6°C). Instead, the nurse told the caller to come to the ED. Or maybe the nurse told a young athlete to come to the ED for an x-ray of an ankle injury.

When the nurse logs such information, the law presumes that it is true because it was written in the course of ordinary business.

Nursing Documentation of Telephone Advice

11/6/2019	1615	Louis Chapman of 123 Elm St., New City, VT, 123-456-7890, phoned asking how big a cut has to be to require stitches. I asked him to describe the injury. He described a 4" gash in his left arm from a fall. I recommended that he apply pressure to the cut and come into the ED to be assessed. ________
		________ **Claire Bowen, RN**

AGAINST MEDICAL ADVICE, DISCHARGE

Patients may leave a health care facility against medical advice (AMA) because they don't understand their condition or treatment, have pressing personal problems, want to exert control over their health care, or have religious or cultural objections to their care.

Although a patient can choose to leave a health care facility AMA at any time, the law requires clear evidence that the patient is mentally competent to make that choice. In most facilities, an AMA form (also known as a *responsibility release form*) serves as a legal document to protect the nurse, the health care providers, and the facility if any problems arise from a patient's unapproved discharge. (See *Patient discharge against medical advice* below.)

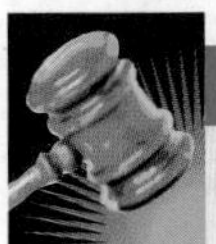

LEGAL CASEBOOK

PATIENT DISCHARGE AGAINST MEDICAL ADVICE

The patient's bill of rights and the laws and regulations based on it give competent adults the right to refuse treatment for any reason without being punished or having their liberty restricted. Some states have turned these rights into law, and the courts have cited the bills of rights in their decisions. The right to refuse treatment includes the right to leave the hospital AMA at any time, for any reason. All the nurse can do in such cases is to try to talk the patient into continuing his or her care.

If a patient still insists on leaving AMA and the facility has a policy on managing the patient who wants to leave, the nurse should follow it exactly. Adhering to policy will help to protect the hospital, coworkers, and the nurse from charges of unlawful restraint or false imprisonment.

The nurse should provide routine discharge care. Even though the patient is leaving AMA, the patient's rights to discharge planning and care are the same as those of a patient who is signed out with medical advice. Therefore, if the patient agrees, escort him or her to the door (in a wheelchair, if necessary), provide information for support services, and offer other routine health care measures. These procedures will protect the facility as well as the patient.

Essential Documentation

The nurse should have the patient sign the AMA form, then clearly document the following:

- patient's reason for leaving AMA
- that the patient knows he or she is leaving AMA
- names of relatives or others notified of the patient's decision and the dates and times of the notifications
- notification of the health care provider, health care provider's visit, and any instructions or orders given
- explanation of the risks and consequences of the AMA discharge, as told to the patient, including the name of the person who provided the explanation
- instructions regarding alternative sources of follow-up care given to the patient
- list of those accompanying the patient at discharge and the instructions given to them
- patient's destination after discharge. (See *Responsibility release form,* page 15.)

The nurse should document any statements and actions reflecting the patient's mental state at the time the patient chose to leave the facility. This will help protect the nurse, the health care providers, and the facility against a charge of negligence. Patients may later claim that their discharge occurred while they were mentally incompetent and that they were improperly supervised while they were in that state.

The nurse should also check the facility's policy regarding incident reports. If the patient leaves without anyone's knowledge or refuses to sign the AMA form, the nurse will probably be required to complete an incident report.

If a patient refuses to sign the AMA form, document this refusal on the AMA form, and enter it in the patient's chart. Use the patient's own words to describe the refusal.

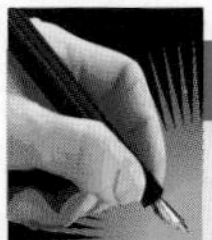

AccuChart

RESPONSIBILITY RELEASE FORM

An AMA form is a medical record as well as a legal document. It is designed to protect the nurse, coworkers, and the institution from liability resulting from the patient's unapproved discharge.

RESPONSIBILITY RELEASE

This is to certify that I, Robert Brown,

a patient in Jefferson Memorial Hospital,

am being discharged against the advice of my doctor and the hospital administration. I acknowledge that I have been informed of the risk involved and hereby release my doctor and the hospital from all responsibility for any ill effects that may result from such a discharge. I also understand that I may return to the hospital at any time and have treatment resumed.

Robert Brown	11/4/19
[Patient's signature]	[Date]
Carl Giordano, MD	11/4/19
[Witness' signature]	[Date]
RE: Robert Brown	Patient identification # 123456
[Name of patient]	

Nursing Documentation Regarding Patient Leaving Against Medical Advice

11/4/2019	1500	**NURSING ASSESSMENT:** Pt. found in room packing his clothes. When asked why he was dressed and packing, he stated, "I'm tired of all these tests. They keep doing tests, but they still don't know what's wrong with me. I can't take anymore. I'm going home." **NURSING INTERVENTION:** Dr. C. Giordano notified and told pt. of possible risks and consequences of his leaving the hospital with headaches and hypertension. Pt. signed AMA form. **PATIENT TEACHING/EDUCATION:** Discussed low Na diet, meds, and appt. with pt. and wife. Pt. states he's going home after discharge. Accompanied pt. in wheelchair to main lobby with wife. Pt. left at 1445. **Lynn Nakashima, RN**

AGAINST MEDICAL ADVICE, OUT OF BED

Even after nurses have told patients that they must not get out of bed alone and that they must call the nurse for help, they may still find patients attempting to climb out of bed or enlisting relatives to help them to the bathroom because they don't want to disturb the nurse. Either scenario puts the patient at risk for a fall and the nurse at risk for a lawsuit. Proper documentation in this situation can protect the nurse in a lawsuit. Some facilities also require the nurse to complete an incident report for a near miss even though no injury has occurred.

Essential Documentation

The nurse should record the date and time of the entry. Clearly document the instructions provided and anything that the patient did in spite of them. Record the names of any visitors or family members present at the time of the instruction. Be sure to include any devices being used to ensure patient safety, such as bed alarms. This shows that the nurse recognized the potential for a fall and initiated fall precautions.

Nursing Documentation Regarding Patient Out of Bed Against Medical Advice		
2/10/2019	0300	**NURSING INTERVENTION:** Assisted pt. to bathroom. Weak, unsteady on feet. States she gets dizzy when she stands. ________ **PATIENT TEACHING:** Instructed pt. to call for assistance to get OOB. Call bell within reach. Pt. demonstrated proper use of the call bell and verbalized that she will call for help when she needs to get OOB. ________ **Joseph Romano, RN**
2/10/2019	0430	Found pt. walking to bathroom on own. Stated she didn't want to bother anyone. Reminded her to call for assistance. ________ **NURSING INTERVENTION:** Told her nurse would check with her every hour to see if she needed to go to bathroom. Pt. agreed she would wait for nurse. ________ **Joseph Romano, RN**

ALCOHOL FOUND AT BEDSIDE

Alcohol at a patient's bedside could pose a threat to the patient, other patients, visitors, or staff members. If nurses observe that patients have alcohol in their possession, they must inform the patients that it cannot be left at the bedside and cannot be consumed without an order from the health care provider. The nurse should further explain that the alcohol must be sent home or locked up and returned to the patient at discharge.

If the health care provider writes an order for alcohol, it may be poured by the nurse and consumed by the patient at the times specified and in the amount prescribed. If the nurse receives an order for alcohol, the nurse should tell the patient that the alcohol must be given from an unopened bottle or can. Explain that already-opened bottles must be discarded. Have another nurse witness the disposal of the liquid contents. If the patient refuses to comply with facility regulations, notify the nursing supervisor, security, and the patient's health care provider. Follow the facility's policy for dealing with patients with alcohol in their possession.

Essential Documentation

If the nurse discovers alcohol in a patient's room or on the patient, the nurse should document the circumstances of the discovery. Describe the appearance of the container, the information on the label, and the smell and color of the liquid. Document the explanation given to the patient about the facility's policy on alcohol, and record the patient's response (e.g., sending the alcohol home, pouring it out under the nurse's observation, or locking it up in a designated hospital storage area). If the alcohol is locked up, then record the following in the chart:

- number of bottles
- description on the label(s)
- color of the liquid
- amount left
- names and departments of the people the notified, any instructions given, and the nurse's actions

Fill out an incident report according to the facility's policy.

If the health care provider writes an order for alcohol, the nurse should document this in the nurse's notes and transcribe the order to the medication record. Record that an explanation of the alcohol order was given to the patient and that the patient was told when the alcohol can be consumed and the amount prescribed. Document that the alcohol was dispensed from an unopened bottle, and record the information from the bottle's label.

Alcohol Found at Bedside

4/25/2019	1000	**NURSING ASSESSMENT:** Found clear bottle filled with clear liquid with label saying "vodka" in pt.'s bedside table. Bottle was unopened. When questioned, pt. stated, "That's vodka. I brought it to the hospital because I enjoy an occasional drink before bed." ______
		PATIENT TEACHING: Explained that alcohol couldn't be kept at the bedside and that he would need to send it home or keep it locked up at the nurses' desk. ______
		NURSING INTERVENTION: Dr. Smith called at 0940 and situation explained. Order given for 11/2 oz of vodka at bedtime, one drink each night, as requested by pt. Vodka bottle locked in medication cart. Also alerted nursing supervisor, Tricia Hamilton, RN, who confirmed that this was within hospital policy. ______
		______ **Kelly Nortan, RN**

ALLERGY TESTING

Allergy testing may be performed on an individual experiencing allergy-type symptoms related to an unidentified cause. A radioallergosorbent test (RAST) is a blood test performed to identify immunoglobulin E reactions to a specific allergy, causing rash, asthma, hay fever, drug reactions, and other atopic complaints. Skin testing is performed to determine specificity and the degree of reactions to allergic agents. With this test, the patient is injected or scratched with various allergens. Identification of the allergic agent will help specify the modality of treatment, such as medications or injections.

A consent form may be required before skin testing, delineating possible adverse effects and benefits. If required, check to see that it is signed before testing and that the patient understands the procedure.

Essential Documentation

The nurse should record the type of test given and the date, time, and route of testing. If required, document that the patient has signed a consent form. If venipuncture is performed, document the site and note whether a hematoma is present. Many facilities have a special form on which this information can be documented and diagrammed.

If skin testing is performed, document the following:

- type of allergen
- strength of solution
- location of injections
- size and type of skin reaction
- frequency and length of time monitored
- signs and symptoms of complications (e.g., tachycardia, wheezing, and difficulty breathing), treatments given, and response

Allergy Testing		
4/23/2019	1200	**NURSING ASSESSMENT:** Allergy testing performed for bee, wasp, and yellow jacket venom for previous allergic reaction to a "bee sting." Solutions of 1/10,000 dilution injected subcutaneously on right lower forearm (bee), right upper forearm (yellow jacket), and right lower forearm (wasp). A 2-cm erythematous area noted on right upper forearm 15 sec. after injection. No reactions noted on right lower forearm and left lower forearm. Pt. denies difficulty breathing. P 72, BP 120/82, RR 16, oral T 97.6°F. No facial edema noted. Pt. c/o intense itching and burning of erythematous site on right upper forearm. ________
		NURSING INTERVENTION: Dr. Brown notified of pt.'s reaction to injections. Hydrocortisone cream 1% ordered and applied to erythematous area. Will recheck pt. in 15 min. ________
		________ **Jane Gordon, RN**

ANAPHYLAXIS

Anaphylaxis, a severe reaction to an allergen after reexposure to the substance, is a potentially fatal response requiring emergency intervention. The nurse should quickly assess the patient for airway, breathing, and circulation and begin cardiopulmonary resuscitation as necessary. Remain with the patient, and monitor vital signs frequently, as indicated. If the cause is immediately evident (e.g., a blood transfusion,), stop the infusion and keep the intravenous (IV) line open with a normal saline solution infusion. Contact the health care provider immediately and anticipate orders such as administering an epinephrine injection. When the patient is stable, perform a thorough assessment to identify the cause of the anaphylactic reaction.

Essential Documentation

The nurse should document the date and time that the anaphylactic reaction started. Record the events leading up to the anaphylactic response. Document the patient's signs and symptoms, such as anxiety, agitation, flushing, palpitations, itching, chest tightness, light-headedness, throat tightness or swelling, or abdominal cramping. Also, document how soon after allergen exposure these findings started. Include the assessment findings, such as arrhythmias, rash, wheals or welts, wheezing, decreased level of consciousness, unresponsiveness, angioedema, decreased blood pressure, weak or rapid pulse, edema, and diaphoresis.

Note the name of the health care provider notified, the time of notification, emergency treatments and supportive care given, and the patient's response. If the allergen is identified, note the allergen on the medical record, medication administration record, nursing care plan, patient identification bracelet, health care provider's orders, and dietary and pharmacy profiles. Document that appropriate departments and individuals were notified, including pharmacy, dietary, risk management, and the nursing supervisor. In addition, the nurse may need to fill out an incident report form.

ANAPHYLAXIS		
9/11/2019	1545	**NURSING ASSESSMENT:** Pt. received Demerol 50 mg I.M. for abdominal incision pain. At 1520 pt. was SOB, diaphoretic, and c/o intense itching "everywhere." Injection site on left buttock has 4-cm erythematous area. Skin is blotchy and upper anterior torso and face are covered with

ANAPHYLAXIS (*continued*)

hives. BP 90/50, P 140 and regular, RR 44 in semi-Fowler's position. I.V. of D5 1/2 NSS infusing at 125 mL/hr in left hand. Exp. wheezes heard bilaterally. O_2 sat. 94% via pulse oximetry on room air. O_2 at 2 L/min via NC started with no change in O_2 sat. Alert and oriented to time, place, and person. Pt. anxious and restless. ______

NURSING INTERVENTION: Dr. J. Brown notified of pt.'s condition at 1525 and orders noted. Fluid challenge of 500 mL NSS over 60 min via left antecubital began at 1535. O_2 changed to 50% humidified face mask with O_2 sat. increasing to 99%. After 15 min of fluid challenge, BP 110/70, P 104, RR 28. Benadryl 25 mg P.O. given. Allergy band placed on pt.'s left hand for possible Demerol allergy. Chart, MAR, nursing care plan, and doctor's orders labeled with allergy information. ______

PATIENT TEACHING: Pt. told he had what appeared to be an allergic reaction to Demerol, that he shouldn't receive it in the future, and that he should notify all health care providers and pharmacies of this reaction. Recommended that pt. wear a medical ID bracelet noting his allergic reaction to Demerol. Medical ID bracelet order form given to pt.'s wife. ______

______ **Pat Sloan, RN**

ARRHYTHMIAS

Arrhythmias occur when abnormal electrical conduction or automaticity changes the heart rate or rhythm, or both. They vary in severity from mild, asymptomatic disturbances requiring no treatment to life-threatening ventricular fibrillation, which requires immediate resuscitation. Arrhythmias are classified according to their origin (ventricular or supraventricular). Their clinical significance depends on their effect on cardiac output and blood pressure. The nurse's prompt detection and response to a patient's arrhythmia can mean the difference between life and death.

Essential Documentation

The nurse should record the date and time of the arrhythmia. Document events before and at the time of the arrhythmia. Record the patient's symptoms and the findings of the cardiovascular assessment, such as pallor, cold and clammy skin, shortness of breath, palpitations, weakness, chest pain, dizziness, syncope, and decreased urine output. Include the patient's vital signs and heart rhythm (if the patient is on a cardiac monitor, place a rhythm strip in the chart). Note the name of the health care provider notified and the time of notification. If ordered, obtain a 12-lead electrocardiogram (ECG) and report the results. Document the interventions and the patient's response. Include any emotional support and education given.

ARRYTHMIAS		
5/24/2019	1700	**NURSING ASSESSMENT:** While assisting pt. with ambulation in the hallway at 1640, pt. c/o feeling weak and dizzy. Pt. said he was "feeling my heart hammering in my chest." Apical rate 170, BP 90/50, RR 24, peripheral pulses weak, skin cool, clammy, and diaphoretic. Denies chest pain or SOB. Breath sounds clear bilaterally. ______ **NURSING INTERVENTION:** Pt. placed in wheelchair and assisted back to bed without incident. O_2 via NC started at 2 L/min. Dr. J. Brown notified at 1645 and orders noted. Lab called to draw stat serum electrolyte and digoxin levels. Stat ECG revealed PSVT at a rate of 180. I.V. infusion of NSS started in left hand at 30 mL/hr with 18G cannula. Placed pt. on continuous cardiac monitoring with portable monitor from crash cart. At 1650 apical rate 180, BP 92/52, and pulses weakened all 4 extremities, lungs clear, skin cool and clammy. Still c/o weakness and dizziness. Dr. Brown notified and patient transferred to ICU for further treatment. Report given to Nancy Powell, RN. ______
		______ **Cathy Doll, RN**

ARTERIAL BLOOD SAMPLING

An arterial blood sample must be collected when arterial blood gas (ABG) analysis is ordered. The sample may be obtained from the brachial, radial, or femoral arteries or withdrawn from an arterial line. Before attempting a radial puncture, an Allen test should be performed. Most ABG samples can be collected by a respiratory therapist or specially trained nurse. However, a health care provider usually performs collection from the radial artery.

ABG analysis evaluates lung ventilation by measuring arterial blood pH and the partial pressure of arterial oxygen and carbon dioxide. ABG samples can also be analyzed for oxygen content and saturation and for bicarbonate values.

Essential Documentation

The nurse should document the teaching provided to the patient about the procedure and why it is being performed as well as the patient's response to the teaching. Record the site of the arterial puncture. If the radial artery is used, record the results of the Allen test. Include the time that the procedure was performed; the patient's temperature, pulse, blood pressure, and respiratory rate; the amount of time pressure was applied to control bleeding; and the type and amount of oxygen therapy the patient was receiving. If the patient is receiving mechanical ventilation, indicate ventilator settings. Record any circulatory impairment, such as swelling, discoloration, pain, numbness, or tingling, in the affected limb and bleeding at the puncture site.

After obtaining an arterial blood sample, fill out a laboratory request for ABG analysis, including the patient's current temperature and respiratory rate, the patient's most recent hemoglobin level, and the fraction of inspired oxygen and tidal volume if the patient is receiving mechanical ventilation. In most facilities, this is entered as a computerized order.

Document the results of the ABG analysis when they become available. Indicate if the health care provider was notified and whether any change in therapy was required.

Arterial Blood Sampling		
3/12/2019	1010	**PATIENT TEACHING:** Procedure and reasons for obtaining arterial blood sample for ABG analysis explained to pt. The pt. indicated that he has undergone this procedure before and had no questions. ________ **NURSING INTERVENTION:** Blood drawn from right radial artery after + Allen's test with capillary refill less than 3 sec. Pressure applied to site for 5 min and pressure dressing applied. ________ **NURSING ASSESSMENT:** No discoloration, bleeding, hematoma, or swelling noted. No c/o pain, numbness, or tingling by pt. right hand pink, warm with 2-sec. capillary refill. Sample for ABGs sent to the lab. Patient on 4 L O_2 by NC. T 99.2°F, P 82, BP 122/74, RR 18, Hgb 10.2. ________ ________ **Pat Toricelli, RN**
3/12/2019	1030	**NURSING ASSESSMENT:** ABG results Pao_2 88 mm Hg, $Paco_2$ 40 mm Hg, pH 7.40, O_2 sat. 94%, HCO_3 24 mEq/L. ________ **NURSING INTERVENTION:** Results reported to Dr. Smith. Oxygen therapy discontinued per doctor's order. ________ ________ **Pat Toricelli, RN**

ARTERIAL LINE INSERTION

An arterial line permits continuous measurement of systolic, diastolic, and mean pressures as well as arterial blood sampling.

After obtaining informed consent, the health care provider uses a preassembled preparation kit to prepare and anesthetize the insertion site. Under sterile technique, the health care provider then inserts the catheter into the artery and attaches the catheter to a fluid-filled pressure tubing that is connected to a monitor.

Direct arterial monitoring is indicated when highly accurate or frequent blood pressure measurements are required.

Essential Documentation

When assisting with the insertion of an arterial line, the nurse should record the health care provider's name; time and date of insertion; insertion site; type, gauge, and length of the catheter; and whether the catheter is sutured in place. Document systolic, diastolic, and mean pressure readings upon insertion, and include a monitor strip of the waveform. Document circulation in the extremity distal to the insertion site by assessing color, pulses, and sensation. Include the amount of flush solution infused every shift. Document emotional support and patient teaching.

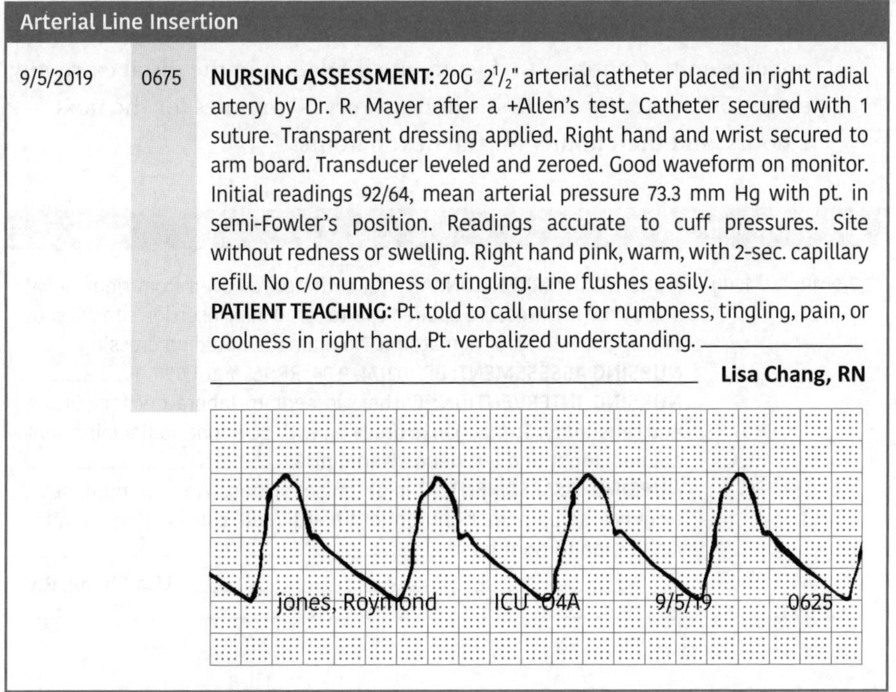

Arterial Line Insertion

9/5/2019 0675 **NURSING ASSESSMENT:** 20G $2\frac{1}{2}$" arterial catheter placed in right radial artery by Dr. R. Mayer after a +Allen's test. Catheter secured with 1 suture. Transparent dressing applied. Right hand and wrist secured to arm board. Transducer leveled and zeroed. Good waveform on monitor. Initial readings 92/64, mean arterial pressure 73.3 mm Hg with pt. in semi-Fowler's position. Readings accurate to cuff pressures. Site without redness or swelling. Right hand pink, warm, with 2-sec. capillary refill. No c/o numbness or tingling. Line flushes easily. ________

PATIENT TEACHING: Pt. told to call nurse for numbness, tingling, pain, or coolness in right hand. Pt. verbalized understanding. ________

________ **Lisa Chang, RN**

ARTERIAL LINE REMOVAL

An arterial line is removed when it is no longer necessary or the insertion site needs to be changed. The nurse should consult the facility's policy and procedures to determine whether registered nurses with specialized training are permitted to perform this procedure. Explain the procedure to the patient, and assemble the necessary equipment. Observe standard precautions, and turn off the monitor alarms. Carefully remove the dressing and sutures if present. Withdraw the catheter using a gentle, steady motion. Apply pressure to the removal site until bleeding stops, and cover the site with an appropriate dressing.

Essential Documentation

When an arterial catheter is removed, the nurse should record the time and date, the name of the person removing the catheter, the length of the catheter, the condition of the insertion site, and the reason why the catheter is being removed. If any catheter specimens were obtained for culture, be sure to document that also. Record how long pressure was maintained to control bleeding. Include the type of dressing applied. Document circulation in the extremity distal to the insertion site, including color, pulses, and sensation, and compare findings to the opposite extremity. Continue to document circulation in the distal extremity every 15 minutes for the first 4 hours, every 30 minutes for the next 2 hours, and then hourly for the next 6 hours.

Arterial Line Removal		
3/7/2019	1200	**NURSING INTERVENTION:** Arterial catheter removed from right radial site by the RN. Pressure applied to site for 10 min. Insertion site without bruising, swelling, or hematoma. No drainage noted on dressing. **NURSING ASSESSMENT:** BP 102/74, P 84, RR 16, oral T 99.7°F. ________ **NURSING INTERVENTION:** Cather tip sent to laboratory for culture and sensitivity. Sterile gauze dressing with povidone-iodine ointment applied. Right and left hands warm, pink. ________ **NURSING ASSESSMENT:** Radial pulse strong. No c/o numbness, tingling, or pain in right or left hand. Will continue to monitor circulation to right hand ________ ________ **Lisa Chang, RN**

ARTERIAL OCCLUSION, ACUTE

Acute arterial occlusion, a potentially life-threatening condition that usually develops abruptly, reduces blood flow and oxygen delivery, leading to ischemia and infarction in distal tissues and organs. The most common cause of acute arterial occlusion is obstruction of a major artery by a clot. The occlusive mechanism may be endogenous, resulting from emboli formation, thrombosis, or plaques, or may be exogenous, resulting from trauma or fracture.

After recognizing the manifestations of acute arterial occlusion, the nurse needs to act quickly to save the limb or life of the patient. Immediately notify the health care provider, and place the patient on complete bed rest. Anticipate orders for heparin to inhibit thrombus growth and reduce the risk of embolization, thrombolytic drugs to dissolve a thrombus, or both. If indicated, prepare the patient for procedures, such as embolectomy or thrombectomy.

Essential Documentation

The nurse should document the patient's signs and symptoms of acute arterial occlusion. Record the presence of any complaints of pain; include the location, intensity, quality, and duration and measures to reduce pain. If the occlusion involves an extremity, document any limb pain, the absence or presence of pulses and their strength, paresthesia, skin color and temperature, capillary refill, and any motor deficits. Assess both limbs, and note any differences. Record whether pulses were present by palpation or Doppler ultrasound. If the occlusion involves a cerebral artery, record signs and symptoms of stroke. For a coronary artery occlusion, include manifestations of acute myocardial infarction. For renal involvement, document urine output.

Record the name of the health care provider notified and the time of notification, and note whether any orders were given. Include any treatments or interventions performed and the patient's response. If the patient requires surgery or other invasive procedures, document the patient teaching as well as the patient's response.

Acute Arterial Occlusion		
11/13/2019	1250	**NURSING ASSESSMENT:** Pt. c/o pain in left leg, rated as 7 on scale of 0 to 10, femoral artery insertion site from cardiac catheterization this morning without hematoma or bruising. Moderate swelling noted in left foot and left lower leg up to knee. Femoral, popliteal, dorsalis pedis, and posterior tibial pulses not palpable on left leg. Strong pulses palpable on right leg and foot. Faint pulses heard by Doppler on left lower extremity. Pt. reports numbness in left foot with decreased sensation to light touch. Normal sensation noted in right leg and foot. Left leg and foot cool and pale, with sluggish capillary refill. Right leg and foot warm, pink, with capillary refill less than 3 sec. Normal strength and ROM to right leg, reduced strength and ROM to left leg. Dr. B. Hampton notified. ________ **Mary Donahue, RN**

Acute Arterial Occlusion (*continued*)		
3/7/2019	1200	**PATIENT TEACHING:** Dr. Hampton in to assess Pt. to undergo embolectomy. Reviewed procedure with pt. and answered his questions. (See pt. education flow sheet for details.) Procedure explained by surgeon, Dr. R. Thomas, including the risks, complications, and alternatives. Informed consent signed and in chart. Preprocedure checklist completed. Pt. scheduled for 1430. ___ ___ **Mary Donahue, RN**

ARTERIAL PRESSURE MONITORING

Used for direct arterial pressure monitoring, an arterial line permits continuous measurement of systolic, diastolic, and mean pressures. It also permits arterial blood sampling.

Direct arterial monitoring is indicated when highly accurate or frequent blood pressure measurements are required, such as for patients with low cardiac output and high systemic vascular resistance or patients who receive titrated vasoactive drugs. Patients who need frequent blood sampling may also benefit from arterial line insertion.

Essential Documentation

The nurse should document systolic, diastolic, and mean arterial pressure readings as indicated for the patient's condition or per unit protocol. Some facilities may use a frequent vital signs assessment sheet for this purpose. Make sure the patient's position is documented when each blood pressure reading is obtained. Describe the appearance of the waveform, and include a monitor strip showing it. A comparison with an auscultated blood pressure should also be included.

Record circulation in the extremity distal to the site by assessing and noting color, warmth, capillary refill, pulses, pain, movement, and sensation. Describe the appearance of the insertion site, noting any evidence of infection or bleeding. If the nurse changes the tubing or flush solution, performs a dressing change and site care, or recalibrates the equipment, the nurse will also need to document these procedures. Include the amount of flush solution infused. Infused flush solution will also need to be recorded on the intake and output record. (See "Intake and output," pages 210 to 212.)

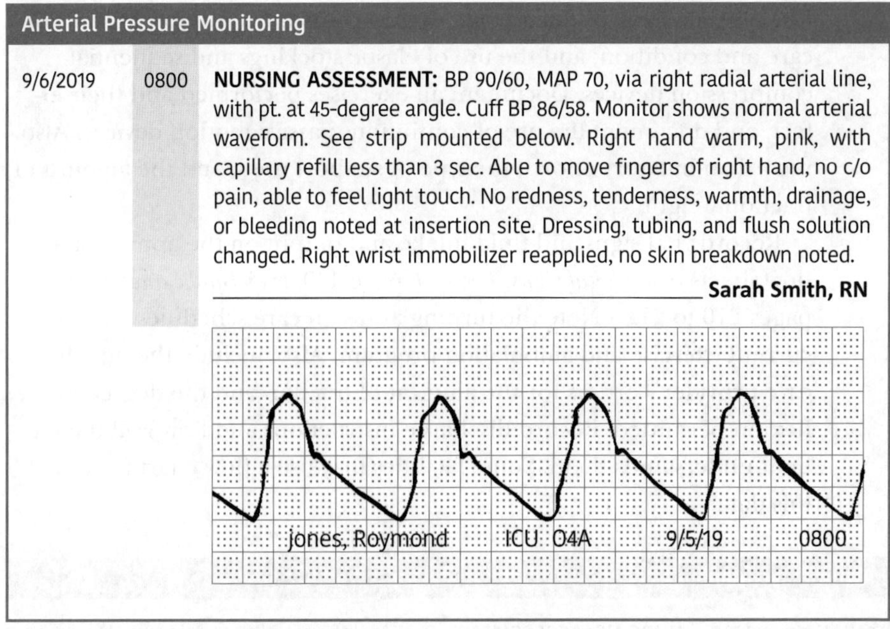

Arterial Pressure Monitoring

9/6/2019	0800	**NURSING ASSESSMENT:** BP 90/60, MAP 70, via right radial arterial line, with pt. at 45-degree angle. Cuff BP 86/58. Monitor shows normal arterial waveform. See strip mounted below. Right hand warm, pink, with capillary refill less than 3 sec. Able to move fingers of right hand, no c/o pain, able to feel light touch. No redness, tenderness, warmth, drainage, or bleeding noted at insertion site. Dressing, tubing, and flush solution changed. Right wrist immobilizer reapplied, no skin breakdown noted.
		________________ **Sarah Smith, RN**

ARTHROPLASTY CARE

Care of the patient after arthroplasty—the rebuilding of joints or the surgical replacement of all or part of a joint—helps restore mobility and normal use of the affected extremity and prevents complications, such as infection, phlebitis, and respiratory problems. Arthroplasty care includes maintaining alignment of the affected joint, assisting with exercises, and providing routine postoperative care. An equally important nursing responsibility is teaching home care and exercises that may continue for several years, depending on the type of arthroplasty performed and the patient's condition. The two most common arthroplastic procedures are knee and hip joint rebuilding or replacement. Other joints, such as the shoulders, elbows, and metacarpals, may also be replaced.

Essential Documentation

The nurse should record the neurovascular status of the affected limb, maintenance of traction (for cup arthroplasty and hip replacement), or knee immobilization (for knee replacement). Describe the patient's position, especially the position of the affected leg; use of positioning devices such as an abductor pillow; skin care and condition; respiratory care and condition; and the use of elastic stockings and sequential compression devices. Document all exercises performed and their effect, and document the use of continuous passive motion devices. Also, record ambulatory efforts, the type of support used, and the amount of traction weight.

Record vital signs and fluid intake and output on the appropriate flow sheets. (See *Vital signs, frequent,* page 430, and *Intake and output,* pages 210 to 212.) Note the turning and skin care schedules and the current exercise and ambulation program. Also, include the health care provider's orders for the amount of traction and the degree of flexion permitted. Record discharge instructions and how well the patient understands them. Some facilities may use a flow chart to record this data.

Arthroplasty Care		
11/12/2019	1800	**NURSING ASSESSMENT:** Dsg to left hip dry and intact. Hemovac drained 30 mL of serosanguineous fluid over last 2 hr. See I/O flowsheet for shift totals. Left pedal pulses strong; foot warm, pink, capillary refill less than 3 sec. Able to move toes, ankle, and knee of left leg and to feel light touch. P 84, BP 140/88, RR 118, oral T 99.4°F. Pt. reports tenderness at incision but no pain elsewhere on left leg or foot. No evidence of warmth, swelling, tenderness, or Homans' sign in either leg. Abductor pillow in place, HOB at 45-degree angle. Pt. using trapeze to shift weight in bed q2hr. No evidence of skin breakdown noted and skin care provided. Understands importance of not bending more than 90 degrees at the hip. ______
		NURSING INTERVENTION: Pt. encouraged to C&DB q1hr while awake. Assisted pt. with incentive spirometer. Able to exhale 850 mL. Lungs clear, cough nonproductive. Elastic hose on right leg removed to wash and lubricate leg; skin intact. Elastic hose reapplied. ______
		PATIENT TEACHING: Reinforced teaching of physical therapist to perform dorsiflexion, plantar flexion, and quadriceps sitting exercises. Call bell within reach. ______
		______ **Thomas Bates, RN**

ASPIRATION, FOREIGN BODY

Aspiration of a foreign body may cause sudden airway obstruction if the foreign body lodges in the throat or bronchus. An obstructed airway causes anoxia, which in turn leads to brain damage and death in 4 to 6 minutes. Abdominal thrusts (Heimlich maneuver) are used to dislodge the foreign body in conscious adults. If the patient is unconscious, cardiopulmonary resuscitation should be initiated. However, an abdominal thrust is contraindicated in pregnant women, markedly obese patients, and patients who have recently undergone abdominal surgery. For such patients, use a chest thrust, which forces air out of the lungs to create an artificial cough.

These maneuvers are contraindicated in a patient with incomplete or partial airway obstruction or when the patient can maintain adequate ventilation to dislodge the foreign body by effective coughing. However, the patient's inability to speak, cough, or breathe demands immediate action to dislodge the obstruction.

Essential Documentation

After the emergency has passed, the nurse should record the date and time of the procedure, the patient's actions before aspirating the foreign body, signs and symptoms of airway compromise, the approximate length of time it took to clear the airway, and the type and size of the object removed. Also, note the patient's vital signs after the procedure, any complications that occurred and nursing actions taken, and the patient's tolerance of the procedure. Include any emotional support and education provided after the event. Document the name of the health care provider notified, the time of notification, and any orders given.

Aspiration Foreign Body		
12/26/2019	1410	**NURSING ASSESSMENT:** While eating dinner, pt. became unable to speak or cough. ———— **NURSING INTERVENTION:** Performed abdominal thrusts X2 and pt. expelled a large piece of chicken. ———— **NURSING ASSESSMENT:** Pt. remained awake and alert. P 82, BP 138/84, RR 24, oral T 97.2°F. Total episode lasted approximately 90 sec. **NURSING INTERVENTION:** Dr. G. Compton notified at 1400. Speech therapist to see pt. to evaluate swallowing. Pt. upset about incident, reassurances given. ———— **Todd Smith, RN**

ASPIRATION, TUBE FEEDING

Tube feedings involve the delivery of a liquid feeding formula directly into the stomach, duodenum, or jejunum. Tube feeding that has been accidentally aspirated into the lungs may result in respiratory compromise, such as pneumonia or acute respiratory distress syndrome. Causes of aspiration include incorrect tube placement, gastroesophageal reflux when the head of the bed is not elevated, and vomiting caused by the patient's inability to absorb or digest the formula.

If the nurse suspects tube-feeding aspiration, the nurse should immediately stop the feeding. Then elevate the head of the bed, and perform tracheal suctioning. Notify the health care provider, and anticipate orders for a chest x-ray and chest physiotherapy. If aspiration pneumonia is suspected, the health care provider may order an ABG analysis, sputum cultures, and antibiotics.

Essential Documentation

The nurse should record the date and time of the aspiration. Include evidence of aspiration, such as vomiting of tube-feeding formula or suctioning of tube feeding from the trachea. Describe the color, odor, and amount of suctioned secretions. Document immediate actions, including stopping the feeding and performing tracheal suctioning, and the patient's response. Document the assessment of the patient's airway, breathing, circulation, and vital signs, including pulse oximetry reading, and any other related signs and symptoms. Check the position of the patient and the placement of the feeding tube, and record the findings. Note the time and name of the health care provider notified, and document new orders and actions, such as removing the feeding tube, obtaining a chest x-ray, administering oxygen, or starting antibiotics. Document emotional support and patient education.

ASPIRATION TUBE FEEDING		
3/2/2019	1400	**NURSING ASSESSMENT:** Called by pt. at 1340. Pt. reported she had just vomited. Found pt. sitting upright in bed with large amount of bile-colored vomitus on gown and noisy respirations. Immediately stopped tube feeding and suctioned small amount of thin, yellow fluid from trachea. P 110, BP 98/64, RR 32, T 100.2°F. Basilar crackles auscultated bilaterally. Skin diaphoretic and pink. O_2 sat. 89% by pulse oximetry on room air. Started O_2 at 4L by NC. Pulse ox increased to 95%. Air bolus confirmed accurate tube placement. ______
		NURSING INTERVENTION: Dr. notified at 1350 and orders received. Tube feedings on hold. NG tube placed to low intermittent suction. I.V. infusion of D5W 1/2 NSS with 20 mEq of KCL at 125 mL/hr started in left antecubital with 18G needle. Radiology called for stat portable CXR. Urine, blood, and sputum cultures obtained and sent to lab. Explained procedures to pt. and answered her questions. ______
		______ **Joanne Wilder, RN**

ASSESSMENT, INITIAL

Also known as a nursing database, the nursing admission assessment form contains the nurse's initial patient assessment data. Completing the form involves collecting information from various sources and analyzing it to assemble a complete picture of the patient. The information obtained can assist with forming nursing diagnoses and creating patient problem lists. The nursing admission form may be configured in a variety of ways, which may differ among facilities and even among departments in the facility.

Essential Documentation

On the nursing admission assessment form, the nurse should record the nursing observations, the patient's perception of his or her health problems, the patient's health history, and the physical examination findings. Include data on the patient's current use of prescription and over-the-counter drugs and herbs; allergies to foods, drugs, and other substances; ability to perform ADLs; support systems; cultural and religious information; the patient's expectations of treatment; and documentation of the patient's advance directive, if the patient has one. Depending on the form, the nurse may fill in blanks, check off boxes, or write narrative notes. Some facilities separate admission information into two forms: an admission history and an admission physical assessment. Most facilities require that this information be documented within the first 24 hours of admission.

For an example of a completed initial assessment, see *Completing the nursing admission assessment* on page 32.

ASTHMA

Asthma is a chronic inflammatory airway disorder characterized by airflow obstruction and airway hyperresponsiveness to various stimuli. It is a type of chronic obstructive pulmonary disease marked by increased airflow resistance. The widespread but variable airflow obstruction seen in asthma is caused by bronchospasm, edema of the airway mucosa, and increased mucus production.

The best treatment for asthma is prevention by identifying and avoiding precipitating factors, such as environmental allergens or irritants, and taking drugs to block the acute obstructive effects of antigen exposure. Usually, such stimuli cannot be removed entirely, so desensitization to specific antigens may be helpful, especially in children. If a patient is

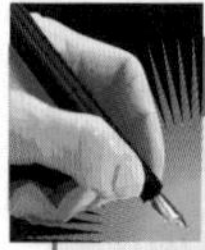

AccuChart

COMPLETING THE NURSING ADMISSION ASSESSMENT

Most health care facilities use a combined checklist and narrative admission form such as the one shown here. The nursing admission assessment becomes a part of the patient's permanent medical record.

ADMISSION DOCUMENT

(To be completed on or before admission by admitting RN)

Name: David Connors
Age: 88
Birth date: 4/15/31
Address: 3401 Elmhurst Ave. Jenkintown, PA
Hospital I.D. No.: 4227
Insurer: Aetna
Policy No.: 605310P
Physician: Joseph Milstein
Admission date: 4/28/19

Preoperative teaching according to standard?
☑ Yes ❑ No

Preoperative teaching completed on 4/28/19

If no, h Surgery not planned
h Emergency surgery

Signature Kate McCauley, RN

T 101°F P 120 R 24
BP (Lying/sitting) Left: 124/66
Right: 120/68
Height 5′7″
Weight 160
Pulses:
L: P Radial P DP P PT
R: P Radial P DP P PT
Apical pulse 120
☑ Regular ❑ Irregular
P = Palpable D = Doppler O = Absent

Admitted from:
❑ Emergency department
☑ Home
❑ Doctor's office
❑ Transfer from ______

Mode:
❑ Ambulatory
☑ Wheelchair
❑ Stretcher
Accompanied by: wife

Signature Kate McCauley, RN

Medical and surgical history

Check (P) if patient or (R) if a blood relative has had any of the following. Check (H) if patient has ever been hospitalized. If it isn't appropriate to question patient because of age or sex, cross out option, for example, ~~infertility~~.

	(R)	(P)	(H)	Interviewer comments
Addictions (e.g.,alcohol, drugs)	❑	❑	❑	
Angina	❑	❑	❑	
Arthritis	❑	❑	❑	
Asthma	❑	☑	☑	lungs clear
Bleeding problems	❑	❑	❑	
Blood clot	❑	❑	❑	
Cancer	❑	❑	❑	
Counseling	❑	❑	❑	
CVA	❑	❑	❑	
Depression	❑	❑	❑	
Diabetes	☑	❑	❑	
Eating disorders	❑	❑	❑	
Epilepsy	❑	❑	❑	
Eye problems (not glasses)	❑	❑	❑	
Fainting	❑	❑	❑	
Fractures	❑	❑	❑	
Genetic condition	❑	❑	❑	
Glaucoma	❑	❑	❑	
Gout	❑	❑	❑	
Headaches	❑	❑	❑	
Hepatitis	❑	❑	❑	
High cholesterol	❑	☑	❑	
Hypertension	❑	❑	❑	
~~Infertility~~	❑	❑	❑	
Kidney disease/ stones	❑	❑	❑	
Leukemia	❑	❑	❑	
Memory loss	❑	❑	❑	
Mood swings	❑	❑	❑	
Myocardial infarction	❑	❑	❑	
Prostate problems	❑	❑	❑	
Rheumatic fever	❑	❑	❑	
Sexually trans. disease	❑	❑	❑	
Thyroid problems	❑	❑	❑	
TB or positive test	❑	❑	❑	
Other	❑	❑	❑	

List any surgeries the patient has had:
Date Type of surgery

Has the patient ever had a blood
transfusion: ❑ Y ☑ N
reaction: ❑ Y ❑ N

COMPLETING THE NURSING ADMISSION ASSESSMENT *(continued)*

UNIT INTRODUCTIO

Patient rights given to patient:	☑ Y	❑ N	Patient valuables:	Patient meds:
Patient verbalizes understanding:	☑ Y	❑ N	☑ Sent home	☑ Sent home
☑Patient ☑Family oriented to:			❑ Placed in safe	❑ Placed in pharmacy
Nurse call system/unit policies:	☑ Y	❑ N	❑ None on admission	❑ None on admission
Smoking/visiting policy/intercom/ siderails/TV channels:	☑ Y	❑ N		

Allergies or reactions

Medications/dyes	☑ Y	❑ N	PCN
Anesthesia drugs	❑ Y	☑ N	
Foods	❑ Y	☑ N	
Environmental (for example, tape, latex, bee stings, dust, pollen, animals, etc.)	☑ Y	❑ N	dust, pollen, cats

Advance Directive Information

1. Does patient have health care power of attorney? ______ ❑ Y ☑ N
   Name ______ Phone ______
   If yes, request copy from patient/family and place in chart. Date done:______ Init. ______
2. Does patient have a living will? ☑ Y ❑ N
3. Educational booklet given to patient/family? ☑ Y ❑ N
4. Advise attending physician if there is a living will or power of attorney ☑ Y ❑ N

Organ and tissue donation

1. Has patient signed an organ and/or tissue donor card? ☑ Y ❑ N
   If yes, request information and place in chart. Date done: 4/28/19
   If no, would patient like to know more about the subject of donation? ❑ Y ❑ N
2. Has patient discussed his wishes with family? ☑ Y ❑ N

Medications

		Reason	Dose	Last time taken
1.	Proventil	asthma	2 puffs q4hr	4/27/19
2.	Tylenol	pain	650 mg	Unknown
3.	Multivitamin	N/A	1 Tablet	4/27/19
4.				

Signature Kate McCauley, RN Date 4/28/19

having an acute asthma attack, the nurse's prompt recognition of respiratory distress is essential to reversing the airway obstruction and possibly preventing death. Expect to administer low-flow humidified oxygen and drugs to decrease bronchoconstriction, reduce bronchial airway edema and inflammation, and increase pulmonary ventilation.

Essential Documentation

The nurse should record the date and time of the entry. Include the assessment findings, such as wheezing, diminished breath sounds, prolonged expiration, coughing, dyspnea, use of accessory respiratory muscles, tachycardia, tachypnea, anxiety, apprehension, and cyanosis. Document vital signs, including pulse oximetry reading.

Document the name of the health care provider notified, the time of the notification, and the orders given, such as supplemental oxygen, bronchodilators, corticosteroids, pulmonary function tests, chest x-rays, and ABG analysis.

Document the nursing actions and the patient's response to these therapies. Use the appropriate flow sheets to record intake and output, vital signs, IV fluids given, positioning, drugs administered, pulse oximetry, and characteristics of cough and breath sounds. Record the patient teaching provided, such as details about the disease process and preventing an acute attack, treatments, drugs, signs and symptoms to report, pursed-lip and diaphragmatic breathing, and the use of respiratory equipment. Include emotional support given to the patient and family.

Asthma		
3/12/2019	0840	**NURSING ASSESSMENT:** Pt. c/o difficulty breathing at 0825 while washing. Pt. sitting upright, using accessory muscles for breathing, nasal flaring and circumoral cyanosis noted. Pt. appeared restless and apprehensive and only able to speak 2 or 3 words at a time. P 124, BP 140/86, RR 36, ax temp 97.2°F, pulse ox. on room air 87%. Breath sounds diminished with expiratory auscultated bilaterally, expiration longer than inspiration. ______
		NURSING INTERVENTION: Dr. F. Cartwright notified of pt.'s respiratory distress and assessment findings at 0830 and came to see pt. and orders given. Humidified O_2 started at 2 L by NC. Albuterol 2.5 mg given via nebulizer. Encouraged slow deep breaths through nose and exhalations through pursed lips. ______
		NURSING ASSESSMENT: Within 10 min, P 92, BP 128/84, RR 24, pulse ox. 96%, lungs clear to auscultation bilaterally. Pt. breathing easier without use of accessory muscles. ______
		PATIENT TEACHING: Reinforced use of diaphragmatic and pursed-lip breathing and use of rescue inhaler for acute attacks. ______
		______ **Pat Coleman, RN**

SELECTED READINGS

American Association of Critical-Care Nurses. (2012). AACN practice alert: Preventing Aspiration. *Critical Care Nurse, 32*(3), 71–73.

Aresti, N., Kassam, J., Bartlett, D., & Kutty, S. (2017). Primary care management of post-operative shoulder, hip, and knee arthroplasty. *BMJ, 359,* j4431. Retrieved from https://www.bmj.com/content/359/bmj.j4431.full

Chang, K. L., & Carlos Guarderas, J. (2018). Allergy testing: Common questions and answers. *American Family Physician, 98*(1), 34–39.

Da Silviera, L., Tomiko, Y., Da Silva, J. M., Pavan Soler, J. M., Yea Ling Sun, C., Tanaka, C., & Fu, C. (2018). Assessing functional status after intensive care unit stay: The Barthel index and the Katz index. *International Journal for Quality in Health Care, 30*(4), 265–270.

Goodwin, B. (2018). AMA discharges: What you may not know: What to do when a patient disregards medical advice. *Urology Times, 46*(11). Retrieved from https://www.urologytimes.com/malpractice-consult/ama-discharges-what-you-may-not-know

Hanson, R. F., & Wallis, E. (2018). Treating victims of child sexual abuse. *American Journal of Psychiatry, 175*(11), 1064–1070.

Hoehn, E. F., Overmann, K. M., Fananapazir, N., Simonton, K., Makoroff, K. L., Bennett, B. L., ... Kurowski, E. M. (2018). Improving emergency department care for pediatric victims of sexual abuse. *Pediatrics, 142*(6), 1–6.

Klauer, K., & Merkrebs, H. M. (2018). Patients leaving against medical advice create liability risk. *Healthcare Risk Management, 40*(9), 97–108.

Leslie, R. A., Gouldson, S., Habib, N., Harris, N., Murray, H., Wells, V., & Cook, T. M. (2013). Management of arterial lines and blood sampling in intensive care: A threat to patient safety. *Anaesthesia, 68*(11), 1114–1119.

Lindgren, B., & Moreta-Sainz, L. (2017). Utilization of arterial blood gases in a medical ICU. *CHEST, 152*(Suppl. 4), A325.

McKibbin, A., & Gill-Hopple, K. (2018). Intimate partner violence: What health care providers should know. *Nursing Clinics of North America, 53*(2), 177–188.

Methangkool, E., Howard-Quijano, K., & Mahajan, A. (2018). Cardiac dysrhythmias: Understanding mechanisms, drug treatments, and novel therapies. *Advances in Anesthesia, 36*(1), 181–199.

Oppenheimer, J. J., & Borish, L. (2018). Asthma yardstick update: Practical recommendations for a sustained step-up in asthma therapy for poorly controlled asthma. *Annals of Allergy, Asthma & Immunology, 121*(6), 660–661.

Pattanaik, D., Lieberman, P., Lieberman, J., Pongdee, T., & Keene, A. T. (2018). The changing face of anaphylaxis in adults and adolescents. *Annals of Allergy, Asthma & Immunology, 121*(5), 594–597.

Shtessel, M., & Tversky, J. (2018). Reliability of allergy skin testing. *Annals of Allergy, Asthma & Immunology, 120*(1), 80–83.

Taylor, C., Lynn, P., & Bartlett, J. (2019). *Fundamentals of nursing* (9th ed.). Philadelphia, PA: Lippincott, Wolters Kluwer.

Van Den Bruele, A. B., Dimachk, M., & Crandall, M. (2019). Elder abuse. *Clinics in Geriatric Medicine, 35*(1), 103–113.

Weathers, E., O'Caoimh, R., Cornally, N., Fitzgerald, C., Kearns, T., Coffey, A., ... O'Sullivan, R. (2016). Advance care planning: A systematic review of randomised controlled trials conducted with older adults. *Maturitas, 91*, 101–109.

Zeanah, C. H., & Humphreys, K. L. (2018). Child abuse and neglect. *Journal of the American Academy of Child & Adolescent Psychiatry, 57*(9), 637–644.

B

BLADDER IRRIGATION, CONTINUOUS

Continuous bladder irrigation can help prevent urinary tract obstruction by flushing out small blood clots that form after prostate or bladder surgery. It may also be used to treat an irritated, inflamed, or infected bladder lining.

This procedure requires the placement of a triple-lumen catheter. One lumen controls balloon inflation, one allows irrigant inflow, and one allows irrigant outflow. The continuous flow of irrigating solution through the bladder also creates a mild tamponade that may help prevent venous hemorrhage. Although typically the catheter is inserted while the patient is in the operating room after prostate or bladder surgery, if the patient is not a surgical patient, the catheter may be inserted at the bedside.

Essential Documentation

Each time a container of solution is completed, the nurse should record the date, time, and type and amount of fluid given on the intake and output record. Include any medications added to the solution. Also, record the time and amount of fluid each time the drainage bag is emptied. Note the appearance of the drainage and any complaints by the patient. Document any changes in the patient's condition (e.g., a distended bladder, clots, or bright red outflow), the name of the health care provider notified and the time of notification, and actions taken. (See *Documenting bladder irrigation,* page 38.)

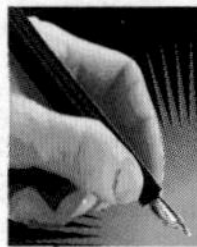

ACCUCHART

DOCUMENTING BLADDER IRRIGATION

As this sample shows, the nurse can monitor the patient's fluid balance by using an intake and output record.

Name: Joseph Klein

Identification #: 49731

Admission date: 8/9/19

INTAKE AND OUTPUT RECORD

	INTAKE						OUTPUT				
	Oral	Tube feeding	Instilled	I.V. and IVPB	TPN	Total	Urine	Emesis Tubes	NG	Other	Total
Date 8/11/19			NSS Bladder irr.								
0700-1500	250		800	1000		2050	2000				2000
1500-2300	200		800	1000		2000	2500				2500
2300-0700	100		800	1000		1900	1500				1500
24hr total	550		2400	3000		5950	6000				6000
Date											
24hr total											
Date											
24hr total											
Date											
24hr total											

Key: IVPB = I.V. piggyback TPN = total parenteral nutrition NG = nasogastric

Standard measures

Styrofoam cup	240 ml	Water (large)	600 ml	Milk (large)	600 ml	Ice cream, sherbet, or gelatin	120 ml
Juice	120 ml	Water pitcher	750 ml	Coffee	240 ml		
Water (small)	120 ml	Milk (small)	120 ml	Soup	180 ml		

Bladder Irrigation

8/11/2019	2300	**NURSING INTERVENTION:** 3000 mL NSS irrigating solution hung at 2250, infusing through intake flow port at 100 drops/min. ________ **NURSING ASSESSMENT:** Drainage bag emptied for 2500 mL of pink-tinged fluid with few small clots. No c/o discomfort. No bladder distention palpated. See I/O record for totals. ________________ **James Black, RN**

BLANK SPACES IN CHART OR FLOW SHEET

Blank spaces should not be left in a patient's chart or flow sheet. The nurse should follow the facility's policy regarding blank spaces on forms. A blank space may imply that the nurse failed to give complete care or assess the patient fully. Because flow sheets and documentation are often complex, nurses may be required to fill in only those fields or prompts that apply to their patient. It is now common for health care facilities to have a written policy on how to complete such forms correctly. Leaving blank spaces in the nurse's notes also allows others to add information to the note. If charting electronically, the computer may not allow the nurse to exit from a particular field unless all spaces are documented.

Essential Documentation

If the information requested on a form does not apply to a particular patient, the facility's policy may require the nurse to write "N/A" (not applicable) or draw a line through empty spaces.

When writing a nurse's notes, the nurse should draw a line through any blank space after the entry and sign his or her name on the far-right side of the column. If the nurse does not have enough room to sign his or her name after the last word in the entry, the nurse should draw a line from the last word to the end of the line. The nurse then should drop down to the next line, draw a line from the left margin almost to the right margin, and sign his or her name on the far-right side.

Blank Spaces in Charting

3/9/2019	1500	**NURSING INTERVENTION:** 20 y.o. male admitted to room 418B by wheelchair. #20 angiocath inserted in left antecubital vein with I.V. of 1000 mL D_5 1/2 NSS infusing at 125 mL/hr. O_2 at 2 L/min via NC. Demerol 50 mg given I.M. for abdominal pain in left ventrogluteal site. Call bell within reach. Nurses should always draw a line through blank spaces; This is not a problem when using electronic health records. ________ ________________________ **David Dunn, RN**

BLOOD TRANSFUSION

A blood transfusion provides whole blood or a blood component, such as packed cells, plasma, platelets, or cryoprecipitates, to replace losses from surgery, trauma, or disease. No matter which blood products are administered, the nurse must use proper identification and crossmatching procedures to ensure that the correct patient receives the correct blood product for transfusion. Be sure to follow facility policy for administering blood products.

Essential Documentation

Before administration of a blood transfusion, the following actions are advised:

- Verify that an order for the transfusion exists.
- Conduct a thorough physical assessment of the patient (including vital signs) to help identify later changes.
- Teach the patient about the procedure's associated risks and benefits, what to expect during the transfusion, signs and symptoms of a reaction, and when and how to call for assistance.
- Patients needing blood transfusions should be told about the risks and benefits of the procedure so that they can give informed consent before it is undertaken.
- Obtain informed consent.
- Check for appropriate and patent vascular access.
- Make sure the necessary equipment is at hand for administering the blood product and managing a reaction, such as an additional free intravenous (IV) line for normal saline solution, oxygen, suction, and a hypersensitivity kit.
- The nurse should be familiar with the specific product to be transfused, the appropriate administration rate, and required patient monitoring. Be aware that the type of blood product and the

patient's condition usually dictate the infusion rate. For example, blood must be infused faster in a trauma victim who is rapidly losing blood than in a 75-year-old patient with heart failure, who may not be able to tolerate rapid infusion.

- Know what personnel will be available in the event of a reaction, and know how to contact them. Resources should include the on-call physician and a blood bank representative.
- Before hanging the blood product, thoroughly double-check the patient's identification and verify the actual product. Check the unit to be transfused against patient identifiers, per facility policy. Have a second licensed health care provider double check the patient's identifying information, type and cross-match data, patient blood group and Rh factor, type and Rh factor of blood to be infused, blood bank identifying information, and expiration date of blood product.
- Infuse the blood product with normal saline solution only, using filtered tubing.

Premedication

Premedication may be prescribed. To help prevent immunologic transfusion reactions, the physician may order such medications as acetaminophen and diphenhydramine before the transfusion begins to prevent fever and histamine release. Febrile nonhemolytic transfusion reactions seem to be linked to blood components, such as platelets or fresh frozen plasma, as opposed to packed red blood cells; thus, premedication may be indicated for patients who will receive these products. Such reactions may be mediated by donor leukocytes in the plasma, causing allosensitization to human leukocyte antigens. Cytokine generation and accumulation during blood component storage may play a contributing role.

Time Frame for Administration

The nurse must confirm the window of time during which the product must be transfused, starting from when the product arrives from the blood bank to when the infusion must be completed. Failing to adhere to these time guidelines increases the risk of such complications as bacterial contamination.

Before administering the blood transfusion, the nurse should clearly document that the product matched the label on the blood product and that the following were verified:

- patient's name
- patient's identification number

- patient's blood group or type
- patient's and donor's Rh factor
- crossmatch data
- blood bank identification number
- expiration date of the product

In addition, the nurse should document that the blood or blood component and the patient were matched by two licensed health care professionals at the patient's bedside according to facility policy, that both of the health care professionals signed the slip that came with the blood, and that both of the health care professionals also verified that the information is correct.

When the nurse has determined that all the information is correct and matches, the consent form has been signed, and the patient's vital signs are within acceptable parameters per the facility's policy, the nurse may administer the transfusion and document the following on the transfusion record:

- date and time that the transfusion was started and completed
- name and credentials of the health care professionals who verified the information
- total amount of the transfusion (at least two health care professionals, registered nurses, or physicians should check to see if all identifying information of the patient and blood type and blood products are accurate and match)
- patient's vital signs before, during, and after the transfusion, according to facility policy
- patient's response to the transfusion

The minimum standards for monitoring patients who are receiving blood transfusion include the following:

- Pulse rate, blood pressure, temperature, and respiratory rate no more than 60 minutes before the blood transfusion is started.
- Pulse rate, blood pressure, and temperature 15 minutes after the start of each blood component. If these readings are significantly different from the baseline observations, the respiratory rate should also be included.
- Pulse rate, blood pressure, and temperature no more than 60 minutes after the end of the transfusion.
- Transfusion reactions can occur immediately, within 24 hours of a transfusion, or more than 24 hours after a transfusion.
- Nurses should know the signs of a transfusion reaction, when to report signs, and how and to whom they should be reported.

In the nurse's notes, provide additional information:

- type and gauge of the catheter
- infusion device used (if any) and its flow rate
- blood-warming unit used (if any)
- amount of normal saline solution used (if any)
- patient teaching regarding transfusion reaction signs and symptoms

If the patient receives autologous blood, document the amount of blood retrieved and reinfused in the intake and output records. Also, monitor and document laboratory data during and after the autotransfusion as well as the patient's pretransfusion and posttransfusion vital signs. Pay particular attention to the patient's coagulation profile, hematocrit and hemoglobin, arterial blood gas, and calcium levels.

Blood Transfusion		
12/16/2019	1015	**NURSING INTERVENTION:** Pt. to be transfused with 1 unit of PRBCs over 4 hr, according to written orders of Dr. M. Richardson. Infusion started at 1025 through 18G catheter in left forearm at 15 mL/hr using blood transfusion tubing. ________ **NURSING ASSESSMENT:** P 82, BP 132/84, RR 16, oral T 98.2° F. Remained with pt. for 1st 15 min. and increased rate to 60 mL/hr after no c/o itching, chills, wheezing, or headache. No evidence of vomiting, swelling, laryngeal edema, or fever noted. ________ **Maryann Belinsky, RN**
12/16/2019	1415	**NURSING ASSESSMENT:** Transfusion of 1 unit PRBCs complete. P 78, BP 130/78, RR 16, oral T 98.0° F. No c/o itching, chills, wheezing, or headache. No evidence of vomiting, swelling, laryngeal edema, or fever noted. ________ **Maryann Belinsky, RN**

BLOOD TRANSFUSION REACTION

During a blood transfusion, the patient is at risk for developing a transfusion reaction. If a reaction develops, immediately take the following steps:

- Stop the transfusion.
- Take down the blood tubing.
- Hang new tubing with normal saline solution running to maintain vein patency.
- Notify the health care provider, and follow facility policy for a blood transfusion reaction.
- Notify the blood bank and laboratory.

Essential Documentation

The nurse should be sure to document the time and date of the reaction, the type and amount of infused blood or blood products, the time the nurse started the transfusion, and the time the nurse stopped it. Also, record clinical signs of the reaction in order of occurrence, the patient's vital signs, urine specimen or blood samples sent to the laboratory for analysis, treatment given, and the patient's response to treatment. Indicate that the nurse sent the blood transfusion equipment (discontinued bag of blood, administration set, attached IV solutions, and all related forms and labels) to the blood bank. Some health care facilities require the completion of a transfusion reaction report that must be sent to the blood bank. (See *Transfusion reaction report,* pages 45 and 46.) Document any follow-up care provided. Be sure to time each note and avoid block charting. Some facilities may also require the completion of an incident report. (See *Avoid block charting,* page 47.)

Blood Transfusion Reaction		
2/13/2019	1350	**NURSING ASSESSMENT:** Pt. reports chills. Cyanosis of lips noted at 1350. Transfusion of packed RBCs stopped. Approximately 100 mL of blood infused. Transfusion started 1215, stopped at 1350. Tubing changed. I.V. of 1000 mL NSS infusing at 30 mL/hr rate in left forearm. **NURSING INTERVENTION:** Notified Dr. Cahill and blood bank. ______ **NURSING ASSESSMENT**: BP 168/88, P 104, RR 25, rectal T 97.6° F. ______ **NURSING INTERVENTION:** Blood samples taken from PRBCs. Two red-top tubes of blood drawn from pt. sent to lab. Urine specimen obtained from catheter. Urine specimen sent to lab for U/A. ______ **NURSING INTERVENTION:** Administered diphenhydramine 50 mg I.M. per order of Dr. Cahill. Two blankets placed on pt. Blood transfusion equipment sent to blood bank. Transfusion reaction report filed. ______
		______ **Maryann Belinsky, RN**
2/13/2019	1415	**NURSING ASSESSMENT:** Pt. reported he's getting warmer. BP 148/80, P 96, RR 20, T 97.6° F. ______
		______ **Maryann Belinsky, RN**
2/13/2019	1430	**NURSING ASSESSMENT:** Pt. no longer complaining of chills. I.V. of 1000 mL NS infusing at 125 mL/hr in right arm. BP 138/76, P 80, RR 18, T 98.4° F. ______
		______ **Maryann Belinsky, RN**

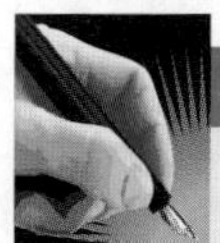

AccuChart

TRANSFUSION REACTION REPORT

If the facility requires a transfusion reaction report, the nurse should include the following types of information.

TRANSFUSION REACTION REPORT

Nursing report

1. Stop transfusion immediately. Keep I.V. line open with saline infusion.
2. Notify responsible physician.
3. Check all identifying names and numbers on the patient's wristband, unit, and paperwork for discrepancies.
4. Record patient's post-transfusion vital signs.
5. Draw posttransfusion blood samples (clotted and anticoagulated) avoiding mechanical hemolysis.
6. Collect posttransfusion urine specimen from patient.
7. Record information as indicated below.
8. Send discontinued bag of blood, administration set, attached I.V. solutions, and all related forms and labels to the blood bank with this form completed.

Clerical errors

☑ None detected
❑ Detected

Vital signs

	Pre-TXN	Post-TXN
Temp.	98.4°	97.6°F
B.P.	120/60	160/88
Pulse	88	104

☑ Urticaria	❑ Nausea	❑ Shock	❑ Hemoglobinuria
❑ Fever	❑ Flushing	❑ Oozing	❑ Oliguria or anuria
☑ Chills	❑ Dyspnea	❑ Back pain	❑ Cyanosis of lips noted
☑ Chest pain	❑ Headache	❑ Infusion site pain	
❑ Hypotension	❑ Perspiration		

Reaction occurred

During administration? Yes
After administration?
How long?
Medications added? No
Previous I.V. fluids? NSS at 30 ml/hr
Blood warmed? No

Specimen collection

Blood: Difficulty collecting? No
Urine: Voided Yes – sent to lab Catheterized

Comments:
Given diphenhydramine 50 mg I.V.

Signature Maryann Belinsky, RN Date 2/13/19

BLOOD BANK REPORT

Unit # 22FM80507
Component Returned Yes
Volume Returned 185 ml

1. Clerical errors
☑ None detected
❑ Detected

Comments:

2. Hemolysis

Note: If hemolysis is present in the posttransfusion sample, a posttransfusion urine sample must be tested for free hemoglobin immediately.

Patient pre-TXN sample	☑ None	❑ Slight	❑ Moderate	❑ Marked
Patient post-TXN sample	☑ None	❑ Slight	❑ Moderate	❑ Marked
Blood Bag	☑ None	❑ Slight	❑ Moderate	❑ Marked
Urine HGB (centrifuged)	❑ None	❑ Slight	☑ Moderate	❑ Marked

(continued)

TRANSFUSION REACTION REPORT *(continued)*

BLOOD BANK REPORT

3. Direct antiglobulin test

Pretransfusion________________ Posttransfusion ________________

If No. 2 and No. 3 are negative, steps 4 through 6 aren't required. Report results to the blood bank physician. Steps 7 and 8 or further testing will be done as ordered by blood bank physician.

4. ABO and Rh Groups

Repeat testing	Cell reaction with							Serum reaction with		ABO/Rh
		Anti-A	Anti-B	Anti-A,B	Anti-D	Cont.	Du	Cont.	CCC	A1 cells	B cells
Pretransfusion											
Posttransfusion											
Unit #											
Unit #											

5. Red cell antibody screen

	Saline/AB					INT
Pretransfusion	Cell	RT	37° C	AHG	CCC	
Date of sample	I					
	II					
By:	Auto					

	Saline/AB					INT
Posttransfusion	Cell	RT	37° C	AHG	CCC	
Date of sample	I					
	II					
By:	Auto					

Specificity of antibody detected:

6. Crossmatch compatibility testing

Use patient pre-TXN and post-TXN serum and the suspected unit red cells obtained from inside the container or from a segment still attached to bag. Observe appearance of blood in bag and administration tubing.

	Albumin				INT
Pretransfusion	RT	37° C	AHG	CCC	
Unit #					
Unit #					

	Albumin				INT
Posttransfusion	RT	37° C	AHG	CCC	
Unit #					
Unit #					

All units on hold for future transfusion must be recrossmatched with the posttransfusion sample.

7. Bacteriologic testing

Pretransfusion________________ Posttransfusion ________________

8. Other testing results

Total bilirubin

Patient pre-TXN ________ mg/dl

Patient 6 hrs. post-TXN _____ mg/dl

Coagulation studies

Urine output studies

Pathologist's conclusions:

Signature ________________ Date________________

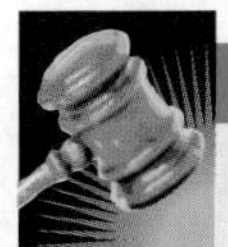

LEGAL CASEBOOK

AVOID BLOCK CHARTING

The nurse's charting should be specific about times, especially the exact time of sudden changes in the patient's condition, significant events, health care provider provider notification, and nursing actions. Do not chart in blocks of time, such as 0700 to 1900. This looks vague, implies inattention to the patient, and makes it hard to determine when specific events occurred. If the patient's chart is used as evidence in a lawsuit, the patient's lawyer may use block charting to show that the nurse did not provide timely nursing care when the patient developed a problem.

These examples show the correct and incorrect ways to chart times.

Correct:

12/16/2019	0600	Pt. complained of nausea, then vomited 300 mL light brown emesis around NG tube. NG tube irrigated with 100 mL NSS 80 mL clear fluid return. ______ **Ann Cook, RN**
11/2/2019	0700	NG tube drained 140 mL light brown fluid over past hr ______ **Ann Cook, RN**

Incorrect:

12/16/2019	0700–1900	Pt. has NG tube in—vomited once—irrigated with NSS 100 mL. No vomiting remainder of shift. ______ **Amy Mars, RN**

BONE MARROW ASPIRATION AND BIOPSY

A specimen of bone marrow—the major site of blood cell formation—may be obtained by aspiration or needle biopsy. The procedure allows evaluation of overall blood composition by studying blood elements and precursor cells as well as abnormal or malignant cells. An aspiration removes cells through a needle inserted into the marrow cavity of the bone; a biopsy removes a small, solid core of marrow tissue through the needle.

Aspirates aid in diagnosing various disorders and cancers, such as oat cell carcinoma, leukemia, and such lymphomas as Hodgkin disease. Biopsies are commonly performed simultaneously to stage the disease and monitor the response to treatment.

Nursing interventions during bone marrow biopsy:

- Reinforce the procedure's purpose with the patient. Explain that there will be some discomfort or pressure and that there may be a crunching sound and a "pop" feeling as the needle penetrates the bone. Make sure informed consent is obtained.
- Assess for bleeding risk: Review the patient's history, coagulation studies, platelet count, anticoagulant therapy, and drugs or supplements that interfere with clotting. Assess for allergies to antiseptic or anesthetic solutions.
- Determine the patient's ability to stay still during the procedure, and explain the importance of doing so. Take baseline vital signs, and administer sedatives as ordered.
- Help the patient to the appropriate position: lateral decubitus or prone if the insertion site will be the posterior iliac crest; supine if the sternum or anterior iliac crest will be used.
- Help the patient maintain position, and offer encouragement to take deep breaths and use relaxation techniques during the procedure. Assess the patient for pallor, diaphoresis, or other changes. Assist the practitioner as needed.
- After aspiration, apply direct pressure over the puncture site according to hospital policy for 5 to 10 minutes until bleeding stops. Cover the site with a sterile dressing.
- Help the patient to a comfortable position. Monitor the patient's vital signs, and assess the puncture site for bleeding.
- Properly label and promptly transport all specimens to the lab.
- Assess postprocedure pain intensity, and provide analgesia as ordered. Teach the patient to watch for signs of infection.
- Do not leave the patient unattended during the procedure.
- Do not let the patient move during the procedure.
- Do not administer analgesics containing aspirin; they may potentiate bleeding.

Essential Documentation

The nurse should document patient education regarding what to expect before and after the procedure and that informed consent has been obtained, if necessary. Many facilities have a separate patient education form for documenting what the nurse teaches and how the patient responds to the teaching. When assisting the health care provider with a bone marrow aspiration or biopsy, document the name of the health care provider performing the procedure and the date and time of the procedure. Also, describe the patient's response to the procedure and the location and condition of the aspiration or biopsy site, including bleeding and drainage as well as any care provided. Record the patient's vital signs before and after the procedure, and observe the site for bleeding and drainage. Document any pertinent information about the specimen sent to the laboratory.

Bone Marrow Biopsy

1/30/2019	1000	**PATIENT TEACHING/EDUCATION:** Explained what to expect before, during, and after bone marrow aspiration and answered pt.'s questions. Refer to pt. education sheet for specific instructions and pt. responses. Informed consent form signed by pt.
		NURSING ASSESSMENT: Preprocedure BP 148/86, P 92, RR 24, oral T 98.6°F.
		NURSING INTERVENTION: Assisted Dr. A. Shelbourne with bone marrow aspiration of left iliac crest at 0915.
		NURSING ASSESSMENT: No bleeding or drainage at site. Pt. denies any discomfort and is resting comfortably. Specimen sent to lab, as ordered. BP 142/82, P 88, RR 22, oral T 98.8°F. Maintaining bed rest. No bruising or bleeding noted at site.
		Margaret Little, RN

BRAIN DEATH

Brain death is commonly defined as the irreversible cessation of all brain functions, including the function of the brainstem. The Uniform Determination of Death Act (1980) established the standards for diagnosing brain death. The American Academy of Neurology (AAN) used these standards to develop practice guidelines in 1995. Other organizations have also published guidelines for diagnosing brain death. Thus, it is important for the nurse to know the state's laws regarding the definition of brain death as well as the facility's policy. (See *Know the state's laws concerning brain death,* page 50.)

The current AAN guidelines recommend that a health care provider examine the patient to confirm the presence of the three cardinal signs of brain death:

- coma or unresponsiveness
- absence of brainstem function (absent pupil reflex to bright light)
- apnea

To make this determination, the health care provider should test the patient for responsiveness or movement, brainstem reflexes (pupillary, corneal, gag/cough, oculocephalic, and oculovestibular), and apnea. The health care provider should also evaluate laboratory and diagnostic test results to eliminate other causes of coma. Although standards may vary by state or facility, the AAN recommends that the health care provider perform the examination twice, at least 6 hours apart.

The AAN checklist for the determination of brain death is presented in Figure B.1.

Essential Documentation

The nurse's note for a patient undergoing testing for brain death should include:

- family teaching and emotional support given
- date and time of the examination
- the name of the person performing the test
- the patient's response and any action taken (If the nurse notified anyone about the test and results, include the date and time of notification, the name of the person notified, the person's response, and any action taken.)
- time of brain and cardiopulmonary death (Include any evidence, such as electrocardiogram [ECG] or electroencephalogram [EEG] strips.)
- notification of organ procurement organization (OPO) prior to cessation of life-support measures

In addition, individuals performing the tests, such as a respiratory therapist, will need to complete their documentation in appropriate sections of the chart.

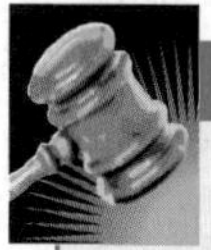

LEGAL CASEBOOK

KNOW THE STATE'S LAWS CONCERNING BRAIN DEATH

In states without laws defining death or without judicial precedents, the common-law definition of death (cessation of circulation and respiration) is still used. In these states, health care providers are understandably reluctant to discontinue artificial life support for brain-dead patients. If nurses are likely to be involved with patients on life-support equipment, they should protect themselves by finding out how the state in which they practice defines death.

Brain Death

6/1/2019	0800	**NURSING ASSESSMENT:** Dr. N. Malone in to speak with pt.'s son, Mark Newton, who has health care POA, about pt.'s condition. Son agreed to tests to determine brain death. **Dawn Silfies, RN**
6/11/2019	0815	**NURSING ASSESSMENT:** Dr. Malone performed clinical exam. See Physician Progress Notes for full report. Son present for exam. Dr. Malone explained results to son. Son states understanding. Pt. also to be seen by Dr. P. Horales for second required testing. Organ donation center notified. **Dawn Silfies, RN**

Checklist for determination of brain death

Date and time____________________

Prerequisites (all must be checked)

- o Coma, irreversible and cause known
- o Neuroimaging explains coma
- o CNS depressant drug effect absent (toxicology screen/serum levels if indicated)
- o No evidence of residual paralytics (electrical stimulation if paralytics used)
- o Absence of severe acid-base, electrolyte, or endocrine abnormality
- o Normothermia or mild hypothermia (core temperature ≥ 36° C/96.8° F)
- o Systolic blood pressure > 100 mmHg
- o No spontaneous respirations

Examination (all must be checked)

- o Pupils nonreactive to bright light
- o Corneal reflex absent
- o Oculocephalic reflex absent (tested only if C-spine integrity ensured)
- o Oculovestibular reflex absent (30-50 mL ice water each ear, observe 1 min, 5 min between ears)
- o No facial movement to noxious stimuli at supraorbital nerve, temporo-mandibular joint
- o Gag reflex absent
- o Cough reflex absent to tracheal suctioning
- o Absence of motor response to noxious stimuli in all 4 limbs (spinally-mediated reflexes are permissible, posturing is not)

Apnea testing (all must be checked)

- o Patient is hemo-dynamically stable and euvolemic
- o Ventilator adjusted to provide normocarbia ($PaCO_2$ 35–45 mmHg)
- o Patient preoxygenated with 100% FiO_2 for > 10 min to PaO_2 > 200 mm Hg
- o Patient well-oxygenated with a PEEP of 5 cm H_2O
- o Provide oxygen via a suction catheter to the level of the carina at 10 L/min or attach T-piece with CPAP at 10 cm H_2O
- o Disconnect ventilator
- o Spontaneous respirations absent
- o ABG drawn at 5 minutes
- o ABG drawn at 10 minutes (reconnect ventilator)
- o $PaCO_2 \geq 60$ mmHg **or** ≥ 20 mmHg rise from baseline

Pre-test ABG: pH___ pCO_2_____ pO_2_____ **Post-test ABG:** pH___ pCO_2_____ pO_2_____@_____min

OR:

- ¤ Apnea test aborted (cardiac ectopy, O_2 sat < 90%, SBP < 100 mmHg)

Ancillary testing (only 1 needs to be performed; to be ordered only if clinical examination cannot be fully performed due to patient factors, or if apnea testing inconclusive or aborted)

- ¤ Cerebral angiogram
- ¤ SPECT
- ¤ EEG
- ¤ TCD

Time of death (MM/DD/YY & 00:00) ________________ **due to**________________ (etiology of coma)

Name of physician and signature

____

- ¤ attending neurologist/neurosurgeon
- ¤ neurocritical care fellow

Figure B.1 Checklist for criteria of brain death determination, excerpt from the Massachusetts General Hospital Brain Death Protocol, most recently revised in March 2011. (Used with permission from Wiener-Kronish, J. P. [Ed.]. 2015. *Critical care handbook of the Massachusetts General Hospital* [6th ed.]. Philadelphia, PA: Lippincott Williams & Wilkins.)

BURNS, ASSESSMENT AND NURSING CARE

Epidemiology

In 2016, more than 200,000 people in the United States were hospitalized with injuries from smoke, fire, or flame exposure; more than 6,000 died. Burns damage skin and underlying tissue, disrupting the skin's regulatory functions. Patients with acute burns require significant and costly interprofessional care that includes nurses, advanced practice nurses, physicians, surgeons, pharmacists, physical and occupational therapists, and social workers.

Nursing History

If the nurse is unable to gather a history from the patient, the nurse should interview family members, friends, or those who were at the scene. In addition to the patient's medical history, record detailed information about the circumstances and mechanism of the injury. Additional questioning will be necessary if the patient was found in an enclosed space, has potential orthopedic injuries associated with the burns, or had clothing on fire. The data collected in these circumstances can significantly change the plan of care. For example, inhalation in closed spaces may involve toxins, which will prompt the provider to order additional tests, and burns to the face may significantly impact the airway. The nurse will also want to gather additional information if an accelerant was used, an explosion was witnessed, the burn is related to a motor vehicle accident, or the reported circumstances are inconsistent with the burn pattern (suspected abuse).

Nursing Assessment

The primary assessment of patients with acute burns starts with airway patency and cervical spine protection (in cases of a suspected spinal cord injury or if the patient is unconscious and there are no other sources of information about the accident). The nurse should assess breathing, central and peripheral circulation, and cardiac status; stabilize any disability, deficit, or gross deformity; and remove clothing to assess the extent of burns and concurrent injuries. Assess vital signs.

Monitoring of vital signs and the color of unburned skin can help the nurse assess the patient's circulatory and cardiac status. Carefully check pulses in any extremity with circumferential burns. These burns can act as tourniquets as burn-associated edema begins, leading to compartment syndrome. In most adult burn patients, the heart rate (HR) will be elevated to 100 to 120 beats per minute (bpm) because of increased circulating catecholamines and hypermetabolism; an HR higher than 120 bpm may indicate hypovolemia from trauma, inadequate oxygenation, or uncontrolled pain and anxiety. Blood pressure and other vital signs in the early stages of burn resuscitation should be the same as the patient's baseline. Arrhythmias may be seen in electrical burn injuries, electrolyte imbalances, or underlying cardiac abnormalities. Begin interventions as ordered to avoid complications.

Essential Documentation

The nurse should assess the level of consciousness and neurologic status. Use the Glasgow Coma Scale to evaluate patient neurologic status throughout resuscitation. Assess patient fluid status, pain level, the percentage of total body surface area (%TBSA) burned, and the depth of the burns.

To determine the extent of the burn, the calculation of the %TBSA can be made using the "rule of nines" (Figure B.2). The size of the

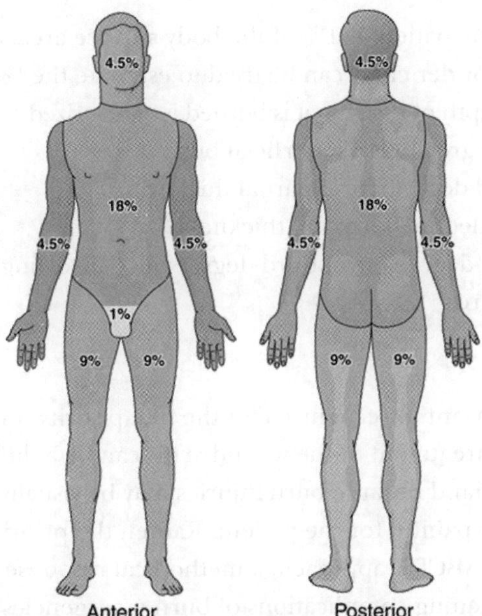

Figure B.2 The rule of nines. The percentage of total body surface area (%TBSA) in the adult is estimated by sectioning the body surface into areas with numerical values related to nine. This method is used to evaluate the extent of skin burns. (Used with permission from Cohen, J. B., & DePetris, A. [Eds.]. 2013. *Medical terminology* [7th ed.]. Philadelphia, PA: Lippincott Williams & Wilkins.)

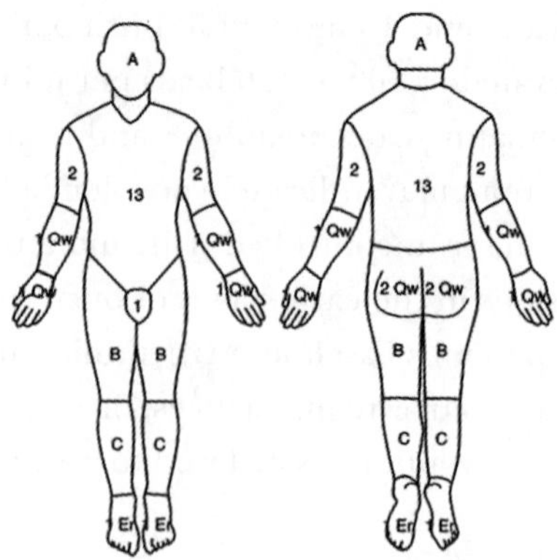

LUND-BROWDER CHART
Relative percentage of body surface area affected by growth

Age in years	0	1	5	10	15	Adult
A—head (back or front)	9 Qw	8 Qw	6 Qw	5 Qw	4 Qw	3 Qw
B—1 thigh (back or front)	2 Er	3 Qr	4	4 Qr	4 Qw	4 Er
C—1 leg (back or front)	2 Qw	2 Qw	2 Er	3	3 Qr	3 Qw

Figure B.3 Lund–Browder tables. (Used with permission from Mattu, A., Chanmugam, S. A., Swadron, S. P., Tibbles, C., Woolridge, D., & Marcucci, L. [Eds.]. 2010. *Avoiding common errors in the emergency department.* Philadelphia, PA: Lippincott Williams & Wilkins.)

palm of the patient is 1% of the body **surface** area. Alternatively, the Lund–Browder chart can be used to estimate the %TBSA (Figure B.3).

The depth of tissue that is burned is categorized as follows (Figure B.4):

- First-degree burn: superficial burn
- Second-degree burn: partial thickness
- Third-degree burn: full thickness
- Fourth-degree burn: third-degree burn involving underlying structures

Nursing Care

It is important to recognize that the first priority for burn patients is *not* the treatment of the wound. This can be a difficult concept to understand because burn injuries may be visually distracting and extremely painful for the patient. Rather, the priority is to implement the ABCDE approach, a methodical response ensuring that the life-threatening complications of burn emergencies are addressed rapidly and effectively.

Never use ice or cold water because it will restrict peripheral circulation locally, increasing the depth of the burn, and it may decrease body

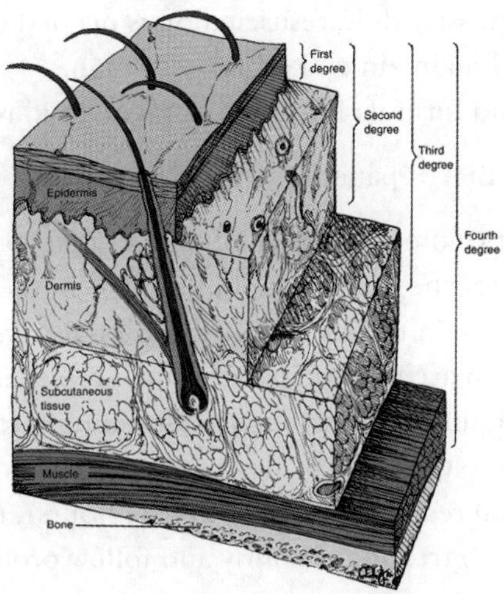

Figure B.4 The depth of injury is commonly classified by the depth of tissue injury (which corresponds to classic burn degree designations) as superficial thickness (first degree), partial thickness (second degree), full thickness (third degree), or subdermal (fourth degree). (Used with permission from Sussman, C., & Bates-Jensen, B. [Eds.]. 2011. *Wound care* [4th ed.]. Philadelphia, PA: Lippincott Williams & Wilkins.)

THE ABCDES OF EMERGENCY BURN CARE

Airway maintenance with cervical spine protection
Breathing and ventilation
Circulation and cardiac status with hemorrhage control
Disability, neurologic deficit, and gross deformity
Exposure to Examine for major associated injuries and maintain warm Environment

Source: American Burn Association. (2011). *Advanced burn life support course provider manual.* Chicago, IL: Author.

temperature. It is imperative to prevent hypothermia in burn patients because body temperatures below 97.7°F (36.5°C) in the first 24 hours are associated with increased mortality. Cover the patient with a clean, dry covering such as a sheet or blanket to prevent evaporative heat loss.

Establishing IV lines using large-bore needles on intact skin areas and starting fluid resuscitation are important in the first few hours after burn injury. The fluid shifting that occurs with large %TBSA burns is a result of shock, which moves the circulating volume into the soft tissue and creates hypovolemia in the first 48 hours after the injury.

Rapid and aggressive fluid resuscitation is needed to replace intravascular volume and maintain end-organ perfusion.

The Parkland formula is used to estimate fluid requirements:

4 mL × %TBSA × patient's weight in kg = total fluid in first 24 hours

After a total volume is calculated, half of that volume is given in the first 8 hours after the time of the injury, 25% in the second 8 hours, and the final 25% in the last 8 hours. Although crystalloids like lactated Ringer's solution are the preferred volume-replacement therapy, some patients will require colloids, such as albumin, to retain as much fluid as possible inside the vessels.

During initial resuscitation (the first 24 hours), reassess the patient's responsiveness to treatment hourly and follow protocols for adjusting fluid based on urine output.

A nasogastric tube may be necessary to alleviate gastric distension, prevent aspiration, and prevent ileus. Insertion of a urinary catheter may be needed.

Burn Wound Care

Burns create a large open wound in which normal skin flora can begin to colonize. Left untreated, this can lead to severe cellulitis or sepsis. Wound care is essential to prevent infection and should be performed immediately after completing primary and secondary assessments and after any life- or limb-threatening conditions are treated. After premedicating the patient with an analgesic agent to reduce pain, the nurse should thoroughly wash the area with water and skin disinfectants or antibacterial soap. Clean away materials found on the wound, and debride large ruptured blisters. Using a strip pattern, apply antibacterial ointment and nonadherent gauze to any open areas. Keep the gauze loose enough to allow for swelling, and secure it with tape.

Additional interventions to prevent infection include:

- Give daily baths with skin disinfectants.
- Perform wound care wearing isolation gown, mask, and surgical cap.
- Implement strict staff and visitor handwashing policies.
- Change linens every few days per institutional policy.
- Minimize the performance of interventions through nonintact skin.

If the patient develops a high fever, he or she may be pancultured and prescribed broad-spectrum antibiotics until a specific organism is identified.

SELECTED READINGS

American Burn Association. (2017). *Advanced burn life support course: Provider manual—2017 update.* Chicago, IL: Author.

American Burn Association. (2017). *Burn incidence and treatment in the United States: 2016.* Retrieved from https://ameriburn.org/who-we-are/media/burn-incidence-fact-sheet/

Battard Menendez, J. (2016). Early identification of acute hemolytic transfusion reactions: Realistic implications for best practice in patient monitoring. *Medsurg Nursing, 25*(2), 88–90, 109.

DeLisle, J. (2018). Is this a blood transfusion reaction? Don't hesitate; check it out. *Journal of Infusion Nursing, 41*(1), 43–51.

Dewar, B., Fedyk, M., & Shamy, M. C. F. (2018). Biological, legal, and moral definitions of brain death. *JAMA: Journal of the American Medical Association, 320*(14), 1494–1495.

Hampe, H. M., Keeling, T., Fontana, M., & Balcik, D. (2017). Impacting care and treatment of the burn patient conversion to electronic documentation. *Critical Care Nursing Quarterly, 40*(1), 8–15.

Heffernan, J. M., & Comeau, O. Y. (2013). Management of patients with burn injury. In J. L. Hinkle & K. H. Cheever (Eds.), *Brunner & Suddarth's textbook of medical-surgical nursing* (13th ed., pp. 1805–1836). Philadelphia, PA: Lippincott Williams & Wilkins.

Hettiaratchy, S., & Papini, R. (2004). Initial management of a major burn: II—assessment and resuscitation. *BMJ, 329*(7457), 101–103.

Nelson, A. (2017). Determining brain death: Basic approach and controversial issues. *American Journal of Critical Care, 26*(6), 496–500.

Onishi, T., Sugino, Y., Shibahara, T., Masui, S., Yabana, T., & Sasaki, T. (2017). Randomized controlled study of the efficacy and safety of continuous saline bladder irrigation after transurethral resection for the treatment of non-muscle-invasive bladder cancer. *BJU International, 119*(2), 276–282.

Passwater, M. (2018). Antibody formation in transfusion therapy. *Journal of Infusion Nursing, 41*(2), 87–95.

Rizvi, T., Batchala, P., & Mukherjee, S. (2018). Brain death: Diagnosis and imaging techniques. *Seminars in Ultrasound, CT and MRI, 39*(5), 515–529.

Rushing, J. (2006). Assisting with bone marrow aspiration and biopsy. *Nursing, 36*(3), 68.

Shepherd, A. J., Mackay, W. G., & Hagen, S. (2017). Washout policies in long-term indwelling urinary catheterisation in adults. *Cochrane Database of Systematic Reviews, 2010*(3), CD004012. https://doi.org/10.1002/14651858.CD004012.pub4

Strauss, S., & Gillespie, G. L. (2018). Initial assessment and management of burn patients. *American Nurse Today, 13*(6), 15–19.

Stupnyckyj, C., Smolarek, S., Reeves, C., McKeith, J., & Magnan, M. (2014). Changing blood transfusion policy and practice. *American Journal of Nursing, 114*(12), 50–59.

Taylor, C., Lynn, P., & Bartlett, J. (2019). *Fundamentals of nursing* (9th ed.). Philadelphia, PA: Lippincott, Wolters Kluwer.

The ABCDEs of emergency burn care. (2015). *American Nurse Today, 10*(10). Retrieved from https://www.americannursetoday.com/abcdes-emergency-burn-care/

Tolich, D. J., Blackmur, S., Stahorsky, K., & Wabeke, D. (2013). Blood management: Best-practice transfusion strategies. *Nursing, 43*(1), 40–47.

Wijdicks, E. F. M., Varelas, P. N., Gronseth, G. S., & Greer, D. M. (2010). Evidence-based guideline update: Determining brain death in adults. Report of the Quality Standards Subcommittee of the American Academy of Neurology. *Neurology, 74*(23). Retrieved from http://n.neurology.org/content/74/23/1911

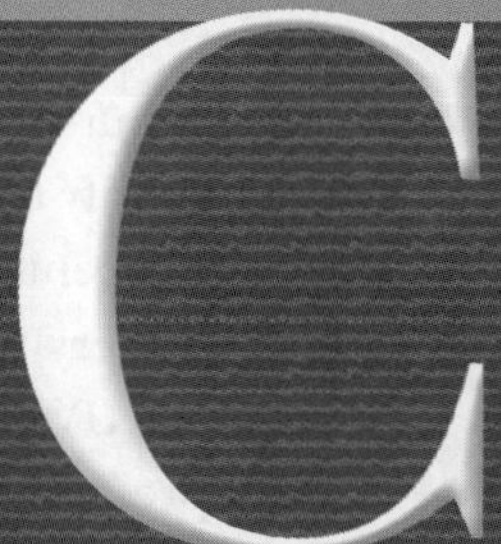

CARDIAC MONITORING (TELEMETRY)

Because it allows continuous observation of the heart's electrical activity, cardiac monitoring is useful not only for assessing cardiac rhythm but also for gauging a patient's response to drug therapy and for preventing complications associated with diagnostic and therapeutic procedures. Like other forms of electrocardiography, cardiac monitoring uses electrodes placed on the patient's chest to transmit electrical signals that are converted into a tracing of cardiac rhythm on an oscilloscope. Cardiac monitoring may be hardwired monitoring, in which the patient is connected to a monitor at the bedside, or telemetry, in which a small transmitter connected to the patient sends an electrical signal to a monitor screen for display.

Essential Documentation

In the nurse's notes, the nurse should document the date and time that monitoring began and the monitoring leads used.

CARDIAC TAMPONADE

With cardiac tamponade, a rapid, unchecked rise in intrapericardial pressure impairs diastolic filling of the heart. The rise in pressure usually results from accumulation blood or fluid in the pericardial sac. If fluid accumulates rapidly, the patient requires emergency lifesaving measures.

Cardiac tamponade may be idiopathic or may result from effusion, hemorrhage trauma or nontraumatic causes, pericarditis, acute myocardial infarction, chronic renal failure, drug reaction, or connective tissue disorders.

If the nurse suspects cardiac tamponade in a patient, the nurse should notify the health care provider immediately and prepare for pericardiocentesis (needle aspiration of the pericardial cavity), emergency surgery (usually a pericardial window), or both. Anticipate intravenous (IV) fluids, inotropic drugs, and blood products to maintain blood pressure until treatment is performed.

Essential Documentation

Include the assessment findings, such as jugular vein distention, decreased arterial blood pressure, pulsus paradoxus, narrow pulse pressure, muffled heart sounds, acute chest pain, dyspnea, diaphoresis, anxiety, restlessness, pallor or cyanosis, rapid and weak pulses, and hepatomegaly. Record the name of the health care provider notified and the time of notification. Make a note of diagnostic tests ordered by the health care provider, such as an electrocardiogram (ECG) or chest x-ray, and the findings. Document treatments and procedures and the patient's response. Note any patient teaching provided. The frequency of vital signs, titration of drugs, and patient responses may be documented on the appropriate flow sheets.

Cardiac Tamponade		
6/5/2019	1320	**NURSING ASSESSMENT:** BP at 1300 90/40 via cuff on right arm. Last BP at 1200 was 120/60. Drop of 17 mm Hg in systolic BP noted during inspiration. P 132 and regular, RR 34, oral T 97.2°F. See frequent vital sign sheet for q15min VS. Neck veins distended with pt. in semi-Fowler's at 45-degrees, heart sounds muffled, peripheral pulses weak. Pt. anxious and dyspneic, skin pale and diaphoretic. Pt. c/o chest pain. Pt. awake, alert, and oriented X3.
6/5/2019	1400	**NURSING INTERVENTION:** Dr. H. Hoffman notified at 1305. Stat portable CXR done. ECG shows sinus tachycardia with rate of 130. 200-mL bolus of NSS given. Dopamine 400 mg in 250 D5W started at 4 mcg/kg/min. Results of CXR called to Dr. Hoffmann. Awaiting Dr. M. May's arrival for pericardiocentesis.
		PATIENT TEACHING: Explained the procedure to pt. and wife and answered their questions.
		Cindy Rogers, RN

CARDIOPULMONARY ARREST AND RESUSCITATION

Guidelines established by the American Heart Association direct the nurse to keep a written, chronological account of a patient's condition throughout cardiopulmonary resuscitation (CPR). If the nurse is the designated recorder, the nurse should document therapeutic interventions and the patient's responses as they occur. The nurse should not rely on memory to record these details later. Writing "recorder" after the nurse's name indicates that the nurse documented the event but did not participate in the code.

The form used to chart a code is the code record. It incorporates detailed information about the nurse's observations and interventions as well as drugs given to the patient. Remember, the code response should follow Advanced Cardiac Life Support guidelines.

Some facilities use a resuscitation critique form to identify actual or potential problems with the resuscitation process. This form tracks personnel responses and response times.

Essential Documentation

The code record is a precise, quick, and chronological recording of the events of the code. (See *The code record*, page 62.) The nurse should document the date and time the code was called. The nurse also needs to record the patient's name, the location of the code, the person who discovered the patient, the patient's condition, and whether the arrest was witnessed or unwitnessed. Document the name of the health care provider running the code, and list other members who participated in the code. Record the exact time for each code intervention, and include vital signs, heart rhythm, laboratory results (e.g., arterial blood gas or electrolyte levels), type of treatment (e.g., CPR, defibrillation, or cardioversion), drugs (name, dosage, and route), procedures (e.g., intubation, temporary or transvenous pacemaker, and central line insertion), and patient response. Record the time that the family was notified. At the end of the code, indicate the patient's status and the time that the code ended. Some facilities require that the health care provider leading the code and the nurse recording the code review the code sheet and sign it.

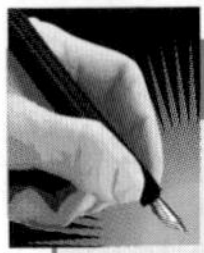

AccuChart

THE CODE RECORD

Here is an example of the completed resuscitation record for inclusion in the patient's chart.

CODE RECORD

Pg. 1 of 1

Arrest Date: 11/9/19
Arrest Time: 0631
Rm/Location: 431-2
Discovered by: C. Brown
☑ RN ☐ MD
☐ Other

Methods of alert:
☐ Witnessed, monitored: rhythm
☐ Witnessed, unmonitored
☑ Unwitnessed, unmonitored
☐ Unwitnessed, monitored; rhythm
Diagnosis: Post anterior wall MI

Condition when needed:
☑ Unresponsive
☐ Apneic
☐ Pulseless
☐ Hemorrhage
☐ Seizure

Ventilation management:
Time: 0635
Method: oral ET tube
Precordial thump:
CPR initiated at: 0631

Previous airway:
☐ ET tube
☐ Trach
☑ Natural

Addressograph

CPR PROGRESS NOTES

VITAL SIGNS						I.V. PUSH			ACTIONS/PATIENT RESPONSE
Time	Pulse CPR	Resp. rate Spont; bag	Blood pressure	Rhythm	Defib (joules)	Atropine	Epinephrine	Other	Responses to therapy, procedures, labs drawn/results
0631	CPR	Bag	0	V fib					
0633	CPR	Bag	0	V fib	360		1 mg		
0635	40	Bag	60 palp	SB PVCs					Oral intubation by Dr. W. Hart
0645	60	Bag	80/40	SB PVCs					ABG drawn Transported to CCU

ABGs & Lab Data

Time Spec Sent	pH	PCO	Po_2	HCO_3^-	Sat%	Fio_2	Other
0640	7.1	76	43	14	80%		

Resuscitation outcome
☑ Successful ☑ Transferred to CCU at 0648
☐ Unsuccessful — Expired at
Pronounced by: MD
Family notified by: S. Quinn, RN
Time: 0645
Attending notified by: S. Quinn, RN Time 0645
Code Recorder S. Quinn, RN
Code Team Nurse B. Mullen, RN
Anesthesia Rep. J. Hanna, RN
Other Personnel B. Russo, RT
MD: Dr. W. Hart

In the nurse's notes, the nurse should record the events leading up to the code, the assessment findings prompting the decision to call a code, who initiated CPR, and other interventions performed before the code team arrived. Include the patient's response to interventions. Document notification of the family and attending physician.

Cardiopulmonary Arrest		
11/9/2019	0650	**NURSING ASSESSMENT:** Summoned to pt.'s room at 0630 by a shout from roommate. Found pt. unresponsive in bed without respirations or pulse. **NURSING INTERVENTION:** Code called at 0630. Initiated CPR with Ann Barrow, RN. Code team arrived at 0632 and continued resuscitative efforts. (See code record.) Pt. transported to CCU, RM 201. Family notified. Dr. R. Stout notified. **Connie Brown, RN**

CARDIOVERSION, SYNCHRONIZED

Used to treat tachyarrhythmias, cardioversion delivers an electric charge to the myocardium at the peak of the R wave. This causes immediate depolarization, interrupting reentry circuits and allowing the sinoatrial node to resume control. Synchronizing the electric charge with the R wave ensures that the current won't be delivered on the vulnerable T wave and thus disrupt repolarization.

Indications for cardioversion include stable paroxysmal atrial tachycardia, unstable paroxysmal supraventricular tachycardia, atrial fibrillation, atrial flutter, and ventricular tachycardia. Cardioversion may be an elective or urgent procedure, depending on how well the patient tolerates the arrhythmia.

Essential Documentation

The nurse should document the date and time of the cardioversion. Record the signing of a consent form and any patient teaching. Include any preprocedure activities, such as withholding food and fluids, withholding drugs, removing dentures, administering a sedative, and obtaining a 12-lead ECG. Document vital signs, and obtain an ECG before starting. Note that the cardioverter was on the synchronized setting, how many times the patient was cardioverted, and the voltage used each time. After the procedure, obtain vital signs, and record that a 12-lead ECG was obtained. Assess and document the patient's level of consciousness, airway patency, respiratory rate and depth, and use of supplemental oxygen until the patient is awake. Indicate the specific time of each assessment, and avoid block charting.

Cardioversion Synchronized

6/18/2019	1800	**PATIENT TEACHING:** Explained procedure to pt. and answered his questions. Pt. states, "I'm very anxious about this cardioversion but I understand why it's necessary." ____
		NURSING INTERVENTION: Consent form signed and placed in chart. Pt. has been NPO for 6 hr. Dentures removed. Started O_2 at 2 L/min via NC. O_2 sat. 94%. ____
		NURSING ASSESMENT: 12-lead ECG shows atrial fibrillation at rate of 130. BP 92/54, RR 28, oral T 96.8°F. Midazolam given I.V. by anesthesiologist, Mark Goodman. Cardioverter set to synchronized setting. Cardioverted X2 with 50 J, followed by 100 J with conversion to NSR at rate of 80. NSR confirmed by 12-lead ECG. BP 102/60, RR 24. Postprocedure rhythm strip attached below. ____
		NURSING ASSESSMENT: Pt. responds with eye opening when name called. O_2 sat. 96% via pulse oximetry. Respirations regular and shallow. Skin color pink, warm, capillary refill less than 3 sec. Breath sounds clear and heard in all lobes. ____
		____ **Susan Banks, RN**

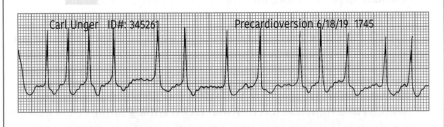

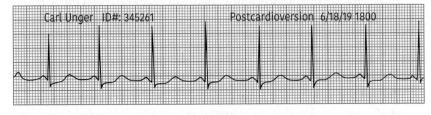

CAREGIVER STRAIN

Illness in a family member commonly takes a toll on other family members and caregivers. In fact, family members under great stress from trying to carry out their own roles while also caring for a sick person are at risk for burnout. If the patient has a long-term illness such as Alzheimer disease, the caregiver could be facing years of hard work. Signs of stress in a caregiver include muscular aches, headache, insomnia, illness, unexplained pain or gastrointestinal complaints, fatigue, weight loss, grinding of the teeth, inability to concentrate, mood swings, use of tranquilizers or alcohol, decreased socialization, depression, forgetfulness, feelings of despair, and thoughts of suicide.

Refer caregivers at risk for or showing signs of strain to social services. Educate caregivers about signs and symptoms of stress to report to their health care provider or nurse. Help them identify support systems and community services that are available.

Essential Documentation

The nurse should record the date and time of the entry. Identify the individual at risk for or experiencing caregiver strain. Describe subjective and objective signs of caregiver strain. Use the caregiver's own words in quotes, when possible. Include education and support given and the caregiver's response. Identify referrals made to services, such as social services, chaplain, support groups, meals-on-wheels, and respite care.

Family education may be documented on a patient education flow sheet, depending on facility policy. Appropriate notes should also be recorded on discharge-planning forms.

Caregiver Strain		
6/2/2019	1830	**NURSING ASSESSMENT:** Pt's. daughter stated concern regarding caring for her father at home. States, "I don't think I can do it myself." **NURSING INTERVENTION:** Social services consulted. Daughter given brochures regarding home care.________________ **Mary Albright, RN**

CARE PLAN, TRADITIONAL

The nursing care plan serves as a written guide to facilitate continuity of care for individual patients. The care plan provides an avenue for communication among health care providers who interact to deliver comprehensive care. Nursing care plans are mainly used in extended care, long-term care, or nursing homes and are not used in acute care facilities.

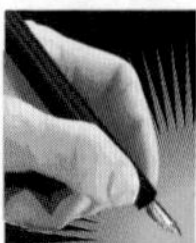

AccuChart

USING A TRADITIONAL CARE PLAN

Here's an example of a traditional care plan. It shows how these forms are typically organized. Remember that a traditional care plan is written specifically for each patient.

DATE	NURSING DIAGNOSIS	EXPECTED OUTCOMES	INTERVENTIONS	REVISION (INITIALS AND DATE)	RESOLUTION (INITIALS AND DATE)
3/8/19	Decreased cardiac output R/T reduced stroke volume secondary to fluid volume overload	Lungs clear on auscultation by 3/10/19 BP will return to baseline by 3/10/19	Monitor for signs and symptoms of hypoxemia, such as dyspnea, confusion, arrhythmias, restlessness, and cyanosis. Ensure adequate oxygenation by placing patient in semi-Fowler's position and administering supplemental O2 as ordered. Monitor breath sounds q4hr. Administer cardiac medications as ordered and document pt.'s response, drugs' effectiveness, and adverse reactions. Monitor and document heart rate and rhythm, heart sounds, and BP. Note the presence or absence of peripheral pulses. KK 3/8/19		

REVIEW DATES		
Date	Signature	Initials
3/8/19	Karen Kramer, RN	KK

The traditional care plan is initiated when the patient is admitted and continues throughout the hospitalization. The patient's problem, expected outcomes, specific interventions, and evaluations, along with the date that the problem was resolved, are typical components of the traditional care plan. The traditional care plan is written from scratch and is rarely used today, except in nursing homes, because of the time required to write one for each patient. It is, however, specific to the patient so that all health care workers understand the precise patient problem, expected outcomes, and individualized interventions.

Essential Documentation

The traditional care plan includes dates for problem identification and resolution, the problem (written as a nursing diagnosis), the expected patient outcomes, individualized nursing interventions, and evaluation of the expected outcome. (See *Using a traditional care plan,* page 66.)

CAST CARE

A cast is a hard mold that encloses a body part, usually an extremity, to provide immobilization without discomfort. It can be used to treat injuries, correct orthopedic conditions, or promote healing after general or plastic surgery, amputation, or neurovascular repair. Care of the cast involves assessment of the limb for neurovascular function, prevention of complications, and patient and family education. Complications include compartment syndrome, palsy, paresthesia, ischemia, ischemic myosis, pressure necrosis, and misalignment or nonunion of fractured bones.

Essential Documentation

Record the date and time of, and the reason for, cast application and the skin condition of the extremity before the cast was applied. Document diagnostic tests performed and the results. Note any contusions, redness, or open wounds. Assess and document the results of neurovascular checks, before and after application, bilaterally. Include the location of special devices, such as felt pads or plaster splints. Document patient education and whether written instructions were given.

Cast Care		
6/5/2019	1400	**NURSING ASSESSMENT:** X-ray shows simple left radial fracture. Fiberglass cast applied to left forearm by Dr. A. Brown at 1330. Before cast application, 5 cm × 10 cm area of bruising at fracture site, no open wounds noted. Radial pulses strong, capillary refill less than 3 sec, hands warm, no finger edema bilaterally. Patient c/o pain at fracture site. No numbness or tingling, able to move fingers and feel light touch in both hands equally. ________
		NURSING INTERVENTION: After cast application, left forearm elevated on 2 pillows. Neurovascular status remains unchanged. ________
		PATIENT TEACHING: Patient and family told to keep left forearm elevated on pillows. Instructed them to call the doctor if pt. is unable to move fingers, if numbness or tingling develops in fingers of left hand, or if pain increases despite taking pain medication as ordered. Explained S/S of infection to report. Advised them not to insert anything into cast. Written discharge instructions for cast care given to pt. and family. All questions answered. Pt. to follow up with orthopedist in 1 week. ________
		________ **Joyce Chow, RN**

CENTRAL VENOUS ACCESS DEVICE INSERTION

A central venous access device (CVAD) is a sterile catheter that is inserted through a major vein, such as the subclavian vein, jugular vein, or femoral vein. CVAD therapy allows for the monitoring of central venous pressure (CVP), which indicates blood volume or pump efficiency. It also permits aspiration of blood samples for diagnostic tests and administration of IV fluids (in large amounts, if necessary) in emergencies or when decreased peripheral circulation causes peripheral veins to collapse. A CVAD helps when prolonged IV therapy reduces the number of accessible peripheral veins, when solutions must be diluted (for large volumes or for irritating or hypertonic fluids such as total parenteral nutrition solutions), and when long-term access is needed to the patient's venous system. A peripherally inserted central catheter (PICC) is inserted in a peripheral vein, such as the basilic vein, and used for infusion and blood sampling only.

Essential Documentation

When assisting the health care provider who inserts a CVAD, the nurse should document the time and date of insertion; type, length, and location of the catheter; solution infused; the health care provider's name;

and the patient's response to the procedure. If the ports are not being used, document that they have needle-free injection caps, and include any orders related to maintaining patency. The nurse also needs to document the time and results of the x-ray performed to confirm placement. Note whether the catheter is sutured in place and the type of dressing applied. For a PICC, record the length of the external catheter.

Central Venous Cather Insertion		
2/24/2019	1100	**PATIENT TEACHING:** Procedure explained to pt. and consent obtained by Dr. S. Chavez. TLC placed by Dr. Chavez on first attempt in right subclavian vein. Cath sutured in place with 3-0 silk, and sterile dressing applied per protocol. Needle-free injection caps placed on all lines. Lines flushed with 100 units heparin. Portable CXR obtained to confirm line placement. Results pending. ______ **NURSING ASSESSMENT:** P 110, BP 90/58, RR 24, oral T 97.9° F. Pt. sitting in semi-Fowler's position and breathing easily, lungs clear bilaterally. ______ **Louise Flynn, RN**
2/24/2019	1150	RN received telephone report from Dr. Turner in radiology confirming proper placement of CV line in superior vena cava. ______ **Joyce Williams, RN**

CENTRAL VENOUS ACCESS DEVICE OCCLUSION

A central venous access device (CVAD) may become occluded because of kinks in the tubing, the presence of a blood clot or fibrin sheath, or crystalline adherence. Signs of occlusion include the inability to draw blood, infuse a solution, or flush the catheter. If CVAD occlusion is suspected, the nurse should check the tubing for kinks. The dressing may need to be removed to check for kinks under it. Ask the patient to cough or change position. Attempt to withdraw blood, or gently flush with normal saline solution. A specialized vascular team should be called to remedy occlusion of a CVAD.

Essential Documentation

The nurse should document the date and time of the occlusion. Record evidence of catheter occlusion. Describe the nursing actions and the results. Include the name of the health care provider notified, the time of notification, and any orders given. Depending on the facility's policy, the nurse may also need to document the occlusion on the IV therapy flow sheet.

Central Venous Device Occlusion		
7/4/2019	1220	**NURSING ASSESSMENT:** Unable to aspirate blood from distal port of TLC. Unable to flush line with NSS. No kinks noted in tubing. Dsg removed, no kinks noted under dsg. Site re-dressed according to protocol. ______ **NURSING INTERVENTION:** Pt. changed from supine to right and left lateral position and asked to cough; still unable to obtain blood return or flush with NSS. Blue distal port labeled "occluded." Dr. S. Brown notified of the occlusion at 1210. ______ ______ **Ruth Clark, RN**

CENTRAL VENOUS ACCESS DEVICE REMOVAL

When a CVAD is no longer necessary, it is removed by the health care provider or by a specialist on the vascular team.

Essential Documentation

After assisting with a CVAD removal, the vascular team should document the interventions.

Central Venous Device Removal		
2/24/2019	1100	**NURSING ASSESSMENT:** CV catheter removed by Dr. C. Romero at 1045 and pressure held for 5 min. ______ **NURSING INTERVENTION:** Catheter tip sent to laboratory for culture. **NURSING ASSESSMENT:** No drainage, redness, or swelling noted at insertion site. Sterile dressing applied. ______ ______ **Louise Flynn, RN**

CENTRAL VENOUS ACCESS DEVICE SITE CARE

CVAD site care and the frequency of care will vary according to the type of catheter and the facility's policy. Site care is performed using aseptic technique. After the access device is inserted, clean the site according to the institution's policies.

The insertion site should be visually inspected and palpated daily through an intact dressing.

When the dressing is removed, inspect the site for signs and symptoms of infiltration or phlebitis, such as discharge, inflammation, and tenderness. The frequency of site care varies from daily to every

48 hours for gauze dressings to every 3 to 7 days for transparent dressings, according to the institution's policy. Dressings should always be changed if they become soiled or lose integrity.

Essential Documentation

After completing the dressing change, the nurse should label the dressing with the time, date, and his or her initials. In the documentation, record the date and time of site care. Depending on facility policy, this documentation may be in the nurse's notes or IV therapy flow sheet. Note the appearance of the insertion site, method of cleaning the site, and type of dressing applied. Describe any drainage on the dressing. If complications are noted, record the name of the health care provider notified, the time of notification, and any orders given.

Central Venous Catheter Care		
9/25/2019	1220	**NURSING INTERVENTION:** Right subclavian TLC dressing removed. Suture intact, insertion site without redness or drainage. Using sterile technique, area and insertion site cleaned with chlorhexidine. Catheter secured with tape and covered with semipermeable transparent dressing. ______
		______ **Nick Cerone, RN**

CENTRAL VENOUS PRESSURE MONITORING

To monitor CVP, the health care provider inserts a catheter through a vein and advances it until the tip lies in or near the right atrium and end-diastolic pressure is seen on the monitor. When connected to a monitoring device, the catheter measures CVP, which is an index of right ventricular function. CVP monitoring helps to assess cardiac function, evaluate venous return to the heart, and indirectly gauge how well the heart is pumping. CVP monitoring may be done intermittently or continuously with a water manometer or pressure-monitoring system, with readings recorded in centimeters of water or millimeters of mercury.

Essential Documentation

The nurse should record CVP readings on a flow sheet or in the nurse's notes, according to the facility's policy. IV fluids may be documented on the IV flow sheet as well.

Central Venous Pressure Monitoring		
10/5/2019	0500	**NURSING INTERVENTION:** Right subclavian CVP attached to monitor with pressure bag setup of 500 mL NSS with 1000 units of heparin added. Line zeroed and calibrated. ______ **NURSING ASSESSMENT:** Normal CVP waveform on monitor shows reading of 4 cm H_2O. Urine output 25 mL in past hr. Mucous membranes dry, skin tents when pinched. P 110, BP 110/72, RR 18, oral T 99.0°F. **NURSING INTERVENTION:** Dr. J. Brown notified of CVP reading and physical assessment findings. Fluid challenge of 500 mL NSS over 1 hr started. ______ ______ **Joanne Nunez, RN**

CHEST PAIN

When the patient complains of chest pain, the nurse needs to act quickly to determine its cause. That's because chest pain may be caused by a disorder as benign as epigastric distress (indigestion) or as serious and life-threatening as acute myocardial infarction.

Essential Documentation

The nurse should record the date and time of the onset of chest pain. Question the patient about the pain, and record the responses using the patient's own words, when appropriate. Include the following:

- Patient's description of the pain: sharp, stabbing, burning, aching, pressure
- What the pain is rated on a scale of 0 to 10
- What the patient was doing when the pain started
- How long the pain lasted, if it had ever occurred before, and whether the onset was sudden or gradual
- Whether the pain radiates and where it radiates to
- Factors that improve or aggravate the pain
- The exact location of the pain. (Ask the patient to point to the pain, and record the patient's response. For example, the patient may vaguely indicate the abdominal area with the hands or may point with one finger to the left chest.)
- Additional signs and symptoms, such as dyspnea, diaphoresis, and nausea

Record the patient's vital signs, cardiac rhythm if available, and the results of a quick assessment of the patient's body systems. Document the time, the name of the health care provider who is notified, and any orders given. Document the nursing actions and the patient's responses. Include any patient education and emotional support provided.

Chest Pain

8/9/2019	0410	Pt. c/o sudden onset of a sharp chest pain that woke him up from sleep. Points to center of chest, over sternum. States, "It feels like an elephant is sitting on my chest." Pain radiates to the neck and shoulders. Rates pain as 7 on a scale of 0 to 10. P 112, BP 90/62, RR 26. Monitor shows ST depressions across V1- V6 chest leads. Lungs have fine crackles in the bases on auscultation. Dr. R. Romano notified and orders received. O_2 at 4 L/min started by NC. Pulse oximetry 94%. NTg S.L. given × 2 with relief of pain. 12-lead ECG and cardiac enzymes. All procedures explained to pt. Reassured pt. that he's being closely monitored. ________ **Martha Wolcott, RN**
8/9/2019	0415	**NURSING INTERVENTION:** Dr. Romano here to see patient. Pt. states pain is now a 1 on a scale of 0 to 10. ECG interpreted by Dr. Romano to show acute ischemia. Pt. prepared for transfer to CCU. ________ **Martha Wolcott, RN**

CHEST TUBE CARE

Inserted into the pleural space, a chest tube allows blood, fluid, pus, or air to drain and allows the lung to reinflate. Chest drainage uses gravity or suction to restore negative pressure and remove material that collects in the pleural cavity. An underwater seal in the drainage system allows air and fluid to escape from the pleural cavity but doesn't allow air to reenter.

Caring for the patient with a chest tube involves maintaining suction; monitoring for and preventing air leaks; monitoring drainage; promoting pulmonary hygiene; promoting patient comfort; performing dressing changes and site care; and preventing, detecting, and treating complications.

Essential Documentation

The nurse will record the date and time of chest tube insertion; chest tube location; type and amount of suction; type, amount, and consistency of drainage; and presence or absence of an air leak. If site care was performed, record the appearance of the site and the type of dressing applied. Document the patient's respiratory status and any pulmonary hygiene performed. Pulmonary hygiene and chest physiotherapy are performed by a respiratory team. Note the patient's level of pain, any comfort measures performed, and the results. Include interventions to prevent complications. If any complications occur, record the nursing interventions and the results. Note the name of the health care provider notified of problems and the time of notification.

Chest Tube Care

5/31/2019	1350	**NURSING ASSESSMENT:** Patient received from recovery room at 1325. Right midaxillary CT to 20 cm of suction. Collection chamber has 100 mL of serosanguineous fluid. No clots noted. Level of drainage dated and timed. No air leak noted. Two rubber-tipped clamps placed at bedside. Dressing dry and intact. No crepitus noted. Breath sounds clear with diminished breath sounds in right lower lobe. P 98, BP 132/82, RR 28 shallow and labored, oral T 99.1°F. Skin pale, warm, and dry, mucous membranes pink. O_2 sat. 97% on 50% face mask. Pt. c/o aching pain at CT site and refused to take deep breaths and cough due to pain. **NURSING INTERVENTION:** Morphine sulfate 2 mg I.V. given at 1335 with relief of pain. Pt. able to C&DB within 15 min after administration. ______________ **Mary Ann Pfister, RN**

CHEST TUBE INSERTION

Insertion of a chest tube permits drainage of air or fluid from the pleural space. Usually performed by a health care provider with a nurse assisting, this procedure requires sterile technique. Insertion sites vary, depending on the patient's condition. For a pneumothorax, the second intercostal space is the usual site because air rises to the top of the intrapleural space. For a hemothorax or pleural effusion, the sixth to the eighth intercostal spaces are common sites because fluid settles to the lower levels of the intrapleural space. For removal of air and fluid, a chest tube is inserted into a high site as well as a low site.

Following insertion, one or more chest tubes are connected to a thoracic drainage system that removes air, fluid, or both from the pleural space and prevents backflow into that space, thus promoting lung reexpansion. Inserting a chest tube requires close observation of the patient and verification of proper placement.

Essential Documentation

The nurse should document the date and time of chest tube insertion. Include the name of the health care provider performing the procedure. Commonly, a flow sheet will be used for documentation about chest tube insertion, drainage, and care. Identify the insertion site and the type of drainage system and suction used. Record the presence of drainage and air leaks. The drainage amount should also be included on the patient's intake and output record. Record the type, amount, and consistency of drainage. Document the patient's vital signs, pulse oximetry reading, auscultation findings, any complications, and nursing actions taken. Record any patient education performed. This may also need to be recorded on a patient teaching record, depending on the facility's policy.

Chest Tube Insertion		
9/30/2019	1100	**PATIENT TEACHING:** Pt. consented to insertion of chest tube after discussing risks and complications with Dr. J. Brown. Informed consent signed. ______
		NURSING ASSESSMENT: Preinsertion P 98, RR 32, BP 118/72, oral T 97.9°F.
		NURSING INTERVENTION: Assisted Dr. Brown with sterile insertion of #22 CT into pt.'s left lower midaxillary area. Tube secured with one suture. CT connected to 20 cm of suction, which immediately drained 100 mL of serosanguineous drainage. No air leaks evident. ______
		NURSING ASSESSMENT: Post insertion P 80, RR 24, BP 120/72. Respirations shallow, unlabored. Slightly decreased breath sounds in left post lower lobe, otherwise breath sounds clear bilaterally. O_2 sat. 99% after CT insertion. On O_2 2 L NC. Equal lung excursion noted. No crepitus palpated. ______
		NURSING INTERVENTION: Petroleum gauze applied to CT insertion site and occlusive dressing applied. ______
		NURSING ASSESSMENT: Pt. reports only minimal discomfort at insertion site. Upright portable CXR obtained. ______
		PATIENT TEACHING: Cough & deep breathing (C&DB) exercises and use of incentive spirometer reviewed with pt. Pt. verbalized understanding and was able to inspire 900 mL of volume. ______
		______ **Carol Slane, RN**

CHEST TUBE REMOVAL

After the patient's lung has reexpanded, the nurse may assist the health care provider in removing the chest tube. In many facilities, other health care professionals, such as advanced practice nurses (clinical nurse specialists or nurse practitioners), are trained to perform chest tube removal.

Essential Documentation

Document the date and time of chest tube removal and the name of the person who performed the procedure. Record the patient's vital signs and the findings of the respiratory assessment before and after chest tube removal. Note whether an analgesic was administered before the removal and how long after administration the chest tube was removed. Describe the patient's tolerance of the procedure. Record the amount of drainage in the collection bottle and the appearance of the wound at the chest tube site. Describe the type of dressing applied. Include any patient education performed.

Chest Tube Removal		
10/9/2019	1300	**PATIENT TEACHING:** Explained to pt. that CT was being removed because left lung is now reexpanded. Explained how to perform Valsalva's maneuver when tube is removed. Pt. was able to give return demonstration. ______
		NURSING INTERVENTION: Administered percocet 2 tabs P.O. 30 min before removal. ______
		NURSING ASSESSMENT: Preprocedure P 88, BP 120/80, RR 18, oral T 97.8°F. O_2 at 2 L via NC, 98% sat. Respirations regular, deep, unlabored. No use of accessory muscles. Full respiratory excursion bilaterally. Breath sounds clear bilaterally. No drainage in collection chamber since 0800. #20 CT removed without difficulty by Dr. M. Smith. CT wound clean. No drainage or redness noted. Petroleum gauze dressing placed over insertion site, covered with 4" × 4" gauze dressing, and secured with 2″ tape. Postprocedure breath sounds remain clear, full respiratory excursion bilaterally, breathing comfortably in semi-Fowler's position, no subcutaneous crepitus noted. P 86, BP 132/84, RR 20. 98% SaO_2 . Pt. without complaints of pain or shortness of breath.
		PATIENT TEACHING: Reminded him of importance of continuing to use incentive spirometer q1hr. CXR ordered for 1400. ______
		______ **Marcy Wells, RN**

CHEST TUBE REMOVAL BY PATIENT

The accidental or intentional removal of a chest tube by the patient can introduce air into the pleural space, leading to the potentially life-threatening complication of pneumothorax. As a precaution, sterile petroleum gauze should be kept at the patient's bedside at all times. Moreover, inappropriate removal of a chest tube can damage the surrounding tissue.

If the patient removes his or her chest tube, the nurse should immediately cover the site with sterile petroleum gauze and tape it in place. Stay with the patient and assess vital signs and respiratory status, and observe for signs and symptoms of pneumothorax. Call for help, and instruct a coworker to notify the health care provider and gather the equipment needed for reinsertion of the chest tube. If the patient is not in respiratory distress, the health care provider may order a chest x-ray to determine if the chest tube needs to be reinserted.

Essential Documentation

The nurse should record the date and time of the entry. Describe how it was discovered that the patient removed the chest tube. Use the patient's own words, if appropriate, to describe what happened. Record the immediate nursing actions and the patient's response. Document vital signs, pulse oximetry reading, and the results of the cardiopulmonary assessment, in particular noting whether the patient has any signs or symptoms of pneumothorax, such as hypotension, distended neck veins, absent breath sounds, tracheal shift, hypoxemia, weak and rapid pulse, dyspnea, tachypnea, diaphoresis, or chest pain. Note the name of the health care provider notified, the time of notification, and any orders given, such as preparing for chest tube reinsertion, administering supplemental oxygen, or obtaining a chest x-ray. Document any support or education given. If the patient requires reinsertion of a chest tube, follow the documentation guidelines for chest tube insertion. (See *Chest tube insertion,* pages 74 and 75.)

Chest Tube Removal by Patient		
4/15/2019	0815	**NURSING ASSESSMENT:** Upon entering room, noted chest tube lying on floor. Pt. stated, "This tube was hurting me so I was rubbing it. Next thing I know it was lying on the floor." ________
		NURSING INTERVENTION: Immediately covered site with petroleum gauze taped in place over left chest wound. ________
		NURSING ASSESMENT: No external trauma to insertion site, no drainage or bleeding noted. Pt. in bed in semi-Fowler's position, breathing comfortably at rate of 22. P 94, BP 110/74. 97% SaO_2. on 3 L NC. Breath sounds clear bilaterally with left lower lobe sounds slightly diminished. Neck veins not distended, no dyspnea noted, trachea in midline, skin warm and dry, no c/o chest pain. Stayed with pt. while Brian Mott, LPN, notified Dr. S. Finnegan at 0745. CXR done, showing left lung inflated. Chest tube to remain out. Repeat CXR ordered for 1000. Pt.'s cardiopulmonary status to be assessed q 5min for 1st hr, then q1hr for next 4 hr, then q4hr thereafter. ________
		PATIENT TEACHING: Reviewed C&DB exercises with pt. and reminded him to do them every hr. ________
		________ **Sarah Clarke, RN**

CLINICAL PATHWAY

A clinical pathway, also known as a *critical pathway,* integrates the principles of case management into nursing documentation. It outlines the standard of care for a specific diagnosis-related group. It incorporates multidisciplinary diagnoses and interventions, such as nursing-related problems, combined nursing and medical interventions, and key events that should occur for the patient to be discharged by a target date.

A clinical pathway is usually organized by categories according to the patient's diagnosis, which dictates the patient's expected length of stay, daily care guidelines, and expected outcomes. These categories, specified for each day, include consultations, diagnostic tests, treatments, drugs, procedures, activities, diet, patient teaching, discharge planning, and anticipated outcomes. Other events or interventions may be added, and the pathway's categories may be presented in various formats and combinations.

Within the managed care system, clinical pathways set the standard for tracking patient progress. They provide the nursing staff with necessary written criteria to guide and monitor patient care.

Essential Documentation

The nurse should record whether the patient's progress follows what is outlined in the clinical pathway by choosing either "variance," if the patient's progress deviates from the standard, or "no variance," if the patient's progress is following the standard. This is recorded for each shift and signed by the nurse. (See *Following a clinical pathway,* pages 79 and 80.)

COLD THERAPY APPLICATION

The application of cold therapy constricts blood vessels; inhibits local circulation, suppuration, and tissue metabolism; relieves vascular congestion; slows bacterial activity in infections; reduces body temperature; and may act as a temporary anesthetic during brief, painful procedures. Because cold therapy also relieves inflammation, reduces edema, and slows bleeding, it may provide effective initial treatment after eye injuries, strains, sprains, bruises, muscle spasms, and burns. However, cold therapy doesn't reduce existing edema because it inhibits reabsorption of excess fluid.

(*Text continues on page 81*)

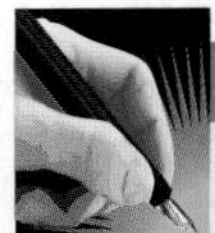

AccuChart

FOLLOWING A CLINICAL PATHWAY

At any point in a treatment course, a glance at the clinical pathway allows the nurse to compare the patient's progress and the nurse's performance as a caregiver with care standards. Below is a sample pathway.

CLINICAL PATHWAY: COLON RESECTION WITHOUT COLOSTOMY

	Patient visit	Presurgery Day 1	O.R. Day	Postop Day 1
Assessments	History and physical with breast, rectal, and pelvic exam Nursing assessment	Nursing admission assessment	Nursing admission assessment on TBA patients in holding area Review of systems assessment*	Review of systems assessment*
Consults	Social services consult Physical therapy consult	Notify referring physician of impending admission	Type and screen for patients in holding area with Hgb < 10	
Labs and diagnostics	Complete blood count (CBC) Coagulation profile ECG Chest X-ray (CXR) Chem profile CT ABD w/wo contrast CT pelvis Urinalysis Barium enema & flex sigmoidoscopy/colonoscopy Biopsy report	Type and screen		CBC
Interventions	Many or all of the above labs/diagnostics will have already been done. Check all results and fax to the surgeon's office.	Check for bowel prep orders Bowel prep* Antiembolism stockings Incentive spirometry Ankle exercises* I.V. access* Routine vital signs (VS)* Sequential compression devices (SCDs)	Shave and prep in O.R. Nasogastric (NG) tube maint.* Intake and output (I/O) VS per routine* Catheter care* Incentive spirometry* SCDs I.V. site care* Head of bed (HOB) 30°* Safety measures* Wound care* Mouth care*	NG tube maintenance* I/O* VS per routine* Catheter care* Incentive spirometry* SCDs I.V. site care* HOB 30°* Safety measures* Wound care* Mouth care* Antiembolism stockings
I.V.s		I.V. fluids, D_5½ NSS @ 75 ml/hr	I.V. fluids, D_5LR @ 125 ml/hr	I.V. fluids, D_5LR @ 125 ml/hr
Medication	Prescribe GoLYTELY/NuLYTELY 10a — 2p Neomycin @ 2p, 3p, and 10p Erythromycin @ 2p, 3p, and 10p	GoLYTELY/NuLYTELY 10a — 2p Erythromycin @ 2p, 3p, and 10p Neomycin @ 2p, 3p and 10p	Preop antibiotics (AB) in holding area Postop AB 2 2 doses PCA (basal rate 0.5 mg) Lovenox Subcut.	PCA (basal rate 0.5 mg) Subcut. heparin
Diet/GI	Clears presurgery day NPO after midnight	Clears presurgery day NPO after midnight	NPO/NG tube	NPO/NG tube
Activity	Preop teaching	Reinforce preop teaching	4 hours after surgery, ambulate with abdominal binder*	Ambulate t.i.d. with abdominal binder* May shower Physical therapy b.i.d. Begin discharge teaching
KEY: * = NSG activities V = Variance N = No variance	1. V (N) 2. V N 3. V N	1. V (N) 2. V (N) 3. V (N)	1. V (N) 2. V (N) 3. V (N)	1. V (N) 2. V (N) 3. V (N)
Signatures:	1. M. Connel, RN 2. ______	1. M. Connel, RN 2. C. Roy, RN	1. L. Singer, RN 2. J. Smith, RN	1. L. Singer, RN 2. J. Smith, RN

(continued)

FOLLOWING A CLINICAL PATHWAY *(continued)*

CLINICAL PATHWAY: COLON RESECTION WITHOUT COLOSTOMY

	Postop Day 2	Postop Day 3	Postop Day 4	Postop Day 5
Assessments	Review of systems assessment*	Review of systems assessment*	Review of systems assessment*	Review of systems assessment*
Consults		Dietary consult		Oncology consult if indicated (or to be done as outpatient)
Labs and diagnostics	Electrolyte 7 (EL-7) CXR	CBC EL-7	Pathology results on chart	CBC EL-7
Interventions	Discontinue NG tube if possible* (per guidelines) I/O* VS per routine* Discontinue catheter* Ambulating* Incentive spirometry* SCDs I.V. site care* HOB 30°* Safety measures* Wound care* Mouth care* Antiembolism stockings	I/O* VS per routine* Incentive spirometry* SCDs I.V. site care* Safety measures* Wound care* Antiembolism stockings SCDs	I/O* VS per routine* Incentive spirometry* I.V. site care* Safety measures* Wound care* Antiembolism stockings	Consider staple removal Replace with Steri-Strips Assess that patient has met discharge criteria*
I.V.s	I.V. fluids D_5½ NSS 20 mcg KCl @ 75 ml/hr	I.V.-Heplock	Heplock	Discontinue Heplock
Medication	PCA	Discontinue PCA P.O. analgesia Resume routine home meds	P.O. analgesia	P.O. analgesia
Diet/GI	Discontinue NG tube per guidelines: (Clamp tube at 8 a.m. if no N/V and residual < 200 ml, Discontinue tube @ 12 noon)* (Check with doctor first)	Clears if pt. has BM/flatus Advance to postop diet if tolerating clears (at least one tray of clears)*	Regular	Regular
Activity	Ambulate q.i.d. with abdominal binder* May shower Physical therapy b.i.d.	Ambulate at least q.i.d. with abdominal binder* May shower Physical therapy b.i.d.	Ambulate at least q.i.d. with abdominal binder* May shower Physical therapy b.i.d.	
Teaching	Reinforce preop teaching* Patient and family education p.r.n.* re: family screening	Reinforce preop teaching* Patient and family education p.r.n.* re: family screening	Reinforce preop teaching* Patient and family education p.r.n.* Discharge teaching re: reportable s/s, F/U and wound care*	Review all discharge instructions and Rx including* follow-up appointments: with surgeon within 3 weeks, with oncologist within 1 month if indicated
KEY: * = NSG activities V = Variance N = No variance	1. V (N) 2. V (N) 3. V (N)	1. V (N) 2. V (N) 3. V (N)	1. V (N) 2. V (N) 3. V (N)	1. V (N) 2. V N 3. V N
Signatures:	1. A. McCarthy, RN 2. R. Mayer, RN	1. A. McCarthy, RN 2. R. Mayer, RN	1. L. Singer, RN 2. J. Smith, RN	1. L. Singer, RN 2.

Essential Documentation

The nurse should record the time, date, and duration of cold application; the site of application; and the type of device used, such as an ice bag or collar, K pad, cold compress, or chemical cold pack. Indicate the temperature or temperature setting of the device if able. Before and after the procedure, record the patient's vital signs and the appearance of the patient's skin. Document any signs of complications, interventions, and the patient's response. Describe the patient's tolerance of treatment.

COLD THERAPY APPLICATION		
11/14/2019	1300	**NURSING ASSESSMENT:** Before cold therapy application, oral T 98.6°F, BP 110/70, P 80, RR 18. Right groin site warm and dry, without redness, edema, or ecchymosis.
		NURSING INTERVENTION: Ice bag applied to right groin for 20 min.
		NURSING ASSESSMENT: Postprocedure T 98.6°F, BP 120/70, P 82, RR 20. Right groin site cool and dry, without redness, edema, graying, mottling, blisters, or ecchymosis. No c/o burning or numbness. Pt. is resting comfortably.
		Greg Pearson, RN

CONFUSION

An umbrella term for puzzling or inappropriate behavior or responses, confusion reflects the inability to think quickly and coherently. Depending on its cause, confusion may arise suddenly or gradually and may be temporary or irreversible. Aggravated by stress and sensory deprivation, confusion commonly occurs in elderly hospitalized patients, in whom it may be mistaken for dementia.

When severe confusion arises suddenly and the patient also has hallucinations and psychomotor hyperactivity, the condition is classified as delirium. Long-term, progressive confusion with the deterioration of all cognitive functions is classified as dementia.

Confusion may result from metabolic, neurologic, cardiopulmonary, cerebrovascular, or nutritional disorders or can result from infection, toxins, drugs, or alcohol. It may also be related to depression.

Essential Documentation

When a patient is confused, the nurse should document how he or she became aware of the patient's confusion. Record the results of the neurologic and cardiopulmonary assessments. Record possible contributing factors, such as abnormal laboratory values, medications, poor nutrition, poor sleep patterns, infection, surgery, pain, sensory overload or deprivation, and the use of alcohol and nonprescription drugs. Record the time and name of the health care provider notified. Note any new orders, such as blood work to assess laboratory values or drug changes. Describe nursing interventions to reduce confusion and to keep the patient safe, and include the patient's response. Document patient teaching and emotional support given.

Confusion		
6/22/2019	0300	**NURSING ASSESSMENT:** Pt. found OOB. Disoriented to time and place. Cooperative. Returned to bed. Pt. received Restoril 5 mg at 0100 CNA assigned to remain with patient. P 100, BP 110/70, RR 20. Pulse oximetry 98% on RA. ________ **Matilda Jennings, RN**

CONTINUOUS RENAL REPLACEMENT THERAPY

Continuous renal replacement therapy (CRRT) is a procedure that filters fluid, solutes, and electrolytes from the patient's blood and infuses a replacement solution. Commonly used to treat unstable patients in acute renal failure, CRRT is also used for treating fluid overload that does not respond to diuretics and for some electrolyte and acid–base disturbances.

CRRT carries a much lower risk of hypotension than conventional hemodialysis because it withdraws fluid more slowly, at about 200 mL/hour. This procedure can be performed in hypotensive patients who require fluid removal but can't undergo hemodialysis. CRRT reduces the risk of other complications and makes maintaining a stable fluid volume and regulating fluid and electrolyte balance easier. CRRT methods vary in complexity and include slow, continuous ultrafiltration (SCUF), continuous arteriovenous hemofiltration (CAVH), and continuous venovenous hemofiltration (CVVH). CRRT is a specialized procedure that's performed by specially trained nurses and requires one-to-one care.

Essential Documentation

When the patient undergoes CRRT, the nurse should record the time that the treatment began and the time it ended and fluid-balance information. Document baseline and hourly vital signs and intake and output. Record laboratory studies, such as electrolytes, coagulation factors, complete blood count, and blood urea nitrogen and creatinine levels.

Weight, vital signs, amount of fluid removed, and laboratory studies may be documented on a specialized flow sheet. Describe the appearance of the ultrafiltrate. Document the inspection of the insertion sites as well as any site care and dressing changes. The nurse should make sure to mark the dressing with the date and time of the dressing change. Record the results of the assessment of circulation in the affected leg if appropriate. Document any medications or blood products given during the procedure. Note any complications, nursing interventions, and the patient's response. Include the patient's tolerance of the procedure.

Continuous Renal Replacment Therapy		
7/27/2019	0815	**NURSING ASSESSMENT:** CAVH started at 0800. See CAVH flow sheet for labs, and hourly VS and I/O. Baseline weight 132.4 lb, P 92, BP 132/74, RR 20, oral T 98.2°F. Ultrafiltrate clear yellow. Left femoral access sites without hematoma, redness, swelling, or warmth. Left foot warm, dorsalis pedis and posterior tibial pulses strong, capillary refill less than 3 sec. ___
		NURSING INTERVENTION: Insertion sites cleaned according to protocol and covered with occlusive dressing. ___
		___ **Tom Costanza, RN**

CORRECTION TO DOCUMENTATION

When the nurse makes a mistake on a chart, he or she should correct it promptly. Never erase, cover, completely scratch out, or otherwise obscure an erroneous entry because this may imply a cover-up. If the chart ends up in court, the plaintiff's attorney will be looking for anything that may cast doubt on the chart's accuracy. Erasures or the use of correction fluid or heavy black ink to obliterate an error are red flags.

Essential Documentation

When the nurse makes a mistake when documenting on the medical record, he or she should correct it by drawing a single line through it and writing the words "mistaken entry" above or beside it. Follow these words with the nurse's initials and the date. If appropriate, briefly explain the necessity for the correction. Make sure the mistaken entry is still readable. This indicates that the nurse is only trying to correct a mistake, not cover it up. For electronic charting systems, an edit selection is available to change documentation. Only the person who entered an entry is permitted to edit it. All changes can be tracked electronically.

Correction to Documentation		
1/19/2019	0900	Mistaken entry. J. M. 1/19/19 ~~Pt. walked to bathroom. States he experienced no difficulty urinating.~~ ________________ ~~**John Mora, RN**~~

CRITICAL TEST VALUES, REPORTING

According to The Joint Commission's National Patient Safety Goals, critical test results must be reported to a responsible licensed caregiver in a timely manner so that immediate action may be taken. Critical test results include diagnostic tests, such as imaging studies, ECGs, laboratory tests, and other diagnostic studies. These critical test results may be reported verbally (including by telephone) and by fax, e-mail, or other technologies. If the results aren't reported verbally, the person sending the results should confirm that they have been received. Critical test values may be reported to another individual (e.g., a nurse, unit secretary, or health care provider's office staff) who will then report the values to the health care provider or licensed caregiver.

Essential Documentation

The nurse should record the date and time of receipt of the critical test result, the person who gave the results to the nurse, the name of the test, and the critical value. Document the name of the health care provider or licensed health care provider notified, the time of the notification, the means of communication used, and any orders given. If the message was not relayed verbally, include confirmation that the critical test result was received by the health care provider. Note any instructions or information given to the patient. If the message was given to a nurse, unit secretary, or office staff personnel include that individual's name.

Reporting Critical Lab Values		
6/4/2019	1000	**NURSING ASSESSMENT:** Annette Lange called from pharmacy at 0945 to report critical PT value of 52 seconds. ________ **NURSING INTERVENTION:** Results reported by telephone to Dr. H. Potter at 0948, orders given to hold warfarin, obtain PT level in a.m., and call Dr. Potter with results. ________ **PATIENT TEACHING:** Pt. informed about elevated PT and the need to hold warfarin until PT levels drop to therapeutic range. Pt. instructed to report any bleeding to nurse. ________ ________________ **Karen Lane, RN**

CULTURAL NEEDS IDENTIFICATION

To provide culturally competent care to the patient, the nurse must remember that the patient's cultural behaviors and beliefs may be different from the nurse's. For example, people in a number of cultures—including Native Americans, Asians, and people from Arab-speaking countries—may find eye contact disrespectful or aggressive. Identifying the patient's cultural needs is the first step in developing a culturally sensitive care plan.

Essential Documentation

The nurse should record the date and time of the assessment. Depending on the facility's policy, the cultural assessment may be part of the admission history form, or there may be a separate, more in-depth cultural assessment tool. (See *Identifying your patient's cultural needs,* pages 86 to 88.)

Assess the patient's communication style. Find out if the patient can speak and read English, his or her ability to read lips, his or her native language, and whether an interpreter is required. Observe the patient's nonverbal communication style for eye contact, expressiveness, and ability to understand common signs. Determine social orientation, including culture, race, ethnicity, family role function, work, and religion. Document the patient's spatial comfort level, particularly in light of his or her conversation, proximity to others, body movement, and space perception. Note the patient's skin color and body structure. Ask about food preferences, family health history, religious and cultural health practices, and definitions of health and illness.

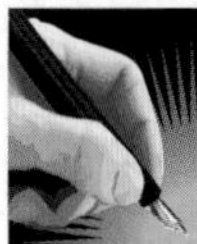

AccuChart

IDENTIFYING YOUR PATIENT'S CULTURAL NEEDS

A transcultural assessment tool can help promote cultural sensitivity in any nursing setting. The nurse should consult the facility's policy on the use of such forms, or incorporate the information included in this sample form when developing the patient's care plan.

Date 3/12/19 Time 1015 Pt name Claudette Valiente Age 34 ❑ M ☑ F

Medical dx: 36 weeks pregnant, states "high sugar in my blood"

Determining your patient's communication needs

Ask the patient

Can you speak English? ☑ Yes ❑ No

Can you read English? ☑ Yes ❑ No with difficulty

What is your native language? Creole

Do you speak or read any other language? No

How do you want to be addressed? ❑ Mr. ❑ Mrs. ❑ Ms. ☑ First name ❑ Nickname

Your observations

How would you characterize the patient's nonverbal communication style? Very open

Eye contact: ❑ Yes ☑ No

Use of interpreter: ❑ Family ❑ Friend ❑ Professional ☑ None

Overall communication style: ☑ Verbally loud and expressive ❑ Quiet, reserved ❑ Silent

Meaning of common signs—O.K., got ya nose, index finger summons, V sign, thumbs up

Understands above signs except "got ya nose"

Determining your patient's social orientation, network, and support system

Ask the patient

Where were you born? Haiti

What setting did you grow up in? ❑ Urban ❑ Suburban ☑ Rural

What is your ethnic identity? Haitian

Who are your major support people? ☑ Family members ❑ Friends ❑ Other

Who is the head of your household? Husband

Who makes major decisions for the family? A family meeting is held

What kind of work did you do in your native country? None What is your present job? None

What level of education did you complete? Finished 6th grade

Is religion important to you? Yes

What is your religious affiliation? Catholic Would you like a chaplain visit? ❑ Yes ☑ No

Do you have any cultural/religious practices/restrictions? Balancing "hot" and "cold," believes in some voodoo passed down from mother and grandmother

Do you celebrate any religious holidays? Easter, Christmas

Do you use a religious healer? No

IDENTIFYING YOUR PATIENT'S CULTURAL NEEDS *(continued)*

Determining your patient's social orientation, network, and support system *(continued)*

Your observations

Interaction with family/significant other — describe Animated, physically close, frequent touch, eye contact with family members

Religious icons on person or in room Keeps cross at bedside

Determining your patient's spatial (space) needs (comfort in conversation, proximity to others, body movement, perception of space and time)

Ask the patient

Are you comfortable with others in the room? Yes

Are you uncomfortable if someone gets in your personal space? Yes, likes people to maintain comfortable, safe distance except for family

What do you consider a proper greeting? Kissing and touch with family, "Hello" to others

Your observations

☑ Tactile relationships, demonstrates affection

❑ Non-contact

Need for personal space Very close with family, maintains 2-3 foot distance from RN

Determining your patient's biological variations (skin color, body structure, genetic and enzymatic patterns, nutritional preferences and deficiencies)

Ask the patient

Do you have any food preferences? Rice, beans, plantains

Is there any food you particularly dislike? Yogurt, cottage cheese

What do you believe promotes health? Good spiritual habits, balancing "hot and "cold," and eating well

What is your family history of disease? Malaria, high blood pressure, "sugar"

Your observations

Skin color Deep brown

Body structure Heavy, large frame

Special dietary concerns Heart healthy diet

Determining your patient's health practices, values, and definitions of health and illness

Ask the patient

What do you think caused your illness? "Ate wrong foods."

Do you know why it started when it did? "No."

What does your illness do to you; how does it work? "I don't think anything is wrong, but the doctor does."

How severe is your illness? How long do you think it will last? "It will go away soon."

(continued)

IDENTIFYING YOUR PATIENT'S CULTURAL NEEDS (*continued*)

Determining your patient's health practices, values, and definitions of health and illness (*continued*)

Ask the patient (continued)

What problems has your sickness caused you? "The doctor says my baby is big. But, a big baby is a strong baby."

What fears do you have about your illness? "I have no fear. I will have a healthy baby."

What kind of treatment do you think you should receive? "Eating healthy."

What are the most important results you hope to receive from this treatment? "A healthy baby."

How does your family get better when they are sick? Uses home remedies such as herbs to treat sickness

What should you do to stay healthy? "Eat well."

Do you do anything to prevent from getting sick? ☐ Yes ☑ No

Do you have any concerns about health and illness? "No."

What types of healing practices do you engage in (hot tea and lemon for cold, copper bracelet for arthritis, magnets)? "Avoiding spices because they bother the baby, balancing hot and cold"

What customs and beliefs concerning major life events are practiced in your native country? "Pregnant women are treated special. Father of the baby doesn't participate in the birth experience; this is "women's business."

Your observations

Appearance and surroundings Patient is clean and neatly groomed. Appears slightly overweight.

History of noncompliance, missed appointments? Often misses appts or arrives late

Signature: Diane Reale, RN

SELECTED READINGS

American Heart Association. (2018). *Highlights of the 2018 focused updates to the American Heart Association guidelines for CPR and ECC: Advanced cardiovascular life support and pediatric advanced life support CPR and emergency cardiac care.* Retrieved from https://eccguidelines.heart.org/index.php/guidelines-highlights/

Carrabba, N., Migliorini, A., Pradella, S., Acquafresca, M., Guglielmo, M., Baggiano, A., ... Valenti, R. (2018). Old and new NICE guidelines for the evaluation of new onset stable chest pain: A real world perspective. *BioMed Research International,* Article ID 3762305. https://doi.org/10.1155/2018/3762305

Dessain, T. E., & Martin, D. (2018). Continuous renal replacement therapy for the critically ill patient. *British Journal of Hospital Medicine, 79*(1), C2–C7.

Evensen, S., Saltvedt, I., Lydersen, S., Wyller, T. B., Taraldsen, K., & Sletvold, O. (2018). Environmental factors and risk of delirium in geriatric patients: An observational study. *BMC Geriatrics, 18*(1), 1–8.

Hoit, B. D. (2018). *Cardiac tamponade.* Retrieved from UpToDate website: https://www.uptodate.com/contents/cardiac-tamponade

Johns Hopkins Medicine. (2018). *Cold therapy (cryotherapy) for pain management.* Retrieved from https://www.hopkinsmedicine.org/healthlibrary/conditions/orthopaedic_disorders/cryotherapy_cold_therapy_for_pain_management_134,95

Kalender, N., & Tosun, N. (2015). Nursing studies about central venous catheter care: A literature review and recommendations for clinical practice. *International Journal of Caring Sciences, 8*(2), 461–477.

Kane, C. J., York, N. L., & Minton, L. A. (2013). Chest tubes in the critically ill patient. *Dimensions of Critical Care Nursing, 32*(3), 111–117.

Laske, R. A., & Stephens, B. A. (2018). Confusion states: Sorting out delirium, dementia, and depression. *Nursing Made Incredibly Easy, 16*(6), 13–16.

National Institute of Health, National Heart, Lung, and Blood Institute. (2018). *Cardioversion.* Retrieved from https://www.nhlbi.nih.gov/health-topics/cardioversion

Nguyen, M. (2009). Nurse's assessment of caregiver burden. *Medsurg Nursing, 18*(3), 147–151.

Nickasch, B. (2016). What do I do next? Nurse confusion and uncertainty in cardiac monitoring. *Medsurg Nursing, 25*(6), 418–422.

Satryb, S. A., Wilson, T. J., & Patterson, M. M. (2011). Casting: All wrapped up. *Orthopaedic Nursing, 30*(1), 37–43.

Taylor, C., Lynn, P., & Bartlett, J. L. (2019). *Fundamentals of nursing: The art and science of person-centered care.* Philadelphia, PA: Lippincott.

Teodorczuk, A., & MacLullich, A. (2018). New waves of delirium understanding. *International Journal of Geriatric Psychiatry, 33*(11), 1417–1419.

D

DEATH OF A PATIENT

After a patient dies, nursing care should include the provision of support to family members and the preparation of the patient for family viewing. This preparation includes the removal of tubes and drains and bathing of the body. Arrangement of transportation to the morgue or funeral home may be done by the nursing supervisor. Identification and disposition of the patient's belongings should be completed in accordance with the family's wishes. Family members should be afforded privacy and given time to remain with their deceased loved one. Emotional support should be provided.

Postmortem care usually begins after the patient's death is certified. If the patient died violently or under suspicious circumstances, postmortem care might be postponed until the medical examiner completes an examination. It is important to be aware of state laws related to notification of organ procurement organizations (OPOs).

Essential Documentation

The death of a patient is pronounced by a physician or nurse practitioner. In some states, registered nurses can pronounce a patient dead. The provider who pronounced the death of the patient should document the date and time of the patient's death. If resuscitation was attempted, indicate the time it started and ended, and refer to the code sheet in the patient's medical record. Note whether the case is being referred to the medical examiner. Include all postmortem care given, noting whether medical equipment was removed or left in place. List all belongings and valuables and the name of the family member who accepted and signed the appropriate valuables or belongings list. Record any belongings left on the patient. If the patient has dentures, note whether they were left in the patient's mouth or given to a family member. (If given to a family member, include the family member's name.) There is a specific form provided by the facility that will be completed by the nurse or other provider regarding the disposition of the patient's body; the name, telephone number, and address of the funeral home; medical examiner office contact; and OPO information. The names of the family members who were present at the time of death should be documented. If the family was not present at the time of death, note the name of the family member and the time notified. Be sure to document any care, emotional support, and education given to the family.

Death of a Patient		
8/22/2019	1420	**NURSING ASSESSMENT:** Called to room by pt.'s daughter, Mrs. Helen Jones, stating pt. not breathing. Pt. found unresponsive in bed at 1345, not breathing, no pulse, no heart or breath sounds auscultated. No code called because pt. has advance directive and DNR order signed in chart. Case not referred to medical examiner. ______
		NURSING INTERVENTION: Death pronouncement made by Dr. Holmes at 1350. NG tube, Foley catheter, and I.V. line in left forearm removed and dressings applied. Pt. bathed and given oral care, dentures placed in mouth. Belongings checked off on belongings list and signed by Mrs. Jones, who will take belongings home with her. Body tagged and sent to morgue at 1415. ______
		PLAN: Mrs. Jones is making arrangements with Restful Funeral Home, 123 Main St., Pleasantville, NY (123) 456-7890. Stayed with daughter throughout her visit. Stated she was OK to drive home. Declined visit by chaplain. ______
		______ **Jeanne Ballinger, RN**

DEHYDRATION, ACUTE

Dehydration refers to the loss of water in the body resulting in a shift in fluid and electrolytes, which can lead to hypovolemic shock, organ failure, and death. Dehydration may be isotonic, hypertonic, or hypotonic. Common causes of dehydration are fever, diarrhea, and vomiting. Other causes include hemorrhage, excessive diaphoresis, burns, excessive wound or nasogastric drainage, and ketoacidosis. Prompt intervention is necessary to prevent complications, which can include death.

Essential Documentation

The nurse should record the date and time of the entry. The date and time are automatically recorded in electronic health records (EHRs).

An EHR and intake–output flow sheet are necessary to document dehydration. Record the results of the physical assessment and any subjective findings. Include laboratory values and the results of any diagnostic tests (e.g., stool culture to identify the cause of excessive diarrhea). Closely monitor and record intake and output on an intake–output flow sheet. (See "Intake and output," pages 210 to 212.) Record the name of the health care provider notified, the time of notification, and any orders given. Document the nursing interventions, such as intravenous (IV) therapy, and the patient's response. Record nursing actions to prevent complications, such as monitoring for IV infiltration and auscultating for breath sounds to detect fluid-volume overload. Also note the patient's level of consciousness.

Dehydration, Acute		
5/25/2019	1300	**NURSING ASSESSMENT:** Pt. admitted to unit from nursing home with increasing lethargy and diarrhea X3 days. Pt. is lethargic, doesn't answer questions, occasionally moans. Skin and mucous membranes dry; tenting occurs when pinched. P 118, BP 92/58, RR 28, rectal T 101.2°F, wt. 102 lb (family reports this is down 3 lb in 3 days). Breath sounds clear, normal heart sounds. Peripheral pulses palpable but weak. No edema. ______
		NURSING INTERVENTION Foley catheter inserted to monitor urine output. Urine sample sent to lab for UA and C&S. Urine color dark amber, specific gravity 1.001. Blood drawn for CBC with diff., BUN, creatinine, and electrolytes. Incontinent of approx. 300 mL of liquid stool, guaiac neg., sample sent for C&S. Dr. S. Holmes in to see pt. and orders written. ______
		Pt. placed on cardiac monitor. Pt. in NSR, no arrhythmias noted. Administering O_2 at 2 L via NC. I.V. infusion started in left upper forearm with 18G catheter of NSS at 100 mL/hr. See I/O record and frequent vital signs assessment sheet for hourly VS and hourly I/O.
		______ **Michelle Pressman, RN**

DEMENTIA

Dementia is considered a syndrome rather than a distinctive disease process. It is a progressive deterioration of cognitive ability characterized by memory loss, inability to perform abstract analysis, lack of judgment, and decline in language skills. Changes in personality and the inability to perform activities of daily living (ADLs) progress over time.

Nursing interventions are focused on helping the patient maintain an optimal level of cognitive performance, preventing physical injury, decreasing anxiety and agitation, increasing communication skills, and promoting the patient's ability to perform ADLs.

Essential Documentation

The nurse should perform a neurologic assessment, as appropriate, including level of consciousness, appearance, behavior, speech, and cognitive function. Record the patient's exact responses. Document measures taken to ensure patient safety, meet personal needs, and promote independence; also document the patient's response. An EHR requires that the nurse document patient safety needs.

Dementia		
3/3/2019	0900	**NURSING ASSESSMENT:** Noted pt. leaving the unit at 0840. When asked where he was going, he stated, "To the store. We need groceries." While assisting pt. back to room, he kept insisting he had to go the store and resisted efforts to bring him back to his room. Pt. oriented to name only. Gait steady. Pt.'s shirt buttoned wrong, shoes mismatched, hair uncombed. Pt. resisting any further neurologic assessment. ____ **NURSING INTERVENTION:** Dr. B. Newmann notified at 0850 of pt.'s wandering, spoke with family, and obtained permission for use of wanderguard alarm. Alarm band placed on pt.'s wrist. Staff will check on pt. frequently and will reorient and redirect pt. as needed. ____ **Charles Bricker, RN**

DIABETIC KETOACIDOSIS

Characterized by severe hyperglycemia, diabetic ketoacidosis (DKA) is a potentially life-threatening condition that occurs most commonly in people with type 1 diabetes. The clinical assessment of the patient with dementia is written on a standardized form, such as the mental-status examination form or other standardized record. An acute insulin deficiency precedes DKA, causing glucose to accumulate in the blood. At the same time, the liver responds to energy-starved cells by converting glycogen to glucose, further increasing blood glucose levels. Because the insulin-deprived cells can't utilize glucose, they metabolize protein, which results in the loss of intracellular potassium and phosphorus and excessive release of amino acids. The liver converts these amino acids into urea and glucose. The result is grossly elevated blood glucose levels and osmotic diuresis, leading to fluid and electrolyte imbalances and profound dehydration. Moreover, the absolute insulin deficiency causes cells to convert fats to glycerol and fatty acids for energy. The fatty acids accumulate in the liver, where they are converted to ketones. The ketones accumulate in blood and urine. Acidosis leads to more tissue breakdown, more ketosis; and eventually, shock, coma, and death.

When caring for a patient with DKA, the nurse should document assessments and interventions in a time frame consistent with institutional policy. Avoid charting in blocks of time.

Essential Documentation

A standardized EHR or flow sheet is used for documentation of the changing condition of a patient experiencing DKA. The nurse should document the patient's hourly blood glucose levels, intake and output, urine glucose levels, mental status, ketone levels, and vital signs. When using an electronic medication administration record (MAR), enter hourly blood glucose levels and treatment with insulin or titration of an insulin drip. Record the clinical manifestations of DKA assessed, such as polyuria, polydipsia, polyphagia, Kussmaul respirations, fruity breath odor, changes in level of consciousness, poor skin turgor, hypotension, hypothermia, warm and dry skin, and mucous membranes. Document all interventions, such as fluid and electrolyte replacement and insulin therapy, and record the patient's response. Record any procedures, such as arterial blood gas analysis, blood samples sent to the laboratory, cardiac monitoring, or insertion of an indwelling urinary catheter. Record results, the names of persons notified, and the time of notification. Include emotional support provided and patient education in the notes.

Diabetic Ketoacidosis		
7/11/2019	0810	**NURSING ASSESSMENT:** Mr. Jones admitted at 0730 with serum blood glucose level of 900. Pt. c/o thirst, nausea, vomiting, and excessive urination. Urine positive for ketones. P 112, BP 94/58, RR 28 deep and rapid, oral T 96.8°F. Skin warm, dry, with tenting when pinched. Mucous membranes dry. Resting with eyes closed. Confused to time and date. **NURSING INTERVENTION:** Blood sample sent to lab for electrolytes, BUN, creatinine, serum glucose, CBC. ABG drawn by respiratory therapist. Urine obtained and sent for UA. O_2 2 L via NC started with O_2 sat. 94% by pulse oximetry. 1000 mL of NSS being infused over 1 hr through I.V. line in right forearm. 25 units I.V. bolus of regular insulin infused through I.V. line in left antecubital followed by a cont. infusion of 100 units regular insulin in 100 mL NSS at 5 units/hr. Monitoring blood glucose with q1hr fingersticks. Next due at 0900. See frequent parameter flow sheet for I/O, VS, and blood glucose results. Notified diabetes educator, Teresa Mooney, RN, about pt.'s admission and the need for reinforcing diabetes regimen. ______ **Louise May, RN**

DISCHARGE INSTRUCTIONS

Hospitals today commonly discharge patients earlier than they did in years past. As a result, the patient is discharged with acute care needs, and family and home health care nurses must change dressings; assess wounds; deal with medical equipment, tube feedings, and IV lines; and perform other functions.

To perform these functions properly, the patient and the caregiver must receive adequate instruction. The nurse is usually responsible for these instructions. If a patient receives improper instructions and injury results, the nurse could be held liable.

Many hospitals distribute printed instruction sheets that adequately describe treatments and home care procedures. The patient's chart should indicate which materials were given and to whom. Generally, the patient or responsible person must sign that he or she received and understood the discharge instructions. EHRs have discharge instructions where documentation of patient teaching is required as well as evidence of teaching efficacy, the patient's willingness to learn, and the patient's ability to "teach back" the information to verify understanding.

Courts typically consider these teaching materials as evidence that instruction took place. However, to support testimony that instructions were given, the materials should be tailored to each patient's specific needs and refer to any verbal or written instructions that were provided. If caregivers practice procedures with the patient and family in the hospital, this should be documented, too, along with the results.

Essential Documentation

Many facilities combine discharge summaries and patient instructions in one discharge summary form. This form contains sections for recording patient assessment, patient education, detailed special instructions, and the circumstances of discharge. (See *The discharge summary form,* page 97.)

When writing a narrative note about discharge instructions, the nurse should include the following information:

- date and time of discharge
- family members or caregivers present for teaching
- treatments, such as dressing changes, or the use of medical equipment

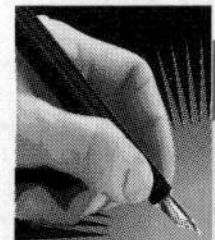

ACCUCHART

THE DISCHARGE SUMMARY FORM

By combining the patient's discharge summary with instructions for care after discharge, the nurse can fulfill two requirements with a single form. When using this documentation method, be sure to give one copy to the patient and keep one for the legal record. Discharge summary and order forms are specific electronic forms used in each facility.

DISCHARGE INSTRUCTIONS

1. Diagnosis Hypertensive crisis

2. Allergies penicillin

3. Medications (drug, dose time) Lopressor 25 mg at 6 a.m. and 6 p.m. by mouth
temazepam 15 mg at 10 p.m. by mouth

4. Diet Low-sodium, low-cholesterol

5. Activity As tolerated

6. Discharged to Home

7. If questions arise, contact Dr. James Pritchett **Telephone No.** (233) 555-1448

8. Special instructions Call doctor with headaches, dizziness

9. Return visit Dr. Pritchett **Place** Health Care Clinic

On Date 12/15/19 **Time** 0845

Tara Nicholas	M. Ambrose, RN	12/8/19
Signature of patient or person responsible for receipt of discharge instructions	**Signature of doctor or nurse reviewing instructions**	**Date**

- signs and symptoms to report to the health care provider
- patient, family, or caregiver understanding of instructions or ability to give a return demonstration of procedures
- whether a patient or caregiver requires further instruction
- health care provider's name and telephone number
- date, time, and location of any follow-up appointments or the need to call the health care provider for a follow-up appointment
- details of instructions given to the patient, including medications, activity, and diet (include any written instructions given to patient)

Discharge Instructions		
12/1/2019	1530	**PATIENT TEACHING/EDUCATION:** Pt. to be discharged today. Reviewed discharge instructions with pt. and wife. Reviewed all medications, including drug name, purpose, doses, administration times, routes, and adverse effects. Drug information sheets given to pt. Pt. able to verbalize proper use of medications. Wife will be performing dressing change to pt.'s left foot. Wife was able to change dressing properly using sterile technique. Pt. and wife were able to state signs and symptoms of infections to report to doctor. Also reinforced low-cholesterol, low-sodium diet and progressive walking guidelines. Wife has many questions about diet and will meet with dietitian before discharge. Pt. understands he's to follow up with Dr. Carney in his office on 12/8/19 at 1400. Wrote doctor's phone number on written instructions. Written discharge instructions given to pt. ________ **Marcy Smythe, RN**

DO-NOT-RESUSCITATE ORDER

When a patient is terminally ill and death is expected, the patient's health care provider and family (and the patient if appropriate) may agree that a do-not-resuscitate (DNR), or no-code, order is appropriate. The health care provider writes the order, and the staff carries it out if the patient goes into cardiac or respiratory arrest.

Because DNR orders are recognized legally, the nurse will incur no liability if he or she does not try to resuscitate a patient and that patient later dies. The nurse may, however, incur liability if he or she initiates resuscitation on a patient who has a DNR order.

Every patient with a DNR order should have a written order on file. Some facilities have specific forms that help define what care the patient or family doesn't wish delivered in the case of a code, such as no CPR or no intubation. The order should be consistent with the facility's policy, which commonly requires that such orders be reviewed every 48 to 72 hours.

Increasingly, patients are deciding in advance of a crisis whether they want to be resuscitated. Health care facilities must provide written information to patients concerning their rights under state law to make decisions regarding their care, including the right to refuse medical treatment and the right to formulate an advance directive.

This information must be provided to all patients upon admission. The nurse must also document that the patient received this information and whether brought a written advance directive with him. (See "Advance directive," pages 8 to 10.) A photocopy of the directive should be placed in the patient's record.

Essential Documentation

If a terminally ill patient without a DNR order tells the nurse that he or she does not want to be resuscitated in a crisis, the nurse should document this statement as well as the patient's degree of awareness and orientation. The nurse should then contact the patient's health care provider and the nursing supervisor and ask for assistance from administration, legal services, or social services.

The nurse has a responsibility to help the patient make an informed decision about continuing treatment. If the patient's wishes differ from those of the patient's family or the health care provider, make sure the discrepancies are thoroughly recorded in the chart. Then document that the charge nurse, nursing supervisor, or legal services staff was notified.

DNR		
6/19/2019	1700	**NURSING ASSESSMENT:** Pt. stated, "If my heart should stop or if I stop breathing, just let me go. I've suffered with this cancer long enough. I've lived a full life and have no regrets." Pt.'s wife was present for this conversation and stated, "I don't want to see him in pain anymore. If he feels he doesn't want any heroic measures, then I stand by his decision." Pt. is alert and oriented to time, place, and person. ______ **NURSING INTERVENTION:** Dr. V. Patel notified of pt.'s wishes concerning resuscitation and stated he'll be in this evening to discuss DNR status with pt. and wife and write DNR orders. Elizabeth Sawyer, charge nurse, notified of pt.'s wishes for no resuscitation. ______ **Joan Byers, RN**

COMPUTERIZED PHYSICIAN ORDER ENTRY (FORMERLY CALLED DOCTOR'S ORDERS)

Computerized physician order entry (CPOE) is the process of a medical professional entering medication orders or other physician instructions electronically instead of on paper charts. A primary benefit of CPOE is that it can help reduce errors related to poor handwriting or the transcription of medication orders. Such forms are especially useful for commonly performed procedures such as cardiac catheterization. As with other standardized documents, blanks are used for information that must be individualized according to the patient's needs.

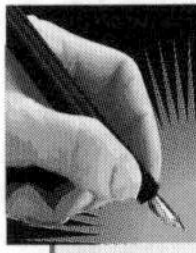

AccuChart

PREPRINTED ORDERS

The following is an example of a preprinted form for charting health care provider's orders. This form specifies the treatment for a patient who's about to undergo cardiac catheterization.

DOCTOR'S ORDERS

Name: Thomas Smith

ID number: 0135467

Allergies: None known

Date/Time	PRECARDIAC CATHETERIZATION ORDERS:
12/7/19 1330	1. NPO after midnight except for medications.
	2. Prep right and left groin areas with medicated soap.
	3. Premedications:
	Benadryl 25 mg; Xanax 0.5 mg } P.O. on call to Cath lab
	4. Have ECG, PT, PTT, creatinine, Hgb, HCT, and platelet count
	on chart before sending the patient to the Cath lab.
	5. Have patient void before leaving for the Cath lab.
	Mona Jones, MD
12/7/19 1400	Susan Smith, RN

Essential Documentation

Before transcribing orders from a preprinted order form, make sure the health care provider has written in the date, time, the patient's full name, and any allergies. Check that all blanks are filled in and individualized to the patient. After reviewing the orders and determining that they are complete, the nurse should record the date and time and sign his or her full name and credentials.

Review *Preprinted orders,* page 100, for an example of documentation.

HEALTH CARE PROVIDER'S ORDERS, TELEPHONE

CPOEs are standard in EHRs. Providers can enter orders remotely. However, when verbal orders are necessary, the provider states the order, and the nurse transcribes the order and reads it back to confirm accuracy. The nurse may then enter the order in the computer and flag it as a verbal order that the provider can sign at a later time. However, when the patient needs immediate treatment and the health care provider is not available to write an order, telephone orders are acceptable. Telephone orders may also be taken to expedite care when new information, such as laboratory data, is available that doesn't require a physical examination.

Essential Documentation

The nurse should record the telephone order on the health care provider's order sheet while the health care provider is still on the telephone. Note the date and time. Write the order verbatim. On the next line, write "T.O." for telephone order. Note that the order was read back to the health care provider and confirmed as correct. The nurse should write the health care provider's name and sign his or her name, along with the note "read back and verified." If another nurse listened to the order, have the other nurse sign the order as well. Draw lines through any blank spaces in the order.

The health care provider should countersign the order within 48 hours. Without the health care provider's signature, the nurse may be held liable for practicing medicine without a license.

Physician Order Telephone		
12/4/2019	0900	Demerol 75 mg and Vistaril 50 mg I.M. now for pain.
		________ **T.O. Dr. White/Cathy Phillips, RN read back and verified.**

HEALTH CARE PROVIDER'S ORDERS, VERBAL

Most patients' health records are computerized, enabling physicians to remotely send orders for patient care via the CPOE system. However, there may be instances in home health care or some extended care facilities that still use verbal physician orders dictated to a nurse. Errors made when interpreting or documenting verbal orders can lead to mistakes in patient care and liability problems for the nurse. Clearly, verbal orders can be a necessity, especially if the nurse is providing home health care. However, in a health care facility, try to take verbal orders only in an emergency, and according to facility policy, when the health care provider can't immediately attend to the patient.

DNR and no-code orders should *not* be given or taken verbally. Carefully follow the facility's policy for documenting a verbal order, and use a special form if one exists.

Essential Documentation

The nurse should write the order out while the health care provider is still present. Read the order back for verification and note it in the chart. Note the date and time, and record the order verbatim. On the following line, write "V.O." for verbal order, followed by "read back and verified." Write the health care provider's name and the name of the nurse who read the order back to the health care provider. The nurse should sign his or her name and draw a line for the health care provider to sign. Draw lines through any spaces between the order and the nurse's verification of the order. Record the type of drug, dosage, time of administration, and any other information the facility's policy requires.

Make sure the health care provider countersigns the order within the time limits set by the facility's policy. Without this countersignature, the nurse may be held liable for practicing medicine without a license.

Physician Verbal Order		
3/23/2019	1500	V.O. by Dr. Blackstone taken for Digoxin 0.125 mg P.O. now and daily in a.m. Furosemide 40 mg P.O. now and daily starting in a.m. ______ ______ **Judith Schilling, RN** read back and verified. ______ ______ **Doctor's signature**

DRUG ADMINISTRATION

There are Joint Commission on Accreditation of Healthcare Organizations (JCAHO) standards now required in terms of the use of abbreviations in documentation; there is a "Do Not Use" list regarding medical charting abbreviations in order to ensure patient safety (see https://www.jointcommission.org/facts_about_do_not_use_list/).

Essential Documentation

Medication administration is a major responsibility of the nurse. Nurses must be cautious and vigilant to be sure the medication is for the correct patient and to ensure that the medication dosage, route, and time of administration are correct. Medications commonly have barcodes that match with the patient's EHR and patient hospital bracelet. The electronic system used by the clinical facility is meant to ensure the safety of the patient. In addition, there are 12 "rights" of medication administration that all nurses should follow:

- Right patient
- Right drug
- Right dose
- Right route
- Right time
- Right response
- Right reason
- Right documentation
- Right assessment and evaluation
- Right client education
- Right to refuse medication
- Right expiration date

When using the MAR, follow these guidelines:

- Know and follow the facility's policies and procedures for recording drug orders and charting drug administration.
- Make sure all drug orders include the patient's full name; the date; and the drug's name, dosage, administration route or method, and frequency. A medication that is ordered for "as needed" or "p.r.n." needs a reason for its use, such as "morphine 2 mg IV q2hr p.r.n. for pain." When appropriate, include the specific number of doses given or the stop date.
- Be sure to include drug allergy information.
- Write legibly.
- Use only standard abbreviations approved by the facility. When doubtful about an abbreviation, write out the word or phrase.
- After administering the first dose, the nurse should sign his or her full name and write his or her licensure status and initials in the appropriate space on the MAR.

- Record drugs immediately after administration so that another nurse doesn't give the drug again.
- When documenting electronically, the nurse should chart the information for each drug immediately after administering it. This is particularly important if the nurse does not use printouts as a backup. Keying in information immediately ensures that all members of the health care team have access to the latest drug administration data for the patient.
- Some scanning computer systems require that both the medication and the barcode on the patient's name band be scanned to ensure the correct medication for the correct patient.
- If a specific assessment parameter must be monitored during administration of a drug, document this requirement on the MAR. For example, when digoxin is administered, the patient's pulse rate needs to be monitored and charted on the MAR. (See *The medication administration record*, pages 105 and 106, for proper documentation of medications).
- The JCAHO "Do Not Use" list:

OFFICIAL "DO NOT USE" LIST

Do Not Use	Potential Problem	Use Instead
U, u (unit)	Mistaken for "0" (zero), the number "4" (four) or "cc"	Write "unit"
IU (International Unit)	Mistaken for IV (intravenous) or the number 10 (ten)	Write "International Unit"
Q.D., QD, q.d., qd (daily) Q.O.D., QOD, q.o.d, qod (every other day)	Mistaken for each other Period after the Q mistaken for "I" and the "O" mistaken for "I"	Write "daily" Write "every other day"
Trailing zero (X. mg) Lack of leading zero (.X mg)	Decimal point is missed	Write X mg Write 0.X mg
MS MSO_4 and $MgSO_4$	Can mean morphine sulfate or magnesium sulfate Confused for one another	Write "morphine sulfate" Write "magnesium sulfate"

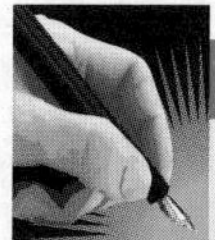

AccuChart

THE MEDICATION ADMINISTRATION RECORD

The MAR contains a permanent record of the patient's medications. The MAR also includes the patient's diagnosis and information about allergies and diet. A sample form is shown below.

NAME: Jack Lemmons MEDICAL RECORD #: 1234567

NURSE'S FULL SIGNATURE, STATUS, AND INITIALS	INIT.		INIT.		INIT.
Roy Charles, RN	RC				
Theresa Hopkins, RN	TH				

DIAGNOSIS: Heart failure, atrial flutter, COPD

ALLERGIES: ASA DIET: Cardiac

ROUTINE/DAILY ORDERS.			DATE: 1/24/19		DATE: 1/25/19		DATE: 1/26/19		DATE: 1/27/19		DATE: 1/28/19		DATE: 1/29/19		DATE: 1/30/19	
ORDER DATE	MEDICATIONS DOSE, ROUTE, FREQUENCY	TIME	SITE	INIT.	SITE	INIT.	SITE	INIT.	SITE	INIT.	SITE	INIT.	SITE	INIT.	SITE	INIT.
1/24/19	digoxin 0.125 mg I.V. daily	0900	right subclavian	RC		(RC)										
1/24/19	furosemide 40 mg I.V. q12hr	0900	right subclavian	RC	right subclavian	RC										
1/24/19	enalaprilat 1.25 mg I.V. q6hr	0511	right subclavian	TH	right subclavian	TH										

(*continued*)

THE MEDICATION ADMINISTRATION RECORD (*continued*)

	P.R.N. MEDICATION
Addressograph	ALLERGIES: ASA

INITIAL	SIGNATURE & STATUS	INITIAL	SIGNATURE & STATUS	INITIAL	SIGNATURE & STATUS	INITIAL	SIGNATURE & STATUS
RC	Roy Charles, RN						
TH	Theresa Hopkins, RN						

YEAR 20 10		P.R.N. MEDICATIONS							
ORDER DATE: 1/24/19 RENEWAL DATE: / DISCONTINUED DATE: /	DATE	1/24/19							
MEDICATION: acetaminophen DOSE: 650 mg	TIME GIVEN	0930							
DIRECTION: p.r.n. mild pain ROUTE: P.O.	SITE								
	INIT.	RC							
ORDER DATE: 1/24/19 RENEWAL DATE: 1/26/19 DISCONTINUED DATE: /	DATE	1/24/19							
MEDICATION: morphine sulfate DOSE: 2 mg	TIME GIVEN	0930							
DIRECTION: 15 min prior to changing right heel dressing ROUTE: I.V.	SITE	right subclavian							
	INIT.	RC							
ORDER DATE: 1/24/19 RENEWAL DATE: / DISCONTINUED DATE: /	DATE	1/24/19							
MEDICATION: Milk of Magnesia DOSE: 30 ml	TIME GIVEN	2115							
DIRECTION: q6hr p.r.n. constipation ROUTE: P.O.	SITE								
	INIT.	TH							
ORDER DATE: 1/25/19 RENEWAL DATE: / DISCONTINUED DATE: 1/25/19	DATE	1/25/19	1/25/19						
MEDICATION: prochlorperazine DOSE: 5 mg	TIME GIVEN	1100	2230						
DIRECTION: q8hr p.r.n. nausea and vomiting ROUTE: P.O.	SITE								
	INIT.	RC	TH						
ORDER DATE: 1/25/19 RENEWAL DATE: / DISCONTINUED DATE: 1/25/19	DATE	1/25/19	X	X	X	X	X	X	X
MEDICATION: fluzone DOSE: 0.5 ml	TIME GIVEN	1100							
DIRECTION: X1 dose only ROUTE: I.M.	SITE	right delt.							
	INIT.	RC							
ORDER DATE: 1/25/19 RENEWAL DATE: / DISCONTINUED DATE: 1/25/19	DATE	1/25/19	X	X	X	X	X	X	X
MEDICATION: furosemide DOSE: 40 mg	TIME GIVEN	1300							
DIRECTION: stat now ROUTE: I.V.	SITE	right subclavian							
	INIT.	RC							
ORDER DATE: / RENEWAL DATE: / DISCONTINUED DATE: /	DATE								
MEDICATION: DOSE:	TIME GIVEN								
DIRECTION: ROUTE:	SITE								
	INIT.								

DRUG ADMINISTRATION, ADVERSE EFFECTS OF

Also called a *side effect*, an adverse drug effect is an undesirable response that may be mild, severe, or life-threatening. Any clinically useful drug can cause an adverse effect.

The nurse plays a key role in reporting adverse drug effect events. Reporting adverse effects helps ensure the safety of drugs regulated by the Food and Drug Administration (FDA). The FDA's Medical Products Reporting Program supplies health care professionals with MedWatch forms on which they can report adverse events. (See https://www.fda.gov/Safety/MedWatch/default.htm.)

A MedWatch form should be completed when it is suspected that a drug is responsible for:

- death
- life-threatening illness
- initial or prolonged hospitalization
- disability
- congenital anomaly
- need for any medical or surgical intervention to prevent a permanent impairment or an injury

Also, promptly inform the FDA of product quality problems, such as:

- defective devices
- inaccurate or unreadable product labels
- packaging or product mix-ups
- intrinsic or extrinsic contamination or stability problems
- particulates in injectable drugs
- product damage

Essential Documentation

When filing a MedWatch form, it should be kept in mind that the nurse is not expected to establish a connection between the drug and the problem. The nurse does not need to include a lot of details; only the adverse event or the problem with the drug needs to be reported.

Furthermore, the nurse does not need to wait until the evidence seems compelling. FDA regulations protect the reporter's identity and the identities of the patient and employer. Send the completed forms to the FDA by using the fax number or mailing address on the form. For voluntary reporting, nurses can also report adverse events online using the MedWatch Voluntary Reporting Online Form. The mandatory reporting MedWatch form may be downloaded, but it cannot be submitted online.

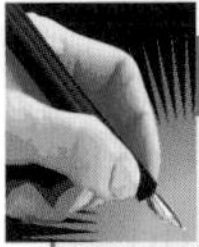

AccuChart

MEDWATCH FORM FOR REPORTING ADVERSE DRUG REACTIONS

MEDWATCH
The FDA Safety Information and Adverse Event Reporting Program

For VOLUNTARY reporting of adverse events, product problems and product use errors

Page __ of __

Form Approved: OMB No. 0910-0291 Expires: 10/31/08
See OMB statement on reverse
FDA Use Only
Triage unit sequence #

PLEASE TYPE OR USE BLACK INK

A. Patient information

1. Patient identifier: 01234 (In confidence)
2. Age at time of event: ____ or Date of birth: 3/11/58
3. Sex: ☑ female ☐ male
4. Weight: ____ lbs or 59 kgs

B. Adverse event or product problem

1. ☐ Adverse event and/or ☑ Product problem (e.g., defects/malfunctions)
2. Outcomes attributed to adverse event (check all that apply)
   - ☐ death ____ (mo/day/yr)
   - ☐ life-threatening
   - ☐ hospitalization – initial or prolonged
   - ☐ disability
   - ☐ congenital anomaly
   - ☐ required intervention to prevent permanent impairment/damage
   - ☐ other: ____
3. Date of event (mo/day/yr): 3/8/19
4. Date of this report (mo/day/yr): 3/8/19
5. Describe Event, Problem or Product Use Error

   After reconstituting 100-mg vial with 10 ml of bacteriostatic water, the drug crystallized and turned yellow.

   Drug wasn't given.
6. Relevant tests/laboratory data, including dates
7. Other relevant history, including preexisting medical conditions (e.g., allergies, race, pregnancy, smoking and alcohol use, hepatic/renal dysfunction, etc.)

C. Product availability

Product available for evaluation? *(Do not send product to FDA)*
☐ yes ☐ no ☐ returned to manufacturer on: ____ (mm/dd/yyyy)

D. Suspect product(s)

1. Name, strength, manufacturer *(from product label)*
   #1 Leucovorin calcium for
   #2 Injection – 100-mg vial
2. Dose, frequency & route used
   #1 100 mg IV X1
   #2
3. Therapy dates (if unknown, give duration) from/to (or best estimate)
   #1 3/8/19
   #2
4. Diagnosis for use (indication)
   #1 Megaloblastic anemia
   #2
5. Event abated after use stopped or dose reduced
   #1 ☐ yes ☐ no ☐ doesn't apply
   #2 ☐ yes ☐ no ☐ doesn't apply
6. Lot # (if known)
   #1 #891
   #2
7. Exp. date (if known)
   #1
   #2
8. Event reappeared after reintroduction
   #1 ☐ yes ☐ no ☐ doesn't apply
   #2 ☐ yes ☐ no ☐ doesn't apply
9. NDC # or Unique ID

E. Suspect medical device

1. Brand name
2. Common device name
3. Manufacturer name, city and state
4. model # ____ catalog # ____ serial # ____ lot # ____ Expiration Date (mm/dd/yyyy) other #
5. Operator or device
   - ☐ health professional
   - ☐ lay user/patient
   - ☐ other: ____
6. If implanted, give date (mo/day/yr)
7. If explanted, give date (mo/day/yr)
8. Is this a Single-use Device that was Reprocessed and Reused on a Patient?
   ☑ yes ☐ no
9. If Yes to Item No. 8, Enter Name and Address of Reprocessor

F. Other (concomitant) medical products

Product names and therapy dates *(exclude treatment of event)*

G. Reporter (see confidentiality section on back)

1. Name & address: Patricia Cohen, 987 Elm Ave., Cincinnati, Ohio
   phone #: (123) 456-7890
   E-mail:
2. Health professional? ☑ yes ☐ no
3. Occupation: RN
4. Also reported to
   - ☐ manufacturer
   - ☐ user facility
   - ☑ distributor/Importer
5. If you do NOT want your identity disclosed to the manufacturer, place an " X " in this box. ☐

FDA Form 3500 1/96) Submission of a report does not constitute an admission that medical personnel or the product caused or contributed to the event.

File a separate MedWatch form for each patient, and attach additional pages if needed. Also, remember to comply with the health care facility's protocols for reporting adverse events associated with drugs.

Product lot numbers are used in product identification, tracking, and product recall; therefore, the lot number should be retained, and the nurse's supervisor should keep a copy of the report on file.

The FDA will report back to the reporter or on the actions it takes and will continue to work to instruct health care professionals about adverse events.

See *MedWatch form for reporting adverse drug reactions*, page 108, for an example of a completed form. (See https://www.fda.gov/Safety/MedWatch/default.htm.)

DRUG ADMINISTRATION, ONE-TIME DOSE

Single-dose medications, which can include a supplemental dose or a stat dose, should be documented not only in the MAR but also in the progress notes.

When transcribing a one-time order to be given on another shift, the nurse must be sure to communicate information to the next shift during report, or use a medication alert sticker to flag the order. A one-time medication order would be included in the electronic MAR and would be documented electronically.

Essential Documentation

A one-time medication order would be included in the electronic MAR or CPOE system. The document should contain the name of the person who gave the drug order, why the order was given, and the patient's response to the drug. Frequent monitoring and documentation show that the nurse monitored the patient for adverse effects, other potential outcomes, and changes in condition.

Drug Administraton One-Time Dose		
6/5/2019	1100	**PATIENT TEACHING:** Pt. agreed to influenza virus vaccine after Dr. J. Moore explained that she was in the high-risk category because of her advanced age and long history of COPD. Dr. Moore also explained risks of vaccine to pt. Pt. denies allergic reaction to eggs, chicken, or chicken feathers or dander. ______ **NURSING ASSESSMENT:** Pt. is afebrile, oral T 97.2°F, and has no active infections. ______ **NURSING INTERVENTION:** Fluzone 0.5 mL I.M. injected in right deltoid. **PATIENT TEACHING:** Explained fever, malaise, and myalgia may occur up to 2 days after vaccination and site may feel tender. ______ ______ **Angela Casale, RN**

DRUG ADMINISTRATION, OPIOID

Whenever an opioid is administered, the nurse must follow stringent federal, state, and institutional regulations concerning administration and documentation. Government regulations are strict and carry heavy penalties for the institution when they're breached. These regulations require opioid drugs to be counted after each nursing shift to ensure an accurate drug count. They also require that a second nurse document the nurse's activity and observe the first nurse if an opioid or part of a dose must be wasted.

Many facilities now use an automated storage system for opioids that eliminates the need for counting the opioids at the end of a shift. This system allows the nurse easy access (via identification and password or fingerprint) to medications, including other drugs and floor stocks for nursing units. Nurses may remove one or more medications by selecting the patient, medication, and amount needed on the keypad. The nurse must then count the amount of the drug remaining in the system and enter it. Each transaction is recorded, and copies are sent to the pharmacy and billing departments. If an inaccurate amount is entered into the system, it's flagged as a discrepancy. Discrepancies should be resolved before each shift ends.

Essential Documentation

Whenever the nurse gives an opioid, it must be documented according to federal, state, and facility regulations. Use the electronic MAR to do the following:

- Sign out the drug on the appropriate form.
- Verify the amount of drug in the container before giving it.
- Have another nurse document the activity and observe the first nurse if part of an opioid dose must be wasted or discarded.

Most health care facilities have a specific electronic system that stores and keeps a count of controlled substances. The drug is retrieved from the system and is scanned before it is administered to the patient.

DRUG ADMINISTRATION, STAT ORDER

A drug that is ordered stat is to be administered to the patient immediately for an urgent medical problem. This single-dose medication should be documented in the electronic MAR.

Essential Documentation

The nurse's documentation should include the name of the person who gave the order, why the order was given, and the patient's response to the drug. In the MAR, write the drug's name, dosage, route, and time given. Stat orders for medications will be entered into the electronic medical record (EMR) and will be flagged or highlighted in a specific color.

Drug Administration Stat Order

2/3/2019	0900	**NURSING ASSESSMENT:** Pt. SOB with crackles auscultated bilaterally in the bases and O_2 sat. decreased to 89% on room air. P 104, BP 92/60, RR 32, and labored. **NURSING INTERVENTION:** Lasix 40 mg P.O. given as per Dr. V. Singh's order **Ann Barrow, RN**
2/3/2019	1000	**NURSING ASSESSMENT:** Pt. responded with urine output of 1500 mL, decreased SOB, and O_2 sat. increased to 97% on room air. P 98, BP 94/60, and RR 16. **Ann Barrow, RN**

DRUG ADMINISTRATION, WITHHOLDING ORDERED DRUG

Under certain circumstances, a prescribed drug cannot or should not be given as scheduled. For example, the nurse may decide to withhold a stool softener for a patient with diarrhea. A patient may be scheduled for a test that requires the patient not to take a certain drug, or a change in the patient's condition may make the drug inappropriate to give. For example, an antihypertensive drug may have been prescribed for a patient who now has low blood pressure. In some circumstances, a patient may refuse a drug. For example, a patient may refuse to take the prescribed cholestyramine because the patient believes it is causing abdominal upset. If a drug is withheld, notify the health care provider.

Essential Documentation

The EHR should document the date and time the drug was withheld, the reason for withholding the drug, the name of the health care provider notified, and the health care provider's response. If the health care provider changed a drug order, record and document the new order and the time it was carried out. Document any actions taken to safeguard the patient.

In an EHR, there is a drop-down menu that allows the nurse to select options such as "patient refused," "parameters not met," or "blood sugar too high or too low," for example. These are prewritten notes that can be selected to document why a drug was held.

Witholding a Drug		
3/3/2019	1800	**NURSING ASSESSMENT/INTERVENTION:** Digoxin 0.125 mg P.O. not given due to HR of 50. Dr. B. Miller notified that medication was witheld. ___ ___ **Betty Griffin, RN**

DRUGS, ILLEGAL

If the nurse observes that the patient has illegal drugs or drug paraphernalia in his or her possession, the nurse should follow the facility's policy and notify the charge nurse, nursing supervisor, security, and the

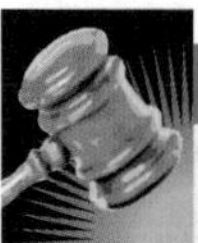

LEGAL CASEBOOK

CONDUCTING A DRUG SEARCH

The nurse who suspects that a patient is abusing drugs has a duty to do something about it. If such a patient harms him- or herself or anyone else, resulting in a lawsuit, the court may hold the nurse liable for the patient's actions.

When the Nurse Knows about Drug Abuse

Suppose the nurse knows for certain that a patient is abusing drugs—for example, an emergency department nurse may find drugs in a patient's clothes or handbag while looking for identification. The facility's policy may obligate the nurse to confiscate the drugs and take steps to ensure that the patient does not acquire more.

When the Nurse Suspects Drug Abuse

When a patient's erratic or threatening behavior makes the nurse suspect the patient is abusing drugs, consult the facility's policy, which may require that the nurse conduct a search. Is the search legal? As a rule of thumb, if the nurse strongly believes the patient poses a threat to him- or herself or others and can document the reasons for searching the patient's possessions, the nurse is probably safe legally.

Guidelines for Searches

Before conducting a search, the nurse should review the facility's guidelines on the matter, then follow the guidelines carefully. Most hospital guidelines will first direct the nurse to contact his or her supervisor and explain why there is a legitimate cause for a search. If the supervisor gives approval for the search, a security guard should be enlisted for help with the search. Besides protecting the nurse, the security guard will serve as a witness if drugs are found. When ready, the nurse should confront the patient, explaining that he or she intends to conduct a search and the reasons for the search.

Depending on the facility's guidelines, the nurse can search a patient's belongings as well as the patient's room. If illegal drugs are found during the search, confiscate them. Remember, possession of illegal drugs is a felony. Depending on the facility's guidelines, the nurse may be obligated to report the patient to the police.

Maintaining Written Records

After completing the search, the nurse should record the findings in an incident report.

patient's health care provider. Depending on the state's guidelines, the nurse may be obligated to report the patient to the police.

Essential Documentation

If the nurse discovers evidence of drugs in the patient's room or on his or her person, the nurse should document the circumstances of the discovery. The nurse should document that the facility's policy on contraband was explained to the patient and note the patient's response. Record the names and departments of the people notified, instructions given, and any actions taken. Document whether a search was performed, who was present during the search, and what was found. When describing what the nurse suspects are illegal drugs, document the form (e.g., pills, liquid, or powder) and the amount, color, and shape. Fill out an incident report, according to the facility's policy.

Conducting a Drug Search

9/1/2019	1000	**NURSING ASSESSMENT:** Clear plastic bag containing white powdery substance, approx. 3 tbsp, with odd odor found in pt.'s bedside stand while retrieving his wash basin at 0930. Upon questioning, pt. stated, "That stuff is none of your business."
		NURSING INTERVENTION: Told pt. that drugs not prescribed by the doctor aren't allowed in the hospital. Security director, Michael Daniels; nursing supervisor, Stacey McLean, RN; and Dr. M. Phillips notified at 0940. Mr. Daniels and Mrs. McLean visited pt. in his room and reinforced hospital policy on contraband. Substance taken by Joseph Smith in security.
		Greg Little, RN

DRUGS, INAPPROPRIATE USE OF

The nurse may suspect that the patient is taking opioids or other drugs when the patient's behavior suddenly changes after he or she has visitors. The nurse who suspects that a patient is abusing drugs has a duty to report this to the nursing supervisor. Follow the facility's policy when drug abuse is suspected.

Essential Documentation

The nurse should record the date and time of the entry. Document how the patient appeared before and after the visitors came to the patient's room. Record any observations and physical assessment findings. Chart the name of the health care provider and the nursing supervisor notified, the time of notification, their instructions, and any actions taken.

Inappropriate Use of Drugs

4/2/2019	1125	**NURSING ASSESSMENT:** Upon entering room, pt. found in bed lethargic. Pupils constricted, speech slurred. P 68, BP 102/58, RR 16. Pt. stated, "My friend gave me something to help with the pain." **NURSING INTERVENTION:** Dr. A. Ettingoff and Ron Howell, RN, nursing supervisor, notified at 1130 and told of lethargy, slurred speech, pinpoint pupils, and pt.'s explanation. Urine specimen sent for drug toxicology. ________ **Eileen Sullivan, RN**
4/2/2019	1130	Dr. Ettingoff in to see pt. Orders written for Narcan. **NURSING INTERVENTION:** Narcan given as ordered. **NURSING ASSESSMENT:** P 72, BP 114/60, RR 20. Speech less slurred, oriented to person, place, and day but not time. Pupils still constricted. ________ **Eileen Sullivan, RN**

DRUGS, PATIENT HIDING

Patients may hide drugs for a variety of reasons: They may think they are not working, they may be saving them for double-dosing at night if they are pain medications, or they may be collecting them for a suicide attempt or to sell. If the patient is hiding medications, the nurse must confront the patient, talk about the situation, and discover the patient's reason for doing it. The patient may need education regarding the function of the medications. If the patient believes the medications are ineffective, discuss that with the health care provider. If the patient is or may be suicidal, call the health care provider and stay with the patient, or have another nurse stay with the patient, until the health care provider arrives. Drugs from the facility should never be left at the bedside. The nurse must always observe patients take their medications, and if the patient will not take them at the time they are delivered, the nurse should take them from the patient and return at a time when the patient will take them. They should never be left at the bedside.

Essential Documentation

If the nurse finds prescribed drugs at the bedside that were not taken by the patient, the nurse should record the date and time. Document how the drugs were found. If the nurse discovers drugs that were not prescribed, the nurse should describe the type of drug (e.g., pills or powders), the amount, and its appearance (e.g., color and shape). If the nurse discovers prescribed drugs, the nurse should record the type of drug and the amount. Record the discussion with the patient about why he or she is hiding medications. Use the patient's own words in quotes whenever possible. Document nursing interventions, such as patient teaching; rescheduling of doses if the patient takes medication at a different time at home; and, if appropriate, removing medications from the patient's room and storing them per the facility's policy. Record the name of the health care provider notified, the time of notification, and any actions taken. Make sure to describe the events in chronological order and note the time.

Patient Hiding Drugs		
5/21/2019	0900	**NURSING ASSESSMENT:** While assisting pt. with her bath at 0800, noted pills in her makeup case. When asked what they were, pt. stated "just some pills." I stated that they looked like her morphine sulfate and she said they were. After some discussion, pt. stated, "My pain is so severe at night, and I want to get a good night's sleep, so I brought some extra pills from home." ________
		PATIENT TEACHING: Discussed with pt. the importance of taking morphine sulfate as prescribed, the dangers of an overdose, and the importance of allowing her health care team to assist in relieving her pain by changing her dose as needed according to her reports of pain relief. ________
		NURSING INTERVENTION: Morphine sulfate pills sent to pharmacy for identification at 0830. Dr. D. Smith notified and came to see pt. Dosage changed with patient input. ________
		PATIENT TEACHING: Pt. instructed to report relief per pain scale and given information sheet on morphine sulfate. Adverse reactions reviewed. Pt. agreed to comply with medication plan and verbalized an understanding of the importance of doing so. ________
		________ **Phillip Stevens, RN**

DRUGS, PATIENT REFUSAL TO TAKE

If a patient refuses to take prescribed drugs, the EHR has a menu where the nurse can enter that the patient refused to take the medication.

Essential Documentation

The EHR will record the date and time of the entry. The nurse should document that the patient refused to take the prescribed drugs and the reason, assuming the patient gives a reason. Record the name of the refused drugs and the time they were due. Include any explanations given on the indications for the drugs and why they were ordered for the patient.

Patient Refusal to Take Medication		
2/15/2019	1015	**NURSING ASSESSMENT:** Pt. refused K-Dur tabs scheduled for 1000, stating that they were too big for her to swallow. ____ **NURSING INTERVENTION:** Dr. P. Boyle notified. K-Dur tabs discontinued. KCL elixir ordered and given. ____ ____ **Kathy Collins, RN**

DYSPNEA

Commonly a symptom of cardiopulmonary dysfunction, dyspnea is the sensation of difficult or uncomfortable breathing. Usually, it's reported as shortness of breath. Dyspnea may arise suddenly or slowly and may subside rapidly or persist for years. Most people usually experience dyspnea when they overexert themselves, and its severity depends on their physical condition. In a healthy person, dyspnea is quickly relieved by rest. Pathologic causes of dyspnea include pulmonary, cardiac, neuromuscular, and allergic disorders. In addition, anxiety may cause shortness of breath.

Whatever the cause of dyspnea, the nurse should place the patient in an upright position, unless contraindicated, and perform a rapid respiratory assessment. Prepare to administer oxygen by nasal cannula or mask. Start an IV line, and begin cardiac monitoring to assess rate and rhythm. Anticipate interventions, such as inserting a chest tube for pneumothorax, giving a diuretic or morphine injection to treat pulmonary edema, or administering breathing treatments for acute asthma or an exacerbation of chronic obstructive pulmonary disease.

Essential Documentation

The EHR records the date and time. "Respiratory assessment" is a section on the EHR. The respiratory assessment includes the patient history. It will allow for documentation of the cardiopulmonary examination, including vital signs and pulse oximetry reading; respiratory rate, depth, and effort; breath and heart sounds; use of accessory muscles; skin color; presence of edema; mental status; chest pain; and diaphoresis. All of these aspects are part of the form for respiratory assessment on the EMR.

The nurse should record the name of the health care provider notified, the time of notification, and any orders given. Describe nursing interventions and results, such as cardiac monitoring, administering oxygen, IV infusions, medications, breathing treatments, and positioning. Document patient education, such as how to perform coughing and deep breathing, pursed-lip breathing, relaxation techniques, and incentive spirometry. Also include any emotional support given.

Dyspnea		
5/3/2019	0900	**NURSING ASSESSMENT:** Pt. c/o SOB after walking from bathroom to bed, approx. 25 feet. ________ **NURSING INTERVENTION:** Assisted pt. back to bed, placed him in high Fowler's position, reattached to O_2 at 2 L/min by NC. ________ **NURSING ASSESSMENT:** Lungs with scattered rhonchi, bilaterally. P 118, BP 132/90, RR 24 labored with use of accessory muscles, axillary T 97.4°F, O_2 sat. by pulse oximetry 87%. Normal heart sounds. Skin pale, +1 edema of both ankles. Alert and oriented to time, place, and person. No c/o chest pain. Pt. states he's been having increasing SOB at home with less and less activity. ________ **NURSING INTERVENTION:** Dr. D. Smith called and came to see pt. Ordered O_2 to be used when out of bed and ambulating. ________ **PATIENT TEACHING:** Pt. instructed to cough and deep-breathe q1hr while awake. Coughed up moderate amount of white sputum. ________ ________ **Sally Jones, RN**
5/3/2019	0920	**NURSING ASSESSMENT:** Pt. denies SOB. P 102, BP 130/88, RR 20, with less effort. O_2 sat. by pulse oximetry 97%. Maintaining O_2 at 2 L/min by NC. ________ ________ **Sally Jones, RN**

SELECTED READINGS

Aronsky, D., Kasworm, E., Jacobson, J. A., Haug, P. J., & Dean, N. C. (2004). Electronic screening of dictated reports to identify patients with do-not-resuscitate status. *Journal of the American Medical Informatics Association, 11*(5), 403–409.

Ashbrook, L., Mourad, M., & Sehgal, N. (2013). Communicating discharge instructions to patients: A survey of nurse, intern, and hospitalist practices. *Journal of Hospital Medicine, 8*(1), 36–41.

Ayumi, S. (2017). Palliative care and nursing support for patients experiencing dyspnea. *International Journal of Palliative* Nursing, *23*(7), 342–351.

Beattie, S. (2009). Hands on help: Post-mortem care. *RN, 69*(10), 24ac1–24ac4.

Burns, J. P., & Truog, R. D. (2016). The DNR order after 40 years. *New England Journal of Medicine, 375*(6), 504–506.

Cole, E. (2018). The toolkit for patients struggling with breathlessness. *Nursing Standard, 33*(5), 36–38.

Collins, M., & Claros, E. (2011). Recognizing the face of dehydration. *Nursing, 41*(8), 26–32.

Davis, A. M., Rivkin-Fish, M., & Love, D. J. (2012). Addressing "difficult patient" dilemmas: Possible alternatives to the mediation model. *American Journal of Bioethics, 12*(5), 13–14.

Ebell, M. H. (2009). Brief screening instruments for dementia in primary care. *American Family Physician, 79*(6), 497–500.

Godshall, M. (2018). Patient safety. Preventing medication errors in the information age. *Nursing, 48*(9), 56–58.

Hand, M. W. (2014). Lasting impressions: Using the perspective of the funeral director to guide post mortem nursing care practice. *Medsurg Nursing, 23*(6), 4–6.

Horwitz, L. I., Moriarty, J. P., Chen, C., Fogerty, R. L., Brewster, U. C., Kanade, S., . . . Krumholz, H. M. (2013). Quality of discharge practices and patient understanding at an academic medical center. *JAMA Internal Medicine, 173*(18), 10. Retrieved from https://www.ncbi.nlm.nih.gov/pmc/articles/PMC3836871/

Jones, J. H., & Trieber, L. A. (2018). Nurses' rights of medication administration: Including authority with accountability and responsibility. *Nursing Forum, 53*(3), 299–303.

Kahn, J. S. (2018). A difficult patient. *Annals of Internal Medicine, 168*(11), 830–831.

Kaldjian, L. C., & Broderick, A. (2011). Developing a policy for do not resuscitate orders within a framework of goals of care. *Joint Commission Journal on Quality & Patient Safety, 37*(1), 11–19.

Kreider, K. E. (2018). Update in the management of diabetic ketoacidosis. *Journal for Nurse Practitioners, 14*(8), 591–597.

Lindner, S. A., Davoren, J. B., Vollmer, A., Williams, B., & Landefeld, C. S. (2007). An electronic medical record intervention increased nursing home advance directive orders and documentation. *Journal of the American Geriatrics Society, 55*(7), 1001–1006.

Lorenzetti, R., Cannarella, M., Jacques, C. H., Donovan, C., Cottrell, S., & Buck, J. (2013). Managing difficult encounters: Understanding physician, patient, and situational factors. *American Family Physician, 87*(6), 419–425.

Mangan, P. (2000). Just hiding drugs or hiding problems too? *Nursing & Residential Care, 2*(9), 413.

McGloin, S. (2015). The ins and outs of fluid balance in the acutely ill patient. *British Journal of Nursing, 24*(1), 14–18.

Mechcatie, E. (2018). Additional screening tool may improve dementia screening. *American Journal of Nursing, 118*(8), 64–65.

Panegyres, P. K., Berry, R., & Burchell, J. (2016). Early dementia screening. *Diagnostics, 6*(1), 6. Retrieved from https://www.ncbi.nlm.nih.gov/pmc/articles/PMC4808821/

Scales, K., & Pilsworth, J. (2008). The importance of fluid balance in clinical practice. *Nursing Standard, 22*(7), 50–55.

Siela, D. (2017). Oxygen requirements for acutely and critically ill patients. *Critical Care Nurse, 37*(4), 58–70.

Simmons, B. B., & DeJoseph, D. (2011). Evaluation of suspected dementia. *American Family Physician, 84*(8), 895–902.

Teo, A. R., Du, Y. B., & Escobar, J. I. (2013). How can we better manage difficult patient encounters? *Journal of Family Practice, 62*(8), 414–421.

Tindale, J. (2012). Community nurses and the electronic discharge summary. *Primary Health Care, 22*(7), 25–27.

Zeng-Treitler, Q., Kim, H., & Hunter, M. (2008). Improving patient comprehension and recall of discharge instructions by supplementing free texts with pictographs. *AMIA Annual Symposium Proceedings Archives,* 849–853. Retrieved from https://www.ncbi.nlm.nih.gov/pmc/articles/PMC2656019/

E

ELOPEMENT FROM A HEALTH CARE FACILITY

If it is discovered that a patient is missing or has left the health care facility without having said anything about leaving (called "elopement"), the unit must be searched immediately, and the nurse manager, the patient's physician, and family must be alerted. The police need to be notified if the patient is at risk of harming self or others.

The legal consequences of a patient leaving the facility without medical permission can be particularly severe, especially if the patient is confused, mentally incompetent, or injured or if death from exposure occurs as a result of that absence.

Essential Documentation

The time of discovering the patient missing, attempts to find the patient, and the people notified of the fact must all be documented. The standard form provided by the facility to record patient elopement should be used.

EMERGENCY TREATMENT, PATIENT REFUSAL OF

A competent adult has the right to refuse emergency treatment. The family cannot overrule that refusal decision, and the health care provider is not allowed to give the expressly refused treatment, even if the patient becomes unconscious.

In most cases, the health care personnel who are responsible for the patient can remain free from legal jeopardy as long as they fully inform the patient about the medical condition and the likely consequences of refusing treatment. The courts recognize a competent adult's right to refuse medical treatment, even when that refusal will clearly result in death. If the patient understands the risks but still refuses treatment, the nurse should notify the nursing supervisor and the patient's health care provider.

The courts recognize several circumstances that justify overruling a patient's refusal of treatment. These include instances when refusing treatment endangers the life of another, when a parent's decision threatens the child's life, or when, despite refusing treatment, the patient makes statements to indicate the desire to live. If none of these grounds exists, then the nurse has an ethical duty to defend the patient's right to refuse treatment and also to attempt to explain the patient's choice to the family, with emphasis on the fact that the decision belongs to the patient as long as the patient is competent.

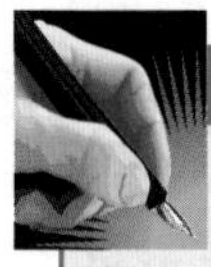

ACCUCHART

REFUSAL-OF-TREATMENT FORM

REFUSAL-OF-TREATMENT RELEASE FORM

I, Thomas Clarke, refuse to allow anyone to
[patient's name]
perform tests to diagnose heart attack & treat for heart attack [insert treatment].

The risks attendant to my refusal have been fully explained to me, and I fully understand the results for this treatment and that if the same isn't done, my chances for regaining my normal health are seriously reduced and that, in all probability, my refusal for such treatment or procedure will seriously affect my health or recovery.

I hereby release Memorial Hospital,
[name of hospital]
its nurses and employees, together with all doctors in any way connected with me as a patient, from liability for respecting and following my expressed wishes and direction.

Melissa Worthing, RN	Thomas Clarke
Witness	Patient or Legal Guardian
1/23/19	3/5/58
Date	Patient's Date of Birth

Essential Documentation

When a patient refuses care, it is important for the nurse to document that he or she has (1) explained the care and the risks involved in not receiving it; (2) documented the patient's understanding of the risks, using the patient's own words; (3) recorded the names of the nursing supervisor and health care provider notified and the time of notification; and (4) documented that the health care provider saw the patient and explained the risks of refusing emergency treatment.

The patient needs to be asked to complete a refusal-of-treatment form as provided by the health care facility. The signed form requires a witnessed signature. (See *Refusal-of-treatment form,* page 122). The signed form indicates that appropriate treatment would have been given had the patient consented. If the patient refuses to sign the release form, the nurse's note should include documentation in the form of writing "refused to sign" on the patient's signature line and adding the nurse's initials and date. For additional protection, the facility may also require the patient's spouse or closest relative to sign a refusal-of-treatment form that indicates who completes it, the spouse or a relative.

END-OF-LIFE CARE

Nurses must meet the physical and emotional end-of-life needs of both the dying patient and those of the family. The dying patient may experience a variety of physical symptoms, including pain, respiratory distress, loss of appetite, nausea and vomiting, and bowel problems. Emotional concerns may include confusion, depression, anxiety, sleep disturbances, and spiritual distress. Nursing interventions should be individualized to the specific needs of the patient.

The nurse can also make the death more comfortable and meaningful for the family. These actions may help:

- if they want to hear about it, telling the family what to expect
- encouraging them to talk to and touch the patient
- allowing them to help with care, if they desire
- providing them with a comfortable environment
- encouraging verbalization of concerns and feelings
- determining whether they would like a member of the clergy to visit

Essential Documentation

The nurse should call the provider and document the time and date of notification, the orders given by the provider, and whether the provider visited the patient. The documentation should include the names of others on the health care team who were notified (note the time called and the response).

The nurse should document interventions that were provided to meet the needs of the family, the names of family members, the teaching provided to the family, and their responses. This may be documented on a standardized teaching record provided by the health care facility.

ENDOTRACHEAL EXTUBATION

When the patient no longer requires endotracheal (ET) intubation, the airway can be removed. The nurse needs to explain this procedure to the patient, and the respiratory therapist needs to be contacted to extubate the patient as ordered by the health care provider. The patient needs to be instructed to cough and breathe deeply after the ET tube is removed and needs to be assessed frequently for signs of respiratory distress.

Essential Documentation

On a flow sheet provided by the facility, the nurse should record the name of the respiratory therapist, the date and time of extubation, the presence or absence of stridor or other signs of upper airway edema, breath sounds, the type and amount of supplemental oxygen administered, any complications and required subsequent therapy, and the patient's tolerance of the procedure. Document patient teaching and support given.

Endotracheal Extubation		
5/26/2019	1700	**PATIENT TEACHING:** Explained extubation procedure to pt. Pt. acknowledged understanding by nodding his head "yes." ______ **NURSING INTERVENTION:** Placed pt. in high Fowler's position and suctioned for scant amount of thin white secretions. ETT removed at 1630. **NURSING ASSESSMENT:** No stridor or respiratory distress noted, breath sounds clear. RR 22, P 92, BP 128/82, oral T 98.4°F. Pulse oximetry 97% on 50% via mask. ______ **PATIENT TEACHING:** Instructed pt. on importance of coughing and deep breathing every hr. Pt. was able to give proper return demonstration. Cough nonproductive. ______ ______ **Margie Egan, RN**

ENDOTRACHEAL INTUBATION

ET intubation involves the oral or nasal insertion of a flexible tube through the larynx into the trachea for the purpose of controlling the airway and mechanically ventilating the patient. Performed by a health care provider, anesthetist, or respiratory therapist, ET intubation usually occurs in emergencies, such as cardiopulmonary arrest, or in diseases such as epiglottitis. However, ET intubation may also occur under more controlled circumstances—for example, just before surgery. In these cases, a consent form will be used and signed by the patient and provider before surgery. The nurse will witness and sign the form to indicate that the patient was given an explanation of the procedure and that the patient verbalized understanding.

ET intubation establishes and maintains a patent airway, protects against aspiration by sealing off the trachea from the digestive tract, permits removal of tracheobronchial secretions in patients who cannot cough effectively, and provides a route for mechanical ventilation.

Essential Documentation

An electronic health record (EHR) will document the indication for the intubation procedure; the success or failure of the procedure will be documented by the health care provider performing the intubation. The type and size of tube, cuff size, amount of inflation, and inflation technique will be recorded by the provider. Information will also be provided by the respiratory therapist, who would also be at the bedside at the time of intubation. The provider or respiratory therapist will indicate whether drugs were administered, and these drugs should be documented on the electronic medication administration record (MAR). Also, the initiation of supplemental oxygen or ventilation therapy will be recorded. The provider or respiratory therapist will record the results of chest auscultation and chest x-ray and note the occurrence of any complications, necessary interventions, and the patient's response. The nurse can document patient education provided on a teaching record that is provided by the health care facility.

Endotracheal Intubation		
3/16/2019	1015	**PATIENT TEACHING:** Pt. informed by Dr. F. Eagan of the need for intubation, the risks, potential complications, and alternatives. Pt. consented to the procedure. ________

Endotracheal Intubation *(continued)*

NURSING INTERVENTION: Pt. given 20 mg etomidate and 100 mg succinylcholine by I.V. and intubated by Dr. B. Langley at 0945 with size 7.5 oral cuffed ETT. Tube taped in place @ #23 at the lip after placement confirmed with CO_2 detector and chest auscultation. Pt. placed on ventilator set at TV 750, FIO_2 45%, 5 cm PEEP, AC of 12. Portable CXR confirms proper placement. __________

NURSING ASSESSMENT: Right lung with basilar crackles and expiratory wheezes. Left lung clear. Pt. opening eyes when name is called. When asked if he's comfortable and in no pain, pt. nods head yes. __________

__________ **Jim Hanes, RN**

ENDOTRACHEAL TUBE, PATIENT REMOVAL OF

Because an ET tube is used to provide mechanical ventilation and maintain a patent airway, the removal of an ET tube by a patient may be an emergency situation. The patient may not have spontaneous respirations, may be in severe respiratory distress, or may suffer trauma to the larynx or vocal cords.

If a patient removes the ET tube, the nurse needs to stay and call for help and assign someone to notify the health care provider while assessing the patient's respiratory status. If the patient is in distress, manual ventilation needs to be performed while others prepare for reinsertion of the ET tube and monitor vital signs. If the patient is alert, the nurse needs to speak calmly and explain the reintubation procedure. If the patient is not in distress, oxygen therapy needs to be provided. If the decision is made not to reintubate the patient, respiratory status and vital signs need to be monitored every 15 minutes for 2 to 3 hours, or as ordered by the health care provider. Some facilities also require that an incident report be completed.

Essential Documentation

An EHR will document the date and time, and the nurse will document the incident regarding the ET tube removal by the patient, the name of the provider and respiratory therapist notified, and the respiratory assessment of the patient. Include documentation of the nursing actions of providing oxygen therapy and the patient response. An incident report will be necessary regarding the patient self-extubation. If the patient needs reintubation, the nurse should complete the EHR used for intubation, noting any patient education provided. (See *Endotracheal intubation,* page 125.)

Patient Removal of Endotracheal Tube		
1/30/2019	0400	**NURSING ASSESSMENT:** Summoned to room by ventilator alarms at 0330. Found pt. in bed with ETT in hand. P 86 and regular, BP 140/70, RR 20 regular and deep. No use of accessory muscles, skin warm, dry, and pink. 100% NRB mask placed. O_2 sat. by pulse oximetry 94%. Lungs clear to auscultation bilaterally. Pt. oriented to time, place, and person. Pt. stated, "I must have been dreaming. And when I woke up, the tube was in my hand." ______
		NURSING INTERVENTION: Dr. N. Smith notified. ETT to remain out. Order to wear O_2 as tolerated while maintaining an O_2 sat. of greater than 92%. CXR and ABG ordered for 0500. ______
		______ **Amy Young, RN**

END-TIDAL CARBON DIOXIDE MONITORING

Monitoring end-tidal carbon dioxide ($ETCO_2$) determines the CO_2 concentration in exhaled gas. With this technique, a photodetector measures the amount of infrared light absorbed by airway gas during inspiration and expiration. A monitor converts this information to a CO_2 value and a corresponding waveform or capnogram.

$ETCO_2$ monitoring provides information about the patient's pulmonary, cardiac, and metabolic status, which aids in patient management and helps prevent clinical compromise. This technique has become standard during anesthesia administration and mechanical ventilation. It may be used to help wean a patient with a stable acid–base balance from mechanical ventilation. It also reduces the need for frequent arterial blood gas (ABG) measurements, especially when combined with pulse oximetry. Other uses for $ETCO_2$ monitoring include assessing resuscitation efforts and identifying the return of spontaneous circulation. Because no CO_2 is exhaled when breathing stops, this technique also detects apnea. When used during ET intubation, $ETCO_2$ monitoring can avert neurologic injury and even death by confirming correct ET tube placement and, because CO_2 is not normally produced by the stomach, by detecting accidental esophageal intubation.

When a patient requires ET intubation, an $ETCO_2$ detector or monitor is usually applied immediately after the tube is inserted. For a nonintubated patient, the adapter is placed near the patient's airway. If a patient is alert, with or without ET intubation, explain the purpose and expected duration of the monitoring.

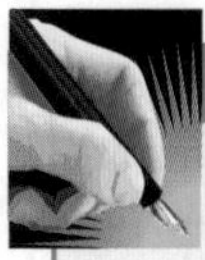

ACCUCHART

DOCUMENTING ETCO_2 ON A FLOW SHEET

								DATE 10/13/19	
		0001	0100	0200	0300	0400	0500	0600	0700
PULMONARY	Ventilator settings	CMV/2 TV 800							
	Peak pressures	/	/	/	/	/	/	/	/
	O_2 /delivery system	35%							
	Oximetry	97%							
	ETCO_2	35%							

Essential Documentation

An EHR will include the date and time, and the nurse should document the initial ETCO_2 value and all ventilator settings. A flow sheet is commonly used to document the waveform from the monitor, ETCO_2 values, and vital signs as changes in patient status occur. Periodically, ABG results should be recorded. ETCO_2 values should also be documented; see "Documenting ETCO_2 on a flow sheet" above for an example of documenting ETCO_2 values.

ENEMA ADMINISTRATION

An enema is a solution introduced into the rectum and colon. Enemas are used to administer medication, clean the lower bowel in preparation for diagnostic or surgical procedures, relieve distention and promote expulsion of flatus, lubricate the rectum and colon, and soften hardened stool for removal. Enema solutions and methods vary to suit the patient's condition or treatment requirements.

Essential Documentation

An enema is considered a medication, and this information would be included in the MAR of the EHR. Documentation of the patient's response/stool will be included in the input/output portion of the flow sheet in the EHR.

EPIDURAL ANALGESIA

Epidural analgesia improves pain relief, causes less sedation, allows patients to do coughing and deep-breathing exercises, and to ambulate earlier after surgery. It is also useful in patients with chronic pain that is not relieved by less invasive methods of pain relief. An epidural catheter is placed by an anesthesiologist in the epidural space outside the spinal cord between the vertebrae. Pain relief with minimal adverse effects is the result of drug delivery so close to the opiate receptors.

Opioids, such as preservative-free morphine (Duramorph) and fentanyl, are administered through the catheter and move slowly into the cerebrospinal fluid to opiate receptors in the dorsal horn of the spinal cord. The opioids may be administered by bolus dose, continuous infusion by pump, or patient-controlled analgesia. They may be administered alone or in combination with bupivacaine (a local anesthetic).

The adverse effects of epidural analgesia include sedation, nausea, urinary retention, orthostatic hypotension, itching, respiratory depression, headache, back soreness, leg weakness and numbness, and respiratory depression. The nurse must monitor the patient for these adverse reactions and notify the health care provider or anesthesiologist if they occur. Most facilities have policies or standards of care that address interventions for adverse effects and monitoring parameters.

Essential Documentation

The nurse will use an EHR and flow sheet to document the date, time, type and dose of drug administered, patient's level of consciousness, pain level (using a 0-to-10 scale), and respiratory rate and quality. Also, record the amount of drug received per hour and the number of dose attempts by the patient if the analgesia is patient controlled. Be sure to include site assessment, dressing changes, infusion bag changes, tubing changes, and patient education. Document complications, such as numbness, leg weakness, and respiratory depression; nursing interventions; and the patient's response.

Most facilities use a flow sheet to document drug dosage, rate, and route; vital signs; respiratory rate; pulse oximetry; pain scale; and sedation scale. The nurse should follow the facility's policy; however, these parameters should be monitored frequently for the first 12 hours, then every 4 hours after that. If the facility does not have a specific flow sheet for epidural documentation, the nurse should use the regular flow sheet and document other as-needed assessments or unusual circumstances in the progress notes.

Epidural Analgesia		
5/22/2019	1500	**NURSING ASSESSMENT:** Pt. received from PACU with epidural catheter in place. Dressing covering site clean, dry, and intact. Pt. receiving bupivacaine 0.125% and fentanyl 5 mcg/mL in 250 mL NSS at rate of 2 mL/hr. Respiratory rate 20 and deep, level of sedation 0 (alert), O_2 sat. by pulse oximetry on O_2 2 L by NC 99%, BP 120/80, P 72. Pt. reports pain as 2 on a scale of 0 to 10. No c/o nausea, itching, H/A, leg weakness, back soreness. Pt. voided 300 mL yellow urine. Bladder scan shows no residual after void. ________
		PATIENT TEACHING: Told pt. to report any pain greater than 3 out of 10, inability to void, and numbness in legs. ________
		NURSING INTERVENTION: Epidural infusion label applied to catheter, infusion tubing, and infusion pump. See flow sheet for frequent monitoring of drug dose, rate, VS, pulse ox., level of pain, and sedation level. ________
		________ **Mary Holmes, RN**

EPIDURAL HEMATOMA

A patient who is receiving or has recently received epidural analgesia is at risk for epidural hematoma, a complication that can lead to lower extremity paralysis. This risk is increased if the patient has received anticoagulants or traumatic or repeated epidural punctures. The nurse should frequently assess for diffuse back pain or tenderness, paresthesia, and bowel and bladder dysfunction, according to unit protocol or the health care provider's orders, to detect signs of epidural hematoma. Prompt assessments and interventions are necessary to avoid paralysis in the patient receiving epidural analgesia.

Essential Documentation

The nurse should use a flow sheet to record the date and time, the frequent patient assessments, the name of the provider notified, the time of notification, provider orders, nursing actions, and the patient's response. Patient education that is provided should be recorded in the EHR.

Epidural Hematoma		
2/23/2019	0925	**NURSING ASSESSMENT:** Called to room by pt. at 0910 for c/o lower back discomfort and numbness in right leg. When asked to point to pain, pt. moved hand around general region of lower back. Pedal pulses palpable with capillary refill less than 3 sec bilaterally. Right foot weaker than left when asked to dorsiflex and plantar flex foot against resistance. Unable to raise right foot off bed. Pt. alert and oriented to time, place, and person. No difficulty urinating, voided 350 mL on bedpan at 0830. ________
		NURSING INTERVENTION: Told pt. to remain in bed, placed call bell within reach, and verified that pt. knows how to use it. Dr. Hoffman, anesthesiologist, notified at 0920 of pt.'s symptoms and will be here to see pt. at 0930. ________
		________ **Julie Robbins, RN**

ESOPHAGEAL TUBE INSERTION (SENGSTAKEN–BLAKEMORE TUBE)

Used to control hemorrhage from esophageal or gastric varices, an esophageal tube is inserted nasally or orally by a health care provider and advanced into the esophagus or stomach. A gastric balloon exerts pressure on the cardia of the stomach, securing the tube and controlling bleeding varices. Most tubes also contain an esophageal balloon to control esophageal bleeding. Usually, gastric or esophageal balloons are deflated after 24 to 36 hours, according to facility policy, to reduce the risk of pressure necrosis.

Essential Documentation

The nurse should document that the patient understands the procedure and that a consent form has been signed. On a flow sheet, the nurse should record the date and time of insertion of the esophageal tube; the name of the provider who performed the procedure; the type of tube used; the type of sedation provided; vital signs before, during, and after the procedure; and patient's tolerance of the procedure.

On the flow sheet, the nurse should also note the esophageal balloon pressure (for Sengstaken–Blakemore and Minnesota tubes), the intragastric balloon pressure (for the Minnesota tube), or the amount of air injected (for Linton and Sengstaken–Blakemore tubes). The flow sheet should include the amount of any fluid used for gastric irrigation and the color, consistency, and amount of gastric return before and after lavage.

Because intraesophageal balloon pressure varies with respirations and esophageal contractions, the flow sheet should include the baseline balloon pressure, which is the most important pressure.

Esophageal Tube (Sengstaken–Blakmore Type) Insertion		
2/11/2019	1210	**PATIENT TEACHING:** Procedure explained to pt. by Dr. M. Fisher. Pt. verbalized understanding of procedure and consent signed. **NURSING ASSESSMENT:** Before procedure P 102, BP 90/60, RR 22, oral T 97.0°F. Sengstaken–Blakemore tube placed w/o difficulty by Dr. Fisher via right nostril. 50 mL air injected into gastric balloon. Abdominal X-ray obtained to confirm placement. Gastric balloon inflated with 500 mL air. Tube secured to football helmet traction. ____ **NURSING ASSESSMENT:** P 102, BP 98/52, RR 28. Large amount of bright red bloody drainage noted. Tube irrigated with 1800 mL of NSS until clear. NG tube placed in left nostril by Dr. Fisher and attached to continuous suction. Esophageal balloon inflated to 30 mm Hg and clamped. Equal breath sounds bilaterally. No SOB. After procedure P 98, BP 92/58, RR 24, oral T 97.0°F. ____ **NURSING INTERVENTION:** Stayed with pt. throughout procedure and provided support. Directed pt. to take slow deep breaths to maintain RR and HR WNL. ____ ____ **Evelyn Sutcliffe, RN**

ESOPHAGEAL TUBE REMOVAL

After gastric or esophageal bleeding has been controlled, the health care provider will remove the esophageal tube by first deflating the esophageal balloon. Then, if bleeding does not recur, traction from the gastric tube is removed, and the gastric balloon is deflated.

Essential Documentation

- On the flow sheet, the nurse should record the removal of the esophageal tube, the date and time, and the provider performing the procedure.

- If esophageal bleeding recurs, record this on the flow sheet.
- Record the deflation of the balloon, vital signs before and after removal of the tube, and patient tolerance of the procedure.

Esophageal Tube Removal

2/12/2019	1100	**NURSING INTERVENTION:** Assisted Dr. M. Fisher with removal of Sengstaken–Blakemore tube.
		NURSING ASSESSMENT: Before removal P 84, BP 102/68, RR 18, oral T 99.1°F. No bleeding noted after deflation of esophageal tube. Gastric balloon deflated. No resistance noted with removal of esophageal tube. After removal P 86, BP 110/68, RR 20, oral T 99.2°F. Pt. stated he was "happy to have the tube out."
		NURSING INTERVENTION: Assisted pt. to brush teeth and rinse with mouthwash. Cleaned crusted nasal secretions with cotton-tipped applicators and warm water.
		Evelyn Sutcliffe, RN

EXPERIMENTAL PROCEDURES

At times, the nurse may participate in administering experimental drugs or procedures to patients or administering established drugs in new ways or at experimental dosage levels. Follow the experimental protocol, and consult with the research coordinator, institutional review board, or human subjects committee. Ensure that the patient has completed the informed-consent process and signed a facility form. The informed-consent process includes the risks and benefits of the procedure, with a clear description of potential discomfort and risks. The patient should be informed that he or she can refuse to participate in the project. Follow the facility procedure regarding patient care during experimental treatment.

Essential Documentation

The nurse needs to do the following:

- Document that the patient has given informed consent for the drug or procedure.
- Obtain a copy of the consent form.
- Use a standardized form provided by the facility to complete all pertinent information about the experimental treatment or procedure.

Experimental Procedures		
10/03/2019	1400	Pt. admitted to unit at 1315. States she's enrolled in a study for an experimental chemotherapy drug and that she wishes to continue with her treatment during this admission. Dr. B. Marks notified of pt.'s admission and participation in a drug trial at 1330. Informed consent for drug trial, name of drug, drug information, study protocol, and contact information faxed to unit and placed in pt.'s chart. Verbal and faxed orders obtained to continue drug protocol. Drug information and orders faxed to pharmacy. Nursing supervisor, Colleen Begacki, RN, notified of situation at 1335. ________ **Lisa Mendocino, RN**

SELECTED READINGS

Aminiahidashti, H., Shafiee, S., Kiasari, A. Z., & Sazgar, M. (2018). Applications of end-tidal carbon dioxide ($ETCO_2$) monitoring in emergency department; a narrative review. *Emergency, 6*(1), 1–6.

Andersen, A. M., Lipkin, P. H., & Law, K. (2016). Elopement patterns and caregiver strategies. *Journal of the American Academy of Child & Adolescent Psychiatry, 55*(10, Suppl.), S108.

Bhorkar, N. M., Dhansura, T. S., Tarawade, U. B., & Mehta, S. S. (2018). Epidural hematoma: Vigilance beyond guidelines. *Indian Journal of Critical Care Medicine, 22*(7), 555–557.

Bloomfield, C., & McNee, B. (2015). Reexamine elopement risk assessment. *Long-Term Living: For the Continuing Care Professional, 64*(6), 28–30.

Feldkamp, J. K. (2015). Implement safety measures to avoid resident elopements. *Caring for the Ages, 16*(5), 14.

Ituk, U., & Wong, C. A. (2018). *Epidural and combined spinal-epidural anesthesia: Techniques.* Retrieved from UpToDate website: http://www.uptodate.com

Janz, D. R., Semler, M. W., Joffe, A. M., Casey, J. D., Lentz, R. J., deBoisblanc, B. P., ... Pragmatic Critical Care Research Group. (2018). A multicenter randomized trial of a checklist for endotracheal intubation of critically ill adults. *Chest, 153*(4), 816–824.

Johnstone, M. (2008). Emergency situations and refusals to care. *Australian Nursing Journal, 15*(9), 21.

Meek, P. D. (2014). Resident and patient elopements: An overview of legal issues and trends. *Journal of Legal Nurse Consulting, 25*(2), 18–21.

Mitchell, J. (2008). Nurses need protection in the workplace. *Australian Nursing Journal, 16*(1), 3.

Ortiz, A. M., Garcia, C. J., Othman, M. O., & Zuckerman, M. J. (2018). Innovative technique for endoscopic placement of Sengstaken-Blakemore tube. *Southern Medical Journal, 111*(5), 307–311.

Pegram, A., Bloomfield, J., & Jones, A. (2008). Safe use of rectal suppositories and enemas with adult patients. ***Nursing** Standard, 22*(38), 39–41.

Pei Chin Cheong, G., Kannan, A., Kwong, F. K., Venkatesan, K., Seet, E., Cheong, G. P. C., & Koh, K. F. (2018). Prevailing practices in airway management: A prospective single-centre observational study of endotracheal intubation. *Singapore Medical Journal, 59*(3), 144–149.

Scammell, J. (2018). Improving end-of-life care. *British Journal of Nursing, 27*(21), 1269.

Seaman, J. B. (2018). Mitigating distress and building resilience: Can we facilitate and sustain intensive care unit nurses' delivery of compassionate end-of-life care? *Annals of the American Thoracic Society, 15*(12), 1400–1402.

Seisa, M. O., Gondhi, V., Demirci, O., Diedrich, D. A., Kashyap, R., & Smischney, N. J. (2018). Survey on the current state of endotracheal intubation among the critically ill. *Journal of Intensive Care Medicine, 33*(6), 354–360.

Sivarajan, V. B., & Bohn, D. (2011). Monitoring of standard hemodynamic parameters: Heart rate, systemic blood pressure, atrial pressure, pulse oximetry, and end-tidal CO_2. *Pediatric Critical Care Medicine, 12*(Suppl.), S2–S11.

Sonneborn, O., & Robers, G. (2018). Nurse-led extubation in the post-anaesthesia care unit. *Journal of Perioperative Practice, 28*(12), 362–365.

F

FAILURE TO PROVIDE INFORMATION

Occasionally, the nurse may encounter patients, their family members, or legal guardians who lack the capacity to provide accurate or complete information about their health history, current medications, or treatments. Most of the time, this is not a willful violation of sincere communication but, rather, a mental status concern. They may be uncooperative for various reasons. They may think that too many caregivers have asked the same questions too many times, they may not understand the significance of the information that is being requested in providing expert care on their behalf, or they may be fearful or disoriented. They may be suspicious of why such personal information needs to be divulged. Alternatively, they may have severe pain, a psychiatric problem, or a language barrier. In such situations, the nurse needs to obtain the information from other sources or forms.

Essential Documentation

The nurse needs to clearly document any trouble encountered in communicating with the patient. Patient responses should be recorded clearly in the patient's own words. Essential documentation in an electronic health record (EHR) is somewhat different because the nurse must seek out a way to include a narrative description of the situation at hand. Checkboxes and filled-in numbers do not "capture" the nature of the situation in a way that others can be made to comprehend the nature of the patient's or other's lack of capacity to participate fully. The nurse's interventions or explanations of the importance of this information in order to provide the patient with the best possible care need to be included. The following also need to be done:

- Document the name of the health care provider notified about the patient's lack of capacity to share information and the time of notification.
- Write down other sources of information, such as family members or previous records.

Narrative notes are becoming scarce with the innovation of EHRs in many health care organizations at all levels of care. However, documenting the full scope of patients' mental and emotional status protects everyone, including the patients, their families, their health care providers, and the care organization, from safety breakdowns. Copying and pasting old information from a previous chart entry is a violation not only of patient safety but also the integrity of the caregiver. This is not tolerated by the nursing profession (American Nurses Association [ANA], 2015).

Failure to Provide Information

2/5/2019	0830	**NURSING ASSESSMENT:** When asked for a list of his current medications, pt. refused. Explained reasons for needing to know about medications, but pt. still refused to share this information. No previous records available. No family members in to visit pt. Pt. won't share names or telephone numbers of family members. Called Dr. T. Raynor at 0815 to report pt. failure to provide information. Dr. will speak with pt. on his rounds this a.m. ________ **Nora Martin, RN**

FALLS, PATIENT

Falls are a major cause of injury and death among older patients. In fact, the older the person, the more likely death will result due to a fall or its complications. In acute care hospitals, 85% of all inpatient incident reports are related to falls; of those who fall, 10% fall more than once, and 10% experience a fatal fall. In nursing homes, approximately 60% of residents fall every year, and about 40% of those residents experience more than one fall. If a patient falls, despite preventive measures, the nurse should:

- Stay with the patient and do not move the patient until a head-to-toe assessment and vital signs check are performed, having assigned another person to notify the health care provider.

- Provide any emergency measures necessary, such as securing an airway, controlling bleeding, or stabilizing a deformed limb.
- Ask the patient or a witness what happened.
- Ask the patient if he or she is in pain, lost consciousness, "saw stars," or hit his or her head. If no problems are detected, return the patient to bed with the help of another person.
- Notify the attending physician.

With the advent of EHRs, more and more organizations that treat people across the life span are including documentation of fall risk management in the initial patient assessment. However, there are many categories of patients who are not perceived to be at a higher fall risk than the general population, and that is a misperception that could create harm for lack of due care. Among those who appear not to be at risk, but may be, are the following: cardiac patients with syncopal (dizziness) episodes, patients with inner ear (vestibular) problems, pregnant women in early pregnancy (dizziness) and later pregnancy (lack of normal balance as the pregnancy progresses), newly walking toddlers due to their proportionately larger head sizes, and the neurologically impaired (patients with seizure disorders, evolving stroke, developing brain tumors, etc.). Such conditions should prompt a fall risk evaluation by the nurse. Including a short fall risk questionnaire for each patient would shed light on these unsuspected conditions. Notably, falls are common among young children without developmental disabilities, and they usually recover rapidly unless they are unattended or experience falls from greater heights than the ground beneath them.

Essential Documentation

If a patient falls despite precautions, the nurse should be sure to:

- File an incident report and chart the event. (See "Incident report," pages 200 to 202.)
- Record how the patient was found and the time discovered.
- Document an objective assessment, avoiding any judgments or opinions.
- Assess the patient and record any bruises, lacerations, or abrasions.
- Describe any pain or deformity in the extremities, particularly the hip, arm, leg, or lumbar spine.
- Record vital signs, including orthostatic blood pressure.
- Start with a head-to-toe assessment, observing for loss of consciousness and neurologic status first.

- Document if the patient had a seizure or a suspected unobserved seizure.
- Document whether the fall was witnessed by others, and if so, include their names.
- Document the patient's neurologic assessment. Include slurred speech, weakness in the extremities, or a change in mental status.
- Record the name of the health care provider and other persons notified, such as family members, and the time of notification.
- Include instructions or orders given.
- Recommend admission or emergency department evaluation for any patient who sustained loss of consciousness, concussion, or head trauma.
- Call the rescue squad if the individual who fell is not already in an inpatient or emergency department facility if indicated.
- Also document any patient education.

Falls		
11/6/2019	1400	**NURSING ASSESSMENT:** Pt. found on floor between bed and chair on left side of bed at 1330. Pt. c/o pain in her right hip area and difficulty moving right leg. No abrasions or lacerations noted. BP elevated at 158/94. P 94, RR 22, oral T 98.2°F. Pt. states, "I was trying to get into the chair when I fell." Pt. alert and oriented to time, place, and person. Speech clear and coherent. Hand grasps strong bilaterally. Right leg externally rotated and shorter than left leg. ________ **NURSING INTERVENTION:** Dr. A. Dayoub notified at 1338. Pt. assisted back to bed with assist of 3, maintaining right hip and leg in alignment. Hip X-ray ordered and showed right hip fracture. Dr. Dayoub aware and family notified. Pt. to be evaluated by orthopedic surgeon. ________ **NURSING INTERVENTION:** Pt. medicated for pain with morphine 4 mg I.V. Maintaining bed rest at present time. ________ **PATIENT TEACHING:** Explaining all procedures to pt. Call bell in hand and understands to call for help with moving. An Incident Report was completed by physician and nurses and placed in chart. ________ ________ **Beverly Kotsur, RN**

FALLS, PRECAUTIONS

Patient falls resulting from slips, slides, knees giving way, fainting, or tripping over equipment can lead to prolonged hospitalization, increased hospital costs, and liability problems. People of all ages fall, notably because they have risks that may not be perceived by direct observation. Among those people are newly walking toddlers, small children, pregnant women, and people with cardiac syncope (dizziness) or neurologic problems that are not visibly detectable (evolving strokes, brain tumors, seizure disorders, etc.). Because falls cause so many problems, the facility may require assessment of each patient for his or her risk of falling and to take measures to prevent falls. (See *Reducing the risk of falls,* page 142.) If the facility requires a risk assessment form for patients, it should be completed and kept in the patient's chart. (See *Risk assessment for falls,* page 143.) Those at risk require a care plan reflecting interventions to prevent falls. (See *Reducing the nurse's liability in patient falls,* page 144.)

Essential Documentation

The nurse's documentation should include the time and date of the nurse's entry that describes the reasons for implementing fall precautions for the patient, such as a high score on an assessment tool that measures risk for falls. Most organizations with EHRs have the capacity to do this within the record, but individuals who do not perceive the patient's risk for falls often do not fill out this form. Documentation of interventions, such as frequent toileting, reorienting the patient to his or her environment, and placing needed objects within patient reach, should be included, as well as the patient's response to these interventions. The nurse should note measures taken to alert other health care professionals of the risk for falls, such as placing a band on the patient's wrist and communicating this risk on the patient's EHR. The nurse needs to record any patient and family teaching and their level of understanding. In some facilities, patient and family education may be documented on an education flow sheet. Recommendations for admission or emergency department evaluation for any patient who sustained loss of consciousness, concussion, or head trauma should be recorded. If not already in an inpatient or emergency department facility, the nurse needs to call the rescue squad indicated by facility policy.

Falls Precautions		
1/26/2019	1000	**NURSING ASSESSMENT:** Score of 13 on admission Risk Assessment for Falls form. High risk for falls communicated to pt. and family. ___
		NURSING INTERVENTION: Risk for falls ID placed on pt.'s L wrist, high-risk for falls checked off on care plan. ___
		NURSING ASSESSMENT: Pt. alert and oriented to time, place, and person. Oriented pt. and family to room and call bell system. ___
		PATIENT TEACHING: Told pt. to call for help before getting out of bed or up from chair on his own. Pt. demonstrated proper use of call bell and verbalized when to use it. Personal items and call bell placed within reach.
		___ **Betty Floyd, RN**

REDUCING THE RISK OF FALLS

There are no foolproof ways to prevent a patient from falling, but The Joint Commission recommends the following steps to reduce the risks of falls and injuries. The nurse should ensure documentation of safety interventions in the appropriate place in the medical record.

Physical Measures

- Provide adequate exercise and ambulation.
- Offer frequent food and liquids.
- Provide regular toileting.
- Evaluate medications (hypnotics, sedatives, analgesics, psychotropics, antihypertensives, laxatives, diuretics, and polypharmacy increase the risk of falling).
- Assess and manage pain.
- Promote normal sleep patterns.

Psychological Measures

- Reorient the patient to his or her environment.
- Communicate with the patient and the family about the risk for falls and the need to call for help before getting up alone.
- Teach relaxation techniques.
- Provide companionship, such as sitters or volunteers.
- Provide diversionary activities.

Environmental Measures

- Orient the patient to his or her environment.
- Use appropriate lighting and noise control.
- Consider a bed alarm.
- Provide a safe space layout (long-term care), such as a low-lying bed or mattress or pads on the floor.
- Place assistive devices within the patient's reach at all times.
- Provide bed adaptations (long-term care).
- Provide accessibility to needed objects at all times.
- Ensure frequent observation of any patient at risk, such as moving the patient closer to the nurses' station and involving family.
- Provide side-rail adaptations and alternatives.
- Use appropriate seating and equipment.
- Provide identifiers of high-risk status, such as an armband or an identifier on the patient's bed or door.

Education

- Provide staff, patient, and family education on identifying and reducing the risk of falls.

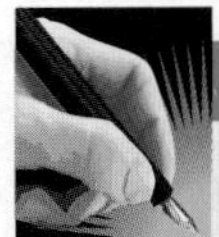

ACCUCHART

RISK ASSESSMENT FOR FALLS

Because falls cause so many problems, the facility may require that a risk assessment be performed every shift and that prevention efforts are documented. For example, if the facility requires a risk assessment form for patients, it should be completed and kept in the patient's chart.

Certain patients have a greater risk of falling than others. The use of a chart, such as the one shown here (which was developed for use with older patients), can help in determining the extent of the risk. The use of the chart requires checking each applicable item and totaling the number of points. A score of 10 or more indicates a risk of falling.

DETERMINING A PATIENT'S RISK OF FALLING

Points	Patient category
	Age
1___	80 or older
2 ✓	70 to 79 years old
	Mental state
0___	Oriented at all times or comatose
2___	Confused at all times
4 ✓	Confused periodically
	Duration of hospitalization
0 ✓	Over 3 days
2___	0 to 3 days
	Falls within the past 6 months
0___	None
2 ✓	1 or 2
5___	3 or more
	Elimination
0 ✓	Independent and continent
1___	Uses catheter, ostomy, or both
3___	Needs help with elimination
5___	Independent and incontinent
1 ✓	**Visual impairment**
3___	**Confinement to chair**
2___	**Blood pressure** Drop in systolic pressure of 20 mm Hg or more between lying and standing positions

Points	Patient category
	Gait and balance Assess gait by having the patient stand in one spot with both feet on the ground for 30 seconds without holding onto something. Then have him walk straight ahead and through a doorway. Next, have him turn while walking.
1___	Wide base of support
1___	Loss of balance while standing
1 ✓	Balance problems when walking
1___	Diminished muscle coordination
1___	Lurching or swaying
1___	Holds on or changes gait when walking through a doorway
1___	Jerking or instability when turning
1___	Needs an assistive device such as a walker
	Medications How many different drugs is the patient taking?
0___	None
1___	1
2 ✓	2 or more

___ Alcohol	___ Cathartics
___ Anesthetics	___ Diuretics
___ Antihistamines	___ Opioids
✓ Antihypertensives	___ Psychotropics
___ Antiseizure drugs	___ Sedative-hypnotics
___ Antidiabetics	___ Other drugs (specify)
✓ Benzodiazepines	

Points	Patient category
1 ✓	Check if the patient has changed drugs, dosage, or both in the past 5 days.
13	**TOTAL**

Signature: Donna Morales, RN
Date/Time: 4/4/19 0800

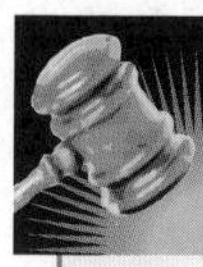

LEGAL CASEBOOK

REDUCING THE NURSE'S LIABILITY IN PATIENT FALLS

Patient falls are a very common area of nursing liability. Patients who are elderly, sedated, or mentally incapacitated are the most likely to fall. The case of *Stevenson v. Alta Bates (1937)* involved a patient who had a stroke and was learning to walk again. As two nurses, each holding one of the patient's arms, assisted her into the hospital's sunroom, one of the nurses let go of the patient and stepped forward to get a chair for her. The patient fell and sustained a fracture. The nurse was found negligent: The court said she should have anticipated the patient's need for a chair and made the appropriate arrangements before bringing the patient into the sunroom.

FALLS, VISITOR OR OTHER

Despite the best efforts to maintain a safe environment, falls may occur. Not only can a patient fall, but family members and other visitors may slip, slide, have knees give way, faint, or trip over equipment as well. When a visitor falls, the event needs to be documented on an incident report. If the visitor requires medical attention, he or she should be taken to the emergency department. The nurse should document safety measures that are present in the environment, such as elevators, railings in hallways and stairwells, lighting in the area where stairs are located, and precautionary signs when there are wet floors in the building.

Essential Documentation

The documentation (including exact location, date, and time as well as name, address, and phone number) of a visitor fall should be made on an incident report, not in the medical record of the patient being visited. (See "Incident report," pages 200 to 202.) The nurse's input should include:

- A description of only what the nurse actually saw and heard and what actions the nurse took to provide care at the scene. Unless actually witnessed, the nurse should write "found on floor" or "as reported by visitor."
- The name of the nursing supervisor who was notified and the time of notification. A narrative description is better than a short description. Because this is not patient data, the visitor's fall information should not be documented in the patient's chart or EHR.
- Assessment of the visitor
- A record of any bruises, lacerations, or abrasions

- A description of any pain or deformity in the extremities, particularly the hip, arm, leg, or lumbar spine
- Documentation of the visitor's neurologic assessment, including slurred speech, weakness in the extremities, or a change in level of consciousness or mental status
- Information regarding transportation to the emergency department or the visitor's refusal to be seen when offered the option

FIREARMS AT BEDSIDE

If the nurse observes or has reason to believe that the patient has a firearm in his or her possession, the facility's policy should be followed, and the security department and nursing supervisor should be contacted immediately. Upon learning of a firearm's presence, the nurse should arrange to remove others from the location quietly and rapidly. Also, additional people (other patients, staff, and visitors) need to be prevented from entering the area. Documentation of the discovery of a visualized weapon should be recorded in the patient's chart or EHR. The nurse must maintain composure throughout and, if necessary, notify area police.

Essential Documentation

These actions must be taken by the nurse:

- Record the date and time of nurse entry.
- Describe the circumstances of the discovery of the weapon and its appearance, including distinguishing marks, color, and approximate size.
- Record the name of the security guard and nursing supervisor notified, the time of notification, their instructions, and nursing actions.
- Document the visits of security and the nursing supervisor to the patient's room and their outcome as well as any police involvement.
- Complete an incident report. (See "Incident report," pages 200 to 202.)

Firearms at Bedside		
8/23/2019	1000	**NURSING ASSESSMENT:** Noted black gun, approx. 6" long in pt.'s bedside table. ________ **NURSING INTERVENTION:** Bedside table moved out of pt.'s reach. Called security at 0931 and reported gun in bedside table to Officer Halliday. Area secured and Mary Delaney, RN, nursing supervisor notified at 0933, Security officer Moore spoke with pt., who produced license to carry gun and turned unloaded gun over to the officer to be locked in hospital safe until discharge. Ms. Delaney reinforced hospital policy on firearms to pt. who stated he understood. Incident Report completed and placed in chart. ________ ________ **Tom O'Brien, RN**

FIREARMS IN THE HOME

Weapons in the home, especially firearms, present a real and frightening threat to the safety and well-being of the patient, family, and the home care team. It is essential to follow the agency's policies and procedures for dealing with firearms in the home.

Above all, the nurse must not allow the patient or family to keep a loaded firearm in the same room where care is being delivered. If a patient refuses to remove a loaded gun from the room, preferably to a locked location, the nurse must discontinue the visit and make it clear why he or she is leaving. Then, the nurse should call the nursing supervisor and the patient's health care provider and let them know about the firearm danger. The agency may have an incident report in which to document the problem. The nurse can request permission to leave the shift, particularly in the belief of being in danger. Unless the nurse's life is in imminent danger, he or she must not touch a firearm in the home.

In addition to considering personal safety in the presence of a loaded gun, the nurse must also consider the safety of the patient and family. The only safe guns are stored in safes with gun locks engaged. Many children have lost their lives due to guns in their own homes or those of friends and relatives. On becoming aware of a gun, one must assess the patient's home situation. Does the gun pose a threat to children in the home? Does anyone in the home have a mental illness? Do any family members have a history of violence? If the nurse thinks that a gun creates an unacceptable risk for someone in the patient's home, he or she must talk with the nursing supervisor about which actions are appropriate.

The ANA (2015) *Code of Ethics for Nurses with Interpretive Statements* stipulates the patient's right to privacy, and this is particularly guaranteed by the US Constitution. One amendment does not override another in how it is applied, but safety is placed above privacy by the Constitution and also the ANA code, and the nurse must act according to judgment in each situation. Approximately 50% of the households in the United States have guns within their walls.

Essential Documentation

The nurse should record any observations of weapons in the home, including location, ownership, and whether a gun is loaded. Document a history of mental illness in the patient or family members. Record whether the weapon is kept under lock and key. If it is possible to determine the presence of a gun lock, try to do so without picking up the weapon. Note whether anyone in the family has a history of violence. If the nurse discontinues the visit and leaves the home because of a firearm, the nurse should describe the reasons for leaving and include the name of the supervisor and health care provider notified. If the nurse feels the home is unsafe for children or other family members, he or she should objectively document the reasons and record the name of the supervisor notified, the directions given, and nursing actions taken.

Firearms in the Home		
4/10/2019	1015	**NURSING ASSESSMENT:** During visit to pt.'s home observed a firearm on the bedside table. Pt. stated it was his weapon and was unloaded. When asked, pt. agreed to remove gun and place it in a locked cabinet. Pt. denies personal or family history of mental illness or suicide attempts. States no problems with violence in family members. No children live in the home, although grandchildren occasionally visit. Pt. verbally agreed to lock up gun in cabinet before home health visits and when grandchildren visit.
		NURSING INTERVENTION: Supervisor, John Bellamy, RN, and Dr. K. Roche alerted to gun in home and pt.'s agreement to lock up gun before home visits.
		Sonja Tjaer, RN

FIREARMS ON FAMILY MEMBER OR VISITOR

If the nurse observes that a family member or visitor has brought a gun to the facility, the facility's policy on dealing with firearms must be followed by immediately contacting the security department and nursing supervisor and calmly diverting all other visitors, staff, and patients away from the area.

Essential Documentation

The nurse should follow these actions:

- Document the occurrence on an incident report.
- Record the visitor's name and relationship to the patient, if known.
- Describe the circumstances of the discovery of the weapon and its appearance, including distinguishing marks, color, and approximate size.

- Record the names of the security guard and nursing supervisor notified, the time of notification, their instructions, and nursing actions.
- Record the visits of security and the nursing supervisor to the patient's room and their outcome.
- Indicate the exact dates and times of the visits.

SELECTED READINGS

American Nurses Association. (2015). *Code of ethics for nurses with interpretive statements.* Silver Spring, MD: Author.

Aumack, T., York, T., & Eyestone, K. (2017). Firearm discharges in hospitals: an examination of data from 2006-2016. *Journal of Healthcare Protection Management,* 33(1), 1–8.

Beil, T. L. (2018). Interventions to Prevent Falls in Older Adults: Updated Evidence Report and Systematic Review for the US Preventive Services Task Force. *JAMA, 319*(16), 1705–1716.

LeLaurin, J. H. & Shorr, R. I. (2019). Preventing Falls in Hospitalized Patients: State of the Science. *Clinics in Geriatric Medicine, 35*(2), 273–283.

McMahon, S. (2017). The Strategies to Reduce Injuries and Develop Confidence in Elders Intervention: Falls Risk Factor Assessment and Management, Patient Engagement, and Nurse Co-management. *Journal of the American Geriatrics Society, 65*(12), 2733–2739.

Ratwani, R. M., Moscovitch, B., & Rising, J. P. (2018). Improving pediatric electronic health record usability and safety through certification. *JAMA Pediatrics, 172*(11), 1007–1008. doi:10:1001/jamapediatrics.2018/2784

Violano, P., Bonne, S., Duncan, T., Pappas, P., Christmas, A. B., Dennis, A., Goldberg, S., ... Crandall M. (2018). Prevention of firearm injuries with gun safety devices and safe storage: An Eastern Association for the Surgery of Trauma Systematic Review. *The Journal of Trauma and Acute Care Surgery, 84*(6), 1003–1011.

G

GASTRIC LAVAGE

After poisoning or a drug overdose, especially in patients who have central nervous system depression or an inadequate gag reflex, gastric lavage is used to flush the stomach and remove ingested substances through a gastric lavage tube. Gastric lavage (GL) is a gastrointestinal decontamination technique that empties the stomach of toxic substances by the sequential administration and aspiration of small volumes of fluid via an orogastric tube. GL used in the past is no longer used routinely in the management of poisoned patients. Less invasive procedures such as adsorption of ingested toxic substances with activated charcoal is commonly used. GL may be used in cooling hyperthermic patients or in upper GI bleeding.

Typically, a physician, performs this procedure in the emergency department or intensive care unit. Correct lavage tube placement is essential for patient safety because accidental misplacement (e.g., in the lungs) followed by lavage can be fatal.

Essential Documentation

The nurse should begin each entry in the clinical record with the date and time of the entry. If possible, document the type of substance ingested, when the ingestion occurred, and how much substance was ingested. The nurse should obtain and record preprocedure vital signs (VS) and level of consciousness (LOC). The date and time of lavage; the size and type of nasogastric tube used; the volume and type of irrigant solution; the method used to verify correct tube placement; and the amount of drained gastric contents, including the color and consistency of drainage, should be recorded by the nurse. The amount of irrigant solution instilled and gastric contents drained should be documented on the intake and output record sheet. The nurse should note whether drainage was sent to the laboratory for analysis as well as any drugs instilled through the tube. The patient's VS should be assessed and recorded every 15 minutes on a frequent VS assessment sheet, and LOC should be assessed and recorded on a Glasgow Coma Scale sheet until the patient is stable. (See "Intake and output," pages 210 to 212; "Level of consciousness, changes in," pages 237 to 239; and "Vital signs, frequent," page 430.) Document the time that the tube was removed and how the patient tolerated the procedure. The nurse should provide and document patient education and emotional support given.

Gastric Lavage		
04/22/2019	2300	**NURSING ASSESSMENT:** A 20-year-old female presented in the emergency room accompanied by a roommate after ingesting an unknown quantity of diazepam. Pt. lethargic, unresponsive to verbal stimuli, but responsive to painful stimuli, gag reflex present, but diminished. Reflexes hypoactive, and PERRL prelavage VS: P 56, BP 90/52, RR 14 and shallow, SpO_2 93%, rectal T 97°F. Single lumen 30 Fr. Ewald tube inserted by Dr. T. Jones at 2315 without difficulty, for gastric lavage. Tube placement verified by pH of aspirant. Lavage performed with 250 mL of NS. Returned content liquid green with small blue flecks and some undigested food. Sample collected and sent to lab for analysis. Postprocedure vitals: P 58, BP 90/54, RR 15 and shallow, SpO_2 93%, rectal T 97.4°F. LOC unchanged. ______ ______ **Lisa Greenwald, RN**
04/22/2019	2315	**NURSING ASSESSMENT:** Lavage repeated ×2 with 500 mL NS each. Gastric return clear after third lavage. Total return 1375 mL. VS: P 60, BP 94/52, RR 15, SpO_2 93%, rectal T 98.6°F. Pt. lethargic, but responsive to verbal stimuli; reflexes remain sluggish. Every 15 min. VS and LOC documented on frequent vital signs and Glasgow Coma Scale sheets. Gastric tube left in place until pt. is fully alert per physician orders. ______ **Lisa Greenwald, RN**

GASTROINTESTINAL HEMORRHAGE

The loss of a large amount of blood from the gastrointestinal (GI) tract is referred to as a GI hemorrhage. Bleeding in the upper GI tract is caused primarily by ulcers, varices, or tears within the GI system, whereas lower GI bleeding may be caused by diverticulitis, polyps, ulcerative colitis, Crohn's disease, or cancer. The nurse's immediate lifesaving interventions focus on stabilizing the cardiovascular system, identifying the bleeding source, and stopping the bleeding.

Essential Documentation

The nurse should begin each entry in the clinical record with the date and time of the entry. After the nurse has provided any necessary lifesaving interventions, the patient and family should be questioned, if possible, about the length of time that blood has been noted in stool or vomitus and the amount and color of blood (e.g., frank red blood, coffee-ground vomitus, or dark-colored or black stool) and documented. The results of the nurse's cardiovascular and GI assessments and immediate interventions taken, such as placing the vomiting patient on his or her side with the head of the bed elevated, are documented. Frequent VS and intake and output may be charted on the frequent VS assessment and intake and output sheets, respectively. (See "Intake and output," pages 210 to 212; "Vital signs, frequent," page 430.) The name of the physician notified, the time of notification, orders given, nursing interventions performed, and the patient's response to them should be noted. The nurse should provide and document patient education and emotional support given.

Gastrointestinal Hemorrhage

05/11/2019	1315	**NURSING ASSESSMENT:** Pt. incontinent of large amount of bloody stool. VS: BP 90/50, P 114, weak and regular, RR 28, SpO_2 92%, oral T 99°F. Skin cool and diaphoretic. Pt. c/o dizziness, but alert and oriented to time, place, and person. Abdomen slightly distended and tender to palpation in right upper and lower quadrants. Bowel sounds hyperactive in four quadrants. Dr. C. Cooper notified. ________ **L. Michelson, RN**
05/11/2019	1330	**NURSING ASSESSMENT:** Dr. Cooper examined pt. and new orders were written. O_2 at 2 L via nasal cannula administered. Lab in to draw blood for CBC and type and crossmatched for 2 units of blood. IV infusion started with 20G catheter in left antecubital fossa; 1,000 mL NS running at 125 mL/hour. Informed consent obtained by Dr. Cooper for colonoscopy. ________ **PATIENT TEACHING:** Reinforced pt. teaching completed regarding what to expect before, during, and after the procedure with pt. and family. Pt. transported to the GI lab for colonoscopy via stretcher and escorted by medical resident. ________ **L. Michelson, RN**

SELECTED READINGS

Benson, B. E., Hoppu, K., Troutman, W. G., Bedry, R., Erdman, A., Höjer, J., Mégarbane, B., ... European Association of Poisons Centres and Clinical Toxicologists. (2013). Position paper update: Gastric lavage for gastrointestinal decontamination. *Clinical Toxicology (Phila), 51*(3), 140–146.

Chapman, W., Siau, K., Thomas, F., Ernest, S., Begum, S., Iqbal, T., & Bhala, N. (2019). Acute upper gastrointestinal bleeding: A guide for nurses. *British Journal of Nursing, 28*(1), 53–59.

Feinman, M., & Haut, E. R. (2014). Upper gastrointestinal bleeding. *The Surgical Clinics of North America, 94*(1), 43–53.

O'Connor, J. P. (2017). Simple and effective method to lower body core temperatures of hyperthermic patients. *American Journal of Emergency Medicine, 35*(6), 881–884.

Rajwani, K., Fortune, B. E., & Brown, R. S. (2018). Critical care management of gastrointestinal bleeding and ascites in liver failure. *Seminars in Respiratory and Critical Care Medicine, 39*(5), 566–577.

Sengupta, N., Cifu, A. S. (2018). Management of patients with acute lower gastrointestinal tract bleeding. *Journal of the American Medical Association, 320*(1), 86–87.

Strate, L. L., & Gralnek, I. M. (2016). ACG Clinical Guideline: Management of patients with acute lower gastrointestinal bleeding. *The American Journal of Gastroenterology, 111*(4), 459–474.

H

HEALTH INSURANCE PORTABILITY AND ACCOUNTABILITY ACT

The Health Insurance Portability and Accountability Act (HIPAA) of 1996 went into effect in the spring of 2003 to strengthen and protect patient privacy. Health care providers (e.g., physicians, nurses, nurse practitioners, physician assistants, pharmacies, hospitals, clinics, and nursing homes), health insurance plans, and government programs (e.g., Medicare and Medicaid) must notify patients about their right to privacy and how their health information will be used and shared. This includes information in the patient's medical record, conversations about the patient's care between health care providers, billing information, health insurers' computerized records, and other health information. Employees must also be taught about privacy procedures.

In 2003, the Security Standards for the Protection of Electronic Protected Health Information were passed. More commonly known as the *Security Rule,* this is a federal regulation that more specifically requires health care organizations to protect the confidentiality, integrity, and availability of electronic patient health information (ePHI). This federal regulation extends to mandating that health care organizations establish technical safeguards for ePHI and regularly monitor the security of ePHI. In addition, it mandates that health care organizations be proactive in pursuing potential threats and resolving breaches in the security of ePHI.

Under HIPAA, patients also have the right to access their medical information, know when health information is shared, and make changes or corrections to their medical records. Patients also have the

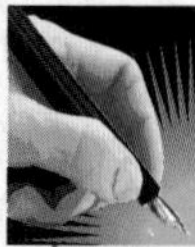

ACCUCHART

DOCUMENTING PATIENT AUTHORIZATION TO USE PERSONAL HEALTH INFORMATION

Most facilities have an authorization form similar to the one shown here to be used for the release of a patient's personal health information for reasons other than routine treatment or billing. The nurse should make sure all the required information is completed before having the patient or legal guardian sign the form.

AUTHORIZATION FORM

By signing, I authorize Community Hospital to use and/or disclose certain protected health information (PHI) about me to Dr. Bedarnz. This authorization permits Community Hospital to use and/or disclose the following individually identifiable health information about me (specifically describe the information to be used or disclosed, such as dates(s) of services, type of services, level of detail to be released, origin of information, etc.):

X-ray films and report, notes on care from 2/6/14 Emergency Department visit

The information will be used or disclosed for the following purpose:

f/u care with Dr. Bedarnz

(If disclosure is requested by the patient, purpose may be listed as "at the request of the individual.")

The purpose(s) is/are provided so that I can make an informed decision whether to allow release of the information. This authorization will expire on 2/7/19.

The practice X will ____ will not receive payment or other remuneration from a third party in exchange for using or disclosing the PHI.

I do not have to sign this authorization in order to receive treatment from Community Hospital. In fact, I have the right to refuse to sign this authorization. When my information is used or disclosed pursuant to this authorization, it may be subject to redisclosure by the recipient and may no longer be protected by the federal HIPAA Privacy Rule. I have the right to revoke this authorization in writing except to the extent that the practice has acted in reliance upon this authorization. My written revocation must be submitted to the Privacy Office at:

Community Hospital
123 Main Street
Oakwood, PA

Marcy Thayer	2/6/19	self
Signed by:	Date:	Relationship to patient:

Marcy Thayer	
Print patient's name	Print name of Legal Guardian, if applicable

right to decide if they want to allow their information to be used for certain purposes, such as marketing or research. Patient records with identifiable health information must be secured so that the records aren't accessible to those who don't have the authorization to view them.

Identifiable health information includes but is not limited to the patient's name, Social Security number, identification number, birth date, admission and discharge dates, and health history.

When patients receive health care, they need to sign an authorization form before protected health information can be used for purposes other than routine treatment or billing. The form should be placed in the patient's medical record. (See *Documenting patient authorization to use personal health information,* p. 154.)

Essential Documentation

The nurse should use the agency's HIPAA authorization form to document the patient's consent for the use and disclosure of protected health information. An authorization form must include a description of the health information that will be used and disclosed, the person authorized to use or disclose the information, the person to whom the disclosure will be made, an expiration date, and the purpose for sharing or using the information. The form is to be signed by the patient or legal guardian and placed in the patient's medical record.

HEARING IMPAIRMENT

Hearing loss occurs in varying degrees that range from the loss of only certain tones to total deafness. Hearing loss is most commonly classified by the cause of the impairment. Conductive loss results from the failure of sound waves to be transmitted through the external ear, middle ear, or both. Sensorineural loss results from pathologic changes in the inner ear, 8th cranial nerve, auditory centers of the brain, or all three. Mixed loss is a combination of conductive and sensorineural loss. Central hearing loss is a result of damage to the brain's auditory pathways or auditory center. A gross or precise assessment can be done to determine the extent of the hearing loss.

Essential Documentation

The nurse should determine the length of time that the patient has had the hearing loss. Describe the patient's degree of hearing loss and whether it is unilateral or bilateral. Note if the increased hearing loss is more significant in one ear. Record whether any hearing aids are being used. Include the effectiveness of hearing aids and the use of secondary modes of communication. Determine what additional methods are currently being used to compensate for the loss, such as lip-reading, sign language, picture boards, or writing pads. Update the nursing care plan to reflect alternative forms of communication with the patient.

Hearing Impairment		
8/06/2019	1000	**NURSING ASSESSMENT:** Pt. states he has had a gradual loss of hearing to both ears due to occupation. He states he has used bilateral hearing aids for 6 years but has used only the right aid for the last 2 months because the left aid isn't fitting well and he hasn't replaced it. He's able to follow conversations and respond appropriately to questions. He states that lip-reading enhances comprehension. ______ **NURSING INTERVENTION:** Care plan amended to include facing pt. when speaking, no gum chewing while speaking with pt., and using a normal tone of voice. Dr. J. Peters notified of ill-fitting hearing aid. Audiologist will meet with pt. tomorrow at 1000 to assess hearing aid fit and function. ______
		______ **Kimberly Sigfried, RN**

HEART FAILURE, DAILY ASSESSMENT

A syndrome characterized by myocardial dysfunction, heart failure leads to impaired pump performance (reduced cardiac output) or to frank heart failure and abnormal circulatory congestion. Congestion of the systemic venous circulation in right-sided heart failure may result in peripheral edema or hepatomegaly; congestion of the pulmonary circulation in left-sided heart failure may cause pulmonary edema, an acute, life-threatening emergency.

Although heart failure may be acute (as a direct result of myocardial infarction), it is generally a chronic disorder associated with the retention of sodium and water by the kidneys. Care for a patient with heart failure centers on symptom management, fluid balance, and prevention and management of complications.

Essential Documentation

The nurse should record the date and time of the entry. Record the patient's subjective symptoms, such as shortness of breath, cough, activity intolerance, chest pain, orthopnea, and fatigue. Document the assessment of the respiratory system (adventitious breath sounds, use of accessory muscles, respiratory rate, pulse oximetry, and signs and symptoms of hypoxia) and cardiovascular system (jugular vein distention, abnormal heart sounds, heart rate, blood pressure, pallor, diaphoresis, cool, clammy skin, hemodynamic monitoring results, cardiac rhythm, the degree and location of edema, urine output, and mental status). Include any new laboratory data, electrocardiogram (ECG) findings, and chest x-rays.

Record interventions, such as daily weight measurements, fluid restriction, intravenous (IV) therapy, and oxygen therapy, and record the patient's response. Chart drugs given during the shift on the medication administration record. Daily intake and output are recorded on the intake and output record. (See "Intake and output," pages 210 to 212.) Record patient education on such topics as energy conservation, disease process, nutrition, fluid restrictions, daily weights, drugs and other treatments, and signs and symptoms to report to the nurse or health care provider. Some facilities may use a patient education record to document any teaching provided (See "Patient teaching," pages 293 to 298.)

Heart Failure

7/8/2019	1500	**NURSING ASSESSMENT:** Pt. is alert and oriented to time, place, and person. BP 136/80, P 88 and regular, RR 20, oral T 98.6°F. O_2 sat. 94% on 2 L NC. Pt. reports SOB with ambulation to the bathroom, approx. 25 feet each way. Denies SOB at rest, no c/o cough or chest pain. Sleeps with 2 pillows. Lungs with scattered rhonchi in posterior fields bilaterally, no use of accessory muscles. Skin is warm and dry, +2 pedal and ankle edema bilaterally, no JVD, S_3 on auscultation. Reports being compliant with 1500 mL fluid restriction with 900 mL taken on this shift. Output this shift 1000 mL clear yellow urine. Wt. #132.5, unchanged from yesterday.
		PATIENT TEACHING: Encouraged pt. to perform ADLs with rest periods as needed. Reviewed 2-gm Na diet and 1500 mL fluid restriction with pt. and wife. They asked many questions and verbalized understanding. See flowsheets for documentation of frequent VS.
		June Lockhart, RN

HEAT THERAPY

Heat therapy is warmth applied directly to the patient's body that raises the tissue temperature and enhances the inflammatory process by causing vasodilation and increasing local circulation. This promotes leukocytosis, suppuration, drainage, and healing. Heat therapy also increases tissue metabolism, reduces pain caused by muscle spasm, and decreases congestion in deep visceral organs. Moist heat softens crusts and exudates and penetrates deeper than dry heat.

Essential Documentation

The nurse should record the date and time of the application; the reason for the use of heat; the site of application; the type of heat used, such as dry or moist; the type of device, such as a K pad, chemical hot pack, or warm compresses; measures taken to protect the patient's skin; and the duration of time the heat was applied. Include the condition of the skin before and after the application of heat therapy, signs of complications, and the patient's response to the treatment. Record any patient education provided.

Heat Therapy		
11/4/2019	0900	**NURSING INTERVENTION:** Warm moist compress applied to lumbar region of the back for 20 min for c/o stiffness and discomfort. ______
		NURSING ASSESSMENT: Skin pink, warm, dry, and intact before application. ______
		PATIENT TEACHING: Told pt. to lay compress over back and not to lie directly on compress. Instructed pt. to call for nurse if he experienced any pain. ______
		NURSING ASSESSMENT: Skin pink, warm, dry, and intact after the procedure. Pt. reports decrease in stiffness and discomfort. ______
		______ **Brian Petry, RN**

HEMODYNAMIC MONITORING

Continuous pulmonary artery pressure (PAP) and intermittent pulmonary capillary wedge pressure (PCWP) measurements provide important information about left ventricular function and preload. This information is useful not only for monitoring but also for aiding diagnosis, refining assessment, guiding interventions, and projecting patient outcomes.

Nearly all acutely ill patients are candidates for PAP monitoring—especially those who are hemodynamically unstable, who need fluid management or continuous cardiopulmonary assessment, or who are receiving multiple or frequently administered cardioactive drugs. PAP monitoring is also crucial for patients with shock, trauma, pulmonary or cardiac disease, or multiorgan disease. It's also used before some major surgeries to obtain baseline measurements.

Current pulmonary artery (PA) catheters have up to six lumens. In addition to distal and proximal lumens used to measure pressures, a balloon inflation lumen inflates a balloon for PCWP measurement, and a thermistor connector lumen allows for cardiac-output measurement. Some catheters also have a pacemaker wire lumen that provides a port for pacemaker electrodes and measures continuous mixed venous oxygen saturation.

The PA catheter is inserted into the heart's right side with the distal tip lying in pulmonary capillary. Fluoroscopy may not be required during catheter insertion because the catheter is flow directed, following venous blood flow from the right heart chambers into the PA.

Essential Documentation

The nurse should document the date and time of catheter insertion. Include the name of the health care provider who performed the procedure. Identify the number of catheter lumens, the catheter insertion site, the pressure waveforms and values of the various heart chambers, and the balloon inflation volume required to obtain a wedge tracing. Note whether any arrhythmias occurred during or after the procedure.

Document any solution infusing through the catheter ports. Record the type of flush solution used and its heparin concentration (if any). Describe the type of dressing applied and the patient's tolerance of the procedure. Chart all site care, dressing changes, tubing, and solution changes.

Hemodynamic Monitoring		
8/19/2019	1300	**PATIENT TEACHING:** PA catheter insertion procedure and need for hemodynamic monitoring explained to pt. and informed consent obtained by Dr. M. Monroe. ________ **NURSING ASSESSMENT:** Four-lumen thermodilution catheter inserted via the right subclavian vein. Pressures on insertion: RV 30/5 mm Hg, PAP 24/10 mm Hg, PCWP 10 mm Hg, and CVP 6 mm Hg. Wedge tracing obtained with 1.5 mL of air for balloon inflation. Portable CXR completed to confirm placement. ________ **NURSING INTERVENTION:** Standard flush solution infusing into distal port. NS infusing at 30 mL/hr into proximal port. Cardiac monitor shows sinus tachycardia with rate of 102; no arrhythmias noted during insertion. Site covered with sterile occlusive dressing. Pt. resting comfortably in bed with HOB at 30°, no c/o pain; breathing unlabored. ________ **Kathy Osborne RN**

HOME CARE, HOME CARE AIDE NEEDS

Aides also provide respite to caregivers.

The registered nurse is responsible for developing the nursing care plan and supervising the home care aide's activities in the patient's home. Most agencies use a standard care plan or duty assignment sheet for this purpose that can be adapted to fit each patient's needs.

To maintain state licensure and certification from The Centers for Medicare and Medicaid and The Joint Commission, the agency must require the home care aide to follow the patient's care plan and to complete a separate home care aide note or entry in the patient's clinical record for every visit.

Essential Documentation

On the home care aide assignment and care plan form, the nurse must itemize every activity that the aide is permitted to provide. This form may consist of a checklist of services and should include the date and time that the plan was initiated. (See *Home care aide assignment care plan*, page 161.) If the care plan was revised, this date and time must also be included. The patient's name and identifying information, the health care providers name, the patient's diagnosis, and short- and long-term goals are also included on the plan.

HOME CARE, INITIAL ASSESSMENT

After the registered nurse receives a referral and orders to begin home care, the nurse then needs to perform a thorough initial assessment of the patient and his or her home environment to set goals and tailor the care to the patient's specific needs. Assessments vary slightly from agency to agency, but the basic information required for completion is the same.

The Conditions of Participation for Home Health Agencies requires that Medicare-certified agencies complete a comprehensive assessment of home care patients using a standardized data set called the Outcome and Assessment Information Set (OASIS). OASIS was developed specifically to measure outcomes for adults who receive home care. Using this instrument, the nurse collects data to measure changes in the patient's health status over time. Typically, the nurse will need to collect OASIS data when a patient starts home care, at the 60-day recertification point, and when the patient is discharged or transferred to another health care facility, such as a hospital or subacute care facility. (See *OASIS—Be careful when charting*, page 162.) The OASIS data are collected using a

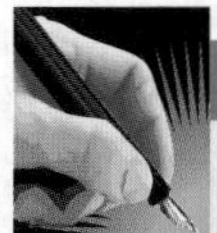

AccuChart

HOME CARE AIDE ASSIGNMENT CARE PLAN

The nurse should use this form to indicate the services to be performed and when the aide should perform them. Also communicate any special details of care on this form.

HOME CARE AIDE ASSIGNMENT AND CARE PLAN

Patient name John Smith Age 39 Date/Time plan initiated 5/01/19 0800
Address 1617 Mulberry Drive, Coopertown, NJ
Primary caregiver Wife, Mary
Diagnosis Multiple trauma Motor Vehicle Accident
Goal — Long term Pt. will return to independent ADLs
Goal — Short term Personal care needs will be met
Additional information Pt has bilateral fracture of tibia and fibula and fracture left humerus. Compare and rate bilateral pulses of dorsalis pedis. Compare and rate left versus right radial pulses.

	Personal Care	Details		Treatments	Details
✓	Bath (Bed, circled)		✓	TPR and Check BM	once a shift
	Shower			Enema	
	Tub			Catheter/tube care	
✓	Mouth care			Special skin care	
	Dentures			Dressings	
✓	Shaving			Intake/output	
	Hair			Oral medication	
✓	Shampoo	3×/week		Assistance (details)	
	Nail care			Exercise program	
✓	Skin care	preventive, lotion		Appliances	
	Positioning/turning	massaging		ADL program	
	Toileting/bedpan				
✓	Commode				
	Toilet				
✓	Dressing		✓	Food serv./household	Prepare breakfast/lunch
	Transfer			Meal planning	
	Ambulation – w/o assist		✓	Preparation	
	w/assist (device)			Serving	
	Feeding			Special diet	
✓	Bedmaking/linen change		✓	Patient laundry	2×/week
				Other	

RN signature Jane Forman, RN

variety of strategies, including observation, interview, review of pertinent documentation when allowed (for example, hospital discharge summaries), discussions with other health care providers where relevant (for example, phone calls to the physician to verify diagnoses), and measurement (for example, intensity of pain).

Essential Documentation

The nurse should use the agency's form to thoroughly and specifically document the assessment of the patient's

- nutritional status
- home environment in relation to safety and supportive services and groups, such as family, neighbors, and community
- knowledge of his or her disease or current condition, prognosis, and treatment plan and
- potential for complying with the treatment plan

When completing the OASIS data set, the nurse will fill in or check off information on more than 80 topics, including:

- sociodemographic data
- physiologic data

OASIS—BE CAREFUL WHEN CHARTING

OASIS was first implemented in 1999 to measure outcomes in home health care. In October of 2000, the OASIS format changed because of the new Medicare payment system for home health care called the Prospective Payment System (PPS). What the nurse documents can have a significant impact on the services the patient receives and the reimbursement the agency collects. The OASIS format was revised again in January 2019 to simplify certification extensions, expand therapy visits, and increase the number of diagnoses that will be a case-mix diagnosis.

A point system is established for certain questions on the OASIS form, and it determines the reimbursement the agency will receive. For example, if the patient has had coronary artery bypass graft surgery and has two wounds, the nurse must document each wound in the appropriate areas of the OASIS form. Failure to document one or both of the wounds could potentially cost the agency a significant amount of money. Wounds are just one of the indicators that govern how much the agency will be reimbursed for patient care.

Problems can also occur when the nurse's assessment on the OASIS form is inconsistent with the health care provider's orders. For example, if the health care provider has ordered gait training and transfers but the nurse documents on the OASIS form that the patient can transfer and ambulate independently, the entire claim may be denied because physical therapy is not needed if the patient is independent.

These OASIS tools are used by Medicare to compare information and review claims. If the nurse has any questions about how to correctly answer OASIS questions in a given circumstance, the nurse should contact his or her supervisor or a continuous quality improvement nurse. Keep in mind that what the nurse documents has a significant impact on the patient and the agency. Read the questions carefully, and be sure of all answers. The nurse does make a difference!

- functional data
- service utilization data
- admission source
- mental, behavioral, and emotional data
- process of care data

HOME CARE, INTERDISCIPLINARY COMMUNICATION IN

Communication between members of the home health care team is essential when caring for a patient at home. Ideally, the team works together toward similar goals to help the patient reach the expected outcomes. Agencies accomplish interdisciplinary communication in various ways. During patient care conferences, the team discusses the patient's care plan and any changes needed in treatment. Between these conferences, team members may communicate with one another verbally, by email, text, or fax. However, the most important form of interdisciplinary communication is the agency's interdisciplinary communication documentation. Surveyors place a great deal of emphasis on this documentation, which shows when, why, and by whom a care plan was changed. It clearly defines deviations from the original care plan. Because the information becomes part of the legal chart, the nurse should follow the guidelines for accurate documentation.

Essential Documentation

When completing interdisciplinary communication documentation, the nurse should be sure to fill in the following:

- patient's name and identification number
- date and time
- nurse's name and title
- name and title of the person to whom the information is being given or from whom the information is being received
- subject matter discussed (e.g., abnormal laboratory results)
- changes to the care plan as a result of this communication
- name of team members notified of the change in the care plan
- outcome of the conversation and any agreements made
- actions taken
- the nurse's signature and title

When the nurse speaks to another member of the home health care team by phone, voicemail, email, text or fax, the same basic information should be documented.

See *Interdisciplinary communication form* for sample documentation, page 164.

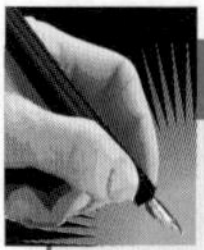

ACCUCHART

INTERDISCIPLINARY COMMUNICATION FORM

Changes concerning the patient or changes to the care plan can be documented on the interdisciplinary communication form.

INTERDISCIPLINARY COMMUNICATION FORM

Date	Time	Discipline	Change in status	Staff Signature
		RN		
		PT		
		OT		
		MSW		
9/21/19	0800	RD	Pt. has lost 5 lb. Increase dietary intake and add Ensure shakes 3×/day	Sue Smith, RD
		HCA		

HOME CARE, PATIENT-TEACHING CERTIFICATION IN

Patient and caregiver teaching are integral parts of almost every care plan. The most common goal is for the patient to have increased knowledge of his or her disease or treatment, and a standardized tool helps achieve that goal in an organized manner. Teaching checklists and certifications help to ensure that information is provided to the patient in a timely manner and in such a way that the patient's and caregiver's level of understanding can be easily evaluated. It also aids in interdisciplinary communication. Patient-teaching guides vary by agency, but the main content of the forms is the same.

Essential Documentation

The patient-teaching certification is a checklist that indicates that the instruction took place. Most documentation begin with the type of therapy or specific disease that will be taught. Then the patient's comprehension level, motivational level, potential barriers to learning, knowledge of the disease or treatment, and skills are assessed. The patient's anticipated outcomes are determined and documented, and the nurse tailors the care plan and teaching plan to the individual needs of the patient or caregiver.

If the agency does not possess a specific patient or caregiver teaching tool, the nurse should document this information in the nurse's notes. Be sure to include all the previously mentioned information, and remember to document clearly on subsequent notes the patient's or caregiver's verbal and nonverbal communication regarding the procedures or instructions, their knowledge, and level of understanding.

Refer to *Patient-teaching certification* for an example of a completed form, page 166.

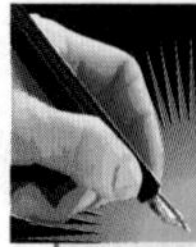

ACCUCHART

PATIENT-TEACHING CERTIFICATION

The model patient-teaching documentation here shows what was taught to a home care patient with an IV line in place. This type of documentation will help the nurse to document the teaching sessions clearly and completely.

PATIENT-TEACHING CHECKLIST/CERTIFICATION OF INSTRUCTION

Patient name Terry Elliott
Caregiver wife
Type of Therapy wound care
Date/Time 07/02/19 0900

CONTENT (Check all that apply; fill in blanks as indicated.)

1. ☑ Reason for Therapy
   Open wound
2. Drug/Solution
   - ❑ Dose
   - ❑ Schedule
   - ❑ Label Accuracy
   - ❑ Storage
   - ❑ Container Integrity
3. Aseptic Technique
   - ☑ Hand Washing
   - ❑ Prepping Caps/Connections
   - ❑ Tubing/Cap/Needle
   - ❑ Needleless Adaptor Changes
4. Access Device Maintenance
   Type/Name ______
   - ❑ Device/Site Inspection
   - ❑ Site Care/Dressing Changes
   - ❑ Catheter Clamping
   - ❑ Maintaining Patency
   - ❑ Saline Flushing
   - ❑ Heparin Locking
   - ❑ Feeding Tube Declogging
   - ❑ Self-Insertion of Device
5. Drug Preparation
   - ❑ Premixed Containers
   - ❑ Compounding
   - ❑ Patient Additives
   - ❑ Piggyback Lipids
6. Method of Administration
   - ❑ Gravity
   - ❑ Pump (name) ______
   - ❑ Continuous ❑ Intermittent
   - ❑ Cycle/Taper
7. Administration Technique
   - ❑ Pump Rate/Calibration
   - ❑ Priming Tubing
   - ❑ Filter
   - ❑ Filling Syringe
   - ❑ Loading Pump
   - ❑ Access Device Hookup/-Disconnect
8. Potential Complications/Adverse Effects
   - ❑ Patient Drug Information Sheet Reviewed
   - ❑ Pump Alarms/Troubleshooting
   - ❑ Phlebitis/Infiltration
   - ❑ Clotting/Dislodgment
   - ☑ Infection
   - ❑ Air Embolus
   - ❑ Breakage/Cracking
   - ❑ Electrolyte Imbalance
   - ❑ Fluid Balance
   - ❑ Glucose Intolerance
   - ❑ Aspiration
   - ❑ Nausea/vomiting/diarrhea/-cramping
   - ❑ Other: ______
9. Self-Monitoring
   - ❑ Weight
   - ☑ Temperature
   - ❑ P ❑ BP
   - ❑ Urine S & A
   - ❑ Fingersticks
   - ❑ Other: ______
10. Supply Handling/Disposal
    - ❑ Disposal of Sharps/Supplies
    - ❑ Opioids
    - ❑ Cleaning Pump
    - ❑ Changing Batteries
    - ❑ Blood/Fluid Precautions
    - ❑ Chemo/Spill Precautions
11. Information Given to Patient Re:
    - ❑ Pharmacy Counseling
    - ❑ Advance Directives
    - ❑ Inventory Checks ______
    - ❑ Deliveries ______
    - ☑ 24-Hour On-Call Staff ______
    - ❑ Reimbursement ______
    - ❑ Service Complaints ______
12. Safety/Disaster Plan
    - ❑ Backup Pump Batteries ______
    - ❑ Emergency Room Use ______
    - ❑ Electrical ______
    - ❑ Disaster ______
    - ❑ Other: ______
13. Written Instructions
    ☑ Yes ❑ No
    If No, Why ______

PATIENT-TEACHING CERTIFICATION *(continued)*

Patient and/or caregiver demonstrates and/or verbalizes competency to perform home infusion therapy.

COMMENTS: Pt. and wife instucted in signs and symptoms of wound infection with good understanding. Pt. and wife able to demonstrate adequate hand- washing technique and he'll check his temperature each evening and record result. Pt. appears motivated to take measures to improve his health. Because of pt.'s fatigue, information needs to be reviewed more than once. Written instructions provided.

Theory/Skill Reviewed/Return Demonstration Completed:

Jane Smith, RN	07/02/19 0900
Signature of RN Educator	Date/Time

CONTENT (Check all that apply; fill in blanks as indicated.)

I agree that I have been instructed as described above and understand that the above functions will be performed in the home by myself and/or caregiver, outside a hospital or medically supervised environment.

John Dougherty	07/02/19 0900
Patient/Caregiver Signature	Date/Time

HOME CARE CERTIFICATION AND CARE PLAN

After the nurse has made the initial visit to the patient and completed the OASIS, the comprehensive care plan needs to be devised. The care plan should be prepared in cooperation with the patient, other health care providers and caregivers. Remember that they may be providing much of the patient's care. Adjust the interventions, patient goals, and teaching accordingly.

Some agencies use a home health certification and care plan form, which is required for Medicare reimbursement, as their official care plan for Medicare patients. This form is also called the Center for Medicare and Medicaid Services (CMS) Form 485. Other agencies use a multidisciplinary, integrated care plan. (See *The home care plan as legal evidence*, page 168.)

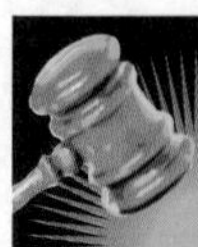

Legal Casebook

THE HOME CARE PLAN AS LEGAL EVIDENCE

The home care plan provides the most direct legal evidence of the nurse's judgment. If the nurse outlines a plan of care and then deviates from it without documenting a rationale for doing so, a court can decide that the nurse strayed from a reasonable standard of care. The nurse should update the care plan routinely so that it accurately reflects clinical judgment about the patient's changing needs.

Essential Documentation

The documentation used for a comprehensive assessment and the information necessary to complete the records may vary from agency to agency. The nurse should record the patient's demographic information and diagnoses. Document drug information, nutritional requirements, use of durable medical equipment and supplies, safety measures, functional limitations, activities, mental status, prognosis, orders for discipline, and treatment. Document the patient's goals, rehabilitation potential, and discharge plans.

Also, include information about the home environment, needed resources, and the emotional states and attitudes of the patient, family, and caregiver. Document physical changes needed in the patient's home to deliver proper care. The nurse should document the assistance given to the patient or family for implementing changes. Describe the primary caregiver, whether he or she lives with the patient, the relationship with the patient, age, physical ability, and willingness to assist the patient. The nurse should document how the patient's strengths and resources are used to enhance the quality of care. Strengths include support systems, good health habits, coping behaviors, a safe and healthful environment, and financial security. Resources include the physician, pharmacy, other health team members, and medical equipment.

If the patient is housebound, the nurse should make sure to document that fact and rationale. (Remember that Medicare requires patients to be housebound to qualify for reimbursement of skilled services at home.)

The nurse should sign the comprehensive assessment and include the date and time the verbal or documented order was obtained to start care. The physician or nurse practitioner must also sign the assessment.

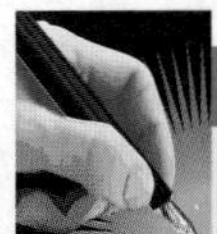

ACCUCHART

HOME HEALTH CERTIFICATION AND CARE PLAN

The form shown here includes space for assessing functional abilities and documenting the care plan. This information is required for Medicare reimbursement.

1. Patient's HI Claim No. 000491675 5
2. Start of Care Date 07/02/19
3. Certification Period From: 07/02/19 To: 09/02/19
4. Medical Record No. 541234
5. Provider No. 0472
6. Patient's Name and Address
Terry Elliot
11 Second Street
Hometown, PA 10981
7. Provider's Name, Address, and Telephone Number
Very Good Home Care
Health Rd
Hometown, PA 10981
8. Date of Birth 07/08/26
9. Sex ☑ M ❑ F
10. Medications: Dose/Frequency/Route (N)ew (C)hanged
Humulin N 24 units subQ every am (c)
Tylenol 325 mg-1000 mg q 4h prn pain
Mom 30 ml at bedtime prn P.O.

		Date
11. IDC-10-CM	Principal Diagnosis	
S91.3	Open Wound Foot	07/01/19
12. IDC-10-CM	Surgical Procedure	
F08L5BZ	Debridement Wound	07/01/19
13. IDC-10-CM	Other Pertinent Diagnoses	
250.03	Type 2 DM uncontrolled	04/01/19
173.9	Perpiheral Vascular Disease	04/01/19

14. DME and Supplies
Walker Wound care Supplies
15. Safety Measures
Correct use of supportive devices
16. Nutritional requirements 20% protein 30% fat
17. Allergies: NKA

18. a. Functional Limitations

1 ☑ Amputation	4 ❑ Hearing	8 ❑ Speech	B ❑ Other
2 ❑ Bowel/Bladder (Incontinence)	5 ❑ Paralysis	9 ❑ Legally Blind	
	6 ☑ Endurance	A ❑ Dyspnea with Minimal Exertion	
3 ❑ Contracture	7 ☑ Ambulation		

18. b. Activities Permitted

1 ❑ Complete Bedrest	5 ❑ Exercises Prescribed	9 ❑ Cane	D ❑ Other (Specify)
2 ❑ Bedrest BRP	6 ☑ Partial Weight Bearing	A ❑ Wheelchair	
3 ❑ Up as Tolerated	7 ☑ Independent At Home	B ☑ Walker	
4 ☑ Transfer Bed/Chair	8 ❑ Crutches	C ❑ No Restrictions	

19. Mental Status

1 ☑ Oriented	3 ☑ Forgetful	5 ❑ Disoriented	7 ❑ Agitated
2 ❑ Comatose	4 ❑ Depressed	6 ❑ Lethargic	8 ❑ Other

20. Prognosis:

1 ❑ Poor	3 ❑ Fair	5 ❑ Excellent
2 ☑ Guarded	4 ❑ Good	

HOME HEALTH CERTIFICATION AND CARE PLAN (*continued*)

21. Orders for Discipline and Treatments (Specify Amount/Frequency/Duration)

SN: Observe/Assess: Cardiopulmonary, respiratory, musculoskeletal, gastrointestinal, and circulatory systems function. Assess: nutritional intake and dietary compliance related to wound healing; skin integrity and peripheral pulses; diabetic home management; and home safety. Instruct pt./caregiver in: diabetic management; signs/symptoms of wound infection; wound care; home safety; and emergency measures. SN to provide: wound care, until pt. is independent: daily wound care to left ankle area = clean area with saline and apply wet to dry saline dressing. SN visits: 5-7/wk × 3 wks; 2-4/wk × 3 wks; 1-3/wk × 3 wks
SN: GOALS: wound healing without infection or further complications, compliance with diabetic home management. Rehab potential to achieve goals: fair. Discharge plan: to family/self when care is independent.

23. Nurse's Signature and Date of Verbal SOC Where Applicable

Jane Smith, RN 07/02/19

25. Date HHA Received Signed POT

07/12/19

24. Physician's Name and Address

Dr. Kyle Stevens
Dr's Medical Center
Hometown, PA 10981

26. I certify/recertify that this patient is confined to his/her home and needs intermittent skilled nursing care, physical therapy and/or speech therapy or continues to need occupational therapy. The patient is under my care, and I have authorized the services on this care plan and will periodically review the plan.

27. Attending Physician's Signature and Date Signed

Kyle Stevens, M.D. 07/07/19

28. Anyone who misrepresents, falsifies, or conceals essential information required for payment of Federal funds may be subject to fine, imprisonment, or civil penalty under applicable Federal laws.

FORM HCFA-485-(C-4) (0-94) (Print Aligned) PROVIDER

The nurse should keep the patient care plan updated. The nurse should document changes in the patient's condition and/or changes in the care needed. Medicare, Medicaid, and certain third-party payers will not reimburse for skilled services that are not reported to the physician.

For sample documentation, see *Home health certification and care plan*, pages 169 and 170.

HOME CARE DISCHARGE SUMMARY

When the patient is ready for discharge, either due to met goals or ineligibility for home care, the nurse needs to prepare a discharge summary for the physician's or nurse practitioner's approval to discharge, notifying reimbursers that services have been terminated and officially

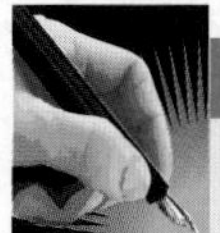

AccuChart

THE HOME CARE DISCHARGE SUMMARY

DISCHARGE SUMMARY

CODE 01
Admission Date 07/02/19
Discharge Date 09/30/19
Medical Record No.: 541234
Phone No.: 881-555-2937
Date of Birth: 07/08/26

Name: Terry Elliot
Address: 11 Second St., Hometown, PA 10981
Primary Diagnosis: Open wound - left foot
Physician: Dr. Kyle Stevens

Services Provided: ☑ Nursing ☐ Occupational Therapy ☐ Speech Therapy ☐ Aide ☐ Physical Therapy ☐ Social Work ☐ Other

Reason for Discharge: ☑ Condition Improved ☐ Died in Hospital ☐ Self/Family Choice ☐ Referred to Hospital ☐ Moved Out of Area ☐ Placed in Long-Term Institution ☐ Referred to Another Agency ☐ Referred, Not Admitted ☐ Died at Home ☐ Other

Physician Notified of Closure: ☑ Yes ☐ No Date/Time: 09/30/19 1300
Family Notified: ☑ Yes ☐ No Date/Time: 09/30/19 1300

Able to verbalize knowledge of the etiology, signs and symptoms, and sequelae/complications of health problem(s).
Patient: ☐ Yes ☑ Partially ☐ No
Family/Caregiver: ☑ Yes ☐ Partially ☐ No

Able to demonstrate knowledge and skills related to the treatment and management of health problem(s).
Patient: ☐ Yes ☑ Partially ☐ No
Family/Caregiver: ☐ Yes ☑ Partially ☐ No

Patient Status:
The patient's condition is: ☐ Stable ☐ Unstable ☑ Improving ☐ Declining ☐ Other

ADL STATUS: ☑ Improving ☐ Unchanged ☐ Declining

	Dependent	Partially Independent	Independent
Bathing			✓
Dressing			✓
Toileting			✓
Transferring			✓
Feeding			✓
Ambulation		✓	
Activity Tolerance	(poor)	(fair) (circled)	(good)

Functional Outcomes:	From	To
Knowledge	poor	fair
Skill	fair	good
Psychosocial	poor	fair
Health Status	poor	fair

SUPPORT SYSTEMS: ☑ Family ☐ Caregiver ☐ Friends ☐ Community Resources ☑ Patient uses support systems appropriately ☐ Support systems inadequate ☐ Patient uses support systems ineffectively ☐ Other

COMMENTS:

Signature: Julie Rose, RN
Date/Time: 9/30/19 1500

(*continued*)

closing the case. The summary is completed on the last visit to the patient. The nurse should use the document provided by the agency for recording the discharge summary. This document may be multidisciplinary and completed via paper or generated within the EMR and sent from the EMR to the care provider.

Essential Documentation

The information included on a discharge summary may vary. The nurse should document the patient's demographic information, admission and discharge dates, the types of services provided, and the reason for discharge. Record the ability of the patient and caregiver to verbalize an understanding of the disease process, signs and symptoms, and complications and to demonstrate the skills necessary to treat and manage the disease. The ability of the patient to perform activities of daily living and to use support systems should also be recorded. In addition to the patient's clinical condition at discharge, also describe the patient's psychological condition. The nurse should provide outcomes attained and recommendations for further care.

Refer to *The home care discharge summary*, page 171, for an example of documentation.

HOME CARE PROGRESS NOTES

In the home setting, as in the acute care setting, the nurse's progress notes document the patient's condition and significant events that occur while under the nurse's care. The nurse needs to write a progress note each time a patient is seen that describes the patient's condition and any skilled services provided during the visit. A skilled service must always be documented in order for the visit to be billable to Medicare. The nurse's notes should also reflect the patient's progress toward goals. Many agencies have the patient sign the progress note to prove that the service was provided on the date and time documented.

The nurse should complete the progress note within 24 hours of the provision of care, and it should be filed in the medical record within 7 days. It is important to remember that Medicare certification reviews can occur without notice, and charts can be audited at any time.

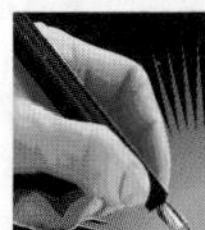

AccuChart

DOCUMENTING IN A HOME CARE PROGRESS NOTE

Progress notes describe—in chronological order—patient problems and needs, nursing observations, reassessments, and interventions. A sample appears here.

❑ Phone Report ❑ Coordination note ☑ Clinical note continuation

Patient Name Terry Elliot ID# 541234 Date/Time: 08/10/19 1100

T = 101°F P = 100 RR = 28 BP = 160/94. Pt. unaware of fever but complaining of increased pain at wound site. (Rates pain as 3 on a scale of 0 to 10. Wound on left ankle = 4 cm × 4.5 cm × 1 cm deep. Open area pink with increased amounts of thick, tan drainage. Wound is foul smelling. Dr. C. Jone's office contacted and pt. to start on cephalexin P.O. SN to increase visits for BID wound care. Pt. denies other complaints. Glucometer FBS = 160 this am. Lungs with diminished breath sounds at bases. Appetite good, bowels regular - had BM today. Began instruction to pt. on cephalexin dose, schedule, and adverse effects. Pt. appears quite anxious about wound condition. Explanation of signs, symptoms, and treatment of wound infection reinforced. Pt. able to repeat explanations. Support offered. SN to return for pm wound care today and check that pt. has started antibiotic therapy. ______________ Jane Smith, RN

Service by (Signature) Title

Essential Documentation

The nurse should complete a progress note each time the patient is seen. If a patient receives more than one skilled nursing visit a day, the nurse must complete a separate note for each visit, outlining the focus of each visit if there is more than one.

Ensure that the progress note provides a chronological accounting of at least the following:

- any changes in the patient's condition
- skilled nursing interventions performed related to the care plan
- the patient's responses to services provided
- the patient's vital signs
- the teaching provided to the patient and caregiver, including a list of written instructional materials and brochures provided

Refer to *Documenting in a home care progress note,* page 173, for an example of progress note documentation.

HOME CARE RECERTIFICATION

To ensure continued home care services for patients who need them, the nurse has to document that the patient still requires such services. Medicare and many managed care plans certify an initial 30-day period during which the agency can receive reimbursement for the patient's home care. When that period is over, the insurer may certify an additional 30-day period based on the nurse's documentation and the physician's or nurse practitioner's agreement that the patient needs continued care. The second 30-day period and every one after that are called recertification periods.

The nurse's documentation requesting recertification must clearly support the patient's need for continued care within the insurer's guidelines. Also a new OASIS must be completed every 60 days. A clinical summary of care must be compiled and sent to the patient's physician or nurse practitioner and then to the insurer. For Medicare, the nurse also needs to prepare a new Certification and Care Plan form 485 for the recertification period. (See *Home health certification and care plan,* pages 169 and 170.) The nurse must return the form to the agency and Medicare before the current 60-day certification period expires. The nurse should make sure the form includes current data as amended by verbal order since the start of care.

Essential Documentation

When preparing a new certification and care plan for recertification, the nurse should make sure the primary diagnosis reflects the patient's current needs, not the original reason for home care. For example, if the patient's primary diagnosis was heart failure but the patient developed a pressure ulcer that requires skilled visits to perform wound care, the nurse will need to change the original primary diagnosis to "open wound." Heart failure may be listed as a secondary diagnosis. (See *Home health certification and care plan,* pages 169 to 170, for full documentation guidelines.)

After the nurse has completed the Certification and Care Plan form, the nurse should review the new orders with the patient's physician or nurse practitioner and sign the "verbal order for start of care" line. This signature serves as a valid verbal order to continue home care services until the physician or nurse practitioner signs the original document.

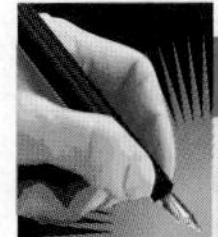

AccuChart

MEDICAL UPDATE AND PATIENT INFORMATION

The home health care agency has to complete this document which provides Medicare with information to support the need for skilled nursing care.

Department of Health and Human Services
Care Financing Administration

Form Approved
OMB No. 0938-0357

MEDICAL UPDATE AND PATIENT INFORMATION

1. Patient's HI Claim No. 000491675
2. SOC Date 07/02/19
3. Certification Period From: 09/02/19 To: 11/02/19
4. Medical Record No. 541234
5. Provider No. 0472
6. Patient's Name and Address Terry Elliot, 11 Second St., Hometown, PA
7. Provider's Name Very Good Home Care
8. Medicare Covered: ☑Y ☐N
9. Date Physician Last Saw Patient: 08/01/19
10. Date Last Contacted Physician: 08/02/19
11. Is the Patient Receiving Care in an 1861 (J)(1) Skilled Nursing Facility or Equivalent? ☐Y ☑N ☐Do Not Know
12. ☐Certification ☑Recertification ☐Modified
13. Dates of Last Inpatient Stay: Admission N/A Discharge N/A
14. Type of Facility: N/A
15. Updated information: New Orders/Treatments/Clinical Facts/Summary from Each Discipline

SN: 08/02/19: Dr. Jones contacted to report temp = 101° F orally, increased amt. thick, tan, foul smelling drainage. Pt. started on cephalexin 500 mg BID po × 10 days, increase wound care to BID and increase SN visits for wound care to 12-14 × 3 wks.

PT: 08/01/19: Verbal order received to increase pt. to ambulation with straight cane. Continue strengthening home exercise program.

SN: 08/08/19: Decrease wound care to daily. Decrease SN visits to 5-7 × 7 wks.

16. Functional Limitations (Expand From 485 and Level of ADL) Reason Homebound/Prior Functional Status

FL: Ambulation, endurance, open, draining wound. RH: Unable to ambulate more than 15 ft. before becoming exhausted. PFS: Independent ambulation.

17. Supplementary Care Plan on File from Physician Other than Referring Physician: ☐Y ☑N
(If Yes, Please Specify Giving Goals/Rehab. Potential/Discharge Plan)

18. Unusual Home/Social Environment

19. Indicate Any Time When the Home Health Agency Made a Visit and Patient was Not Home and Reason Why if Ascertainable N/A

20. Specify Any Known Medical and/or Non-Medical Reason the Patient Regularly Leaves Home and Frequency of Occurrence

Doctor's office visits as needed.

21. Nurse or Therapist Completing or Reviewing Form Jane Smith, RN
Date (Mo., Day, Yr.) 08/02/19

HCFA-486 (C3) (02-94) (Print Aligned) PROVIDER

The clinical summary that the nurse includes with the new Certification and Care Plan form must contain a summary of all disciplines represented on the patient's care team, including the home health nursing assistant, along with updated treatments and goals and the frequency and duration of visits. Also, the nurse should include what has already been accomplished in addition to realistic goals for continued treatment. (See *Medical update and patient information*, page 175.)

HOME CARE REFERRAL

Before the nurse begins caring for a patient at home, the agency will receive information about that patient on a referral, or intake, form. The agency will use this form to make sure the patient is eligible for home care and that the agency can provide the services needed before taking the new case.

To meet Medicare's criteria for home care reimbursement, the patient will need to meet the following conditions:

- The patient must be confined to the home.
- The patient must need skilled services.
- The patient must need skilled services on an intermittent basis.
- The care must be reasonable and medically necessary.
- The patient must be under the care of a physician.

Essential Documentation

The nurse should document the patient's demographic information, including the name and telephone number of the physician and primary caregiver, and insurance information. Record orders and services required, specifying the amount, frequency, and duration. Note the patient's functional limitations and activities permitted. List drug orders and allergy information. Record advance directive information. Include the patient's medical and psychosocial histories, cultural and religious considerations, environmental assessment, vital signs, and physical assessment findings. Date and sign the entry.

See *Referral for home care*, pages 177 and 178, for sample documentation.

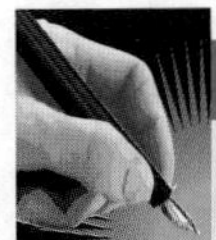

AccuChart

REFERRAL FOR HOME CARE

Also called the intake form, the nurse uses this form to document a new patient's needs when beginning the evaluation. Use the following form as a guide.

EPISODE (1) 2 3 4

Date of Referral: 07/01/19 Branch ______ Chart#: 0001234 H ______

Info Taken By: Jane Smith, RN Admit Date: 07/02/19

Patient's Name: Terry Elliot

Address: 11 Second St.

City: Hometown State: PA Zip: 10981

Phone: 881-555-2937 Date of Birth: 07/08/26

Primary Caregiver Name & #: Susan Elliot 881-555-2937

Insurance Name: Medicare Ins.#: 123-45-6789A

Is this a managed care policy (HMO): No

Primary Dx: (Code S91.00) Open wound Foot/Complications (Onset) Date: 07/11/19

(Code E11.9) Type 2 DM Uncontrolled (Exac.) Date: 07/11/19

(Code 173.9) Periph Vascular Disease (Exac.) Date: 07/11/19

Procedures: (Code F08L5BZ) Debridement Wound (Onset) Date: 07/11/19

Referral Source: Doctor's office Phone: 881-555-6900

Physician Name & Phone #: (UPIN 22222) Dr. Kyle Stevens

Phone: 881-555-6900

Physician Address: Dr's Medical Center, Hometown, PA 10981

Hospital N/A Admit N/A Discharge N/A

Functional Limitations: Pain Management, Pain, ambulation dysfunction

ORDERS/SERVICES (specify amount, frequency, and duration):

SN: 5-7 visits/wk × 9 wks for assessment and wound care left foot: Saline wet to dry drsg

AI: 3-5 visits/wk × 9 wks for assistance with ADLs and personal care

PT, OT, ST: PT 1-3 visits/wk × 9 wks to assess mobility and safety, and develop home exercise program.

MSW: 1-2 visits × 1 mo. for financial assessment and long-term planning

Spiritual Coordinator: N/A Counselor: N/A

Volunteer: N/A

Other Services Provided: N/A

Goals: Wound healing without complications.

Equipment: walker and dressing supplies

Company & Phone #: Best Med Equip. Co 881-260-1026

Safety Measures: Correct use of supportive devices Nutritional Req: 20% protein 30% fat

FUNCTIONAL LIMITATIONS: (Circle Applicable)			ACTIVITIES PERMITTED: (Circle Applicable)		
(1) Amputation	5 Paralysis	9 Legally Blind	1. Complete Bedrest	5. Partial Wgt Bearing	A. Wheelchair
2 Bowel/Bladder	(6) Endurance	A Dyspnea With Minimal Exer	2. Bedrest BRP	6. Independent at Home	(B) Walker
3 Contracture	(7) Ambulation	B Other	3. Up as Tolerated	7. Crutches	C. No Restriction
4 Hearing	8 Speech		(4) Transfer Bed/ Chair	8. Cane	D. Other — specify

(continued)

REFERRAL FOR HOME CARE (*continued*)

Accessibility to Bath Y (N) Shower Y (N) Bathroom (Y) N Exit (Y) N

Mental Status: (Circle) (Oriented) Comatose (Forgetful) Depressed Disoriented Lethargic Agitated Other

Allergies: NKA

• Hospice Appropriate Meds • Med company: N/A

MEDICATIONS: Humulin N 24 units subQ every am changed
Tylenol 325-1000 mg q4hr prn pain P.O. unchanged
Darvocet N 100 one tab q4hr prn pain P.O. new
MOM 30 ml at bedtime prn P.O. unchanged

Living Will Yes ___ No X Obtained ___ Family to mail to office ___

Guardian, POA, or Responsible Person: wife

Address & Phone Number: same

Other Family Members: N/A

ETOH: 0 Drug Use: X Smoker 1-2 ppd × 25 yrs

HISTORY: Chronic peripheral vascular disease with periodic open wounds of feet and legs. Seen by doctor in office 04/01/19 and new wound of left foot debrided.

Social History (place of birth, education, jobs, retirement, etc.): Korean War veteran retired (× 18 yrs) construction worker

ADMISSION NOTES: VS: T 99|F orally AP 88 RR 22 BP 150/82

Lungs: diminished bilat. at bases Extremities: right BKA, left foot pale, DP and PT pulses +.

Wgt: 155 lb Recent wgt loss/gain of denies

Admission Narrative: Pt. independent in Insulin administration and instructed in Insulin dosage change with good understanding. Wound of Ø ankle-outer malleolar area = 4 cm × 5 cm × 1 cm deep; open with beefy red appearance, wound edges pink, moderate amount serosanguineous drainage present. Wound care performed by RN per care plan. Pain controlled with Darvocet prn.

Psychosocial Issues N/A

Environmental Concerns None

Are there any cultural or spiritual customs or beliefs of which we should be aware before providing Hospice services?
N/A

Funeral Home: N/A Contact made YES ___ NO

DIRECTIONS: 1 block before intersection of Main St, on Second St.

Agency Representative
Signature: Jane Smith, RN Date: 07/02/19

HOME CARE TELEPHONE ORDERS

Typically, a physician's order to change some aspect of home care for the patient will come by telephone or email, fax, or text. Either the nurse or the physician may initiate this conversation for various reasons. No matter who originated the contact or how it came about, it's the nurse's responsibility to immediately read back and document any orders received. The nurse needs to use the appropriate verbal order form and send it to the physician or nurse practitioner for a signature.

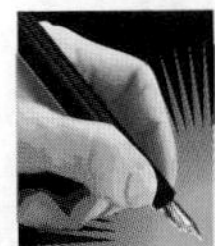

AccuChart

HOME CARE TELEPHONE ORDER FORM

Here's an example of a form used by one agency to fulfill the documentation requirements for telephone orders. The health care provider must sign the order within 48 hours.

Facility name		**Address**	
Very Good Home Care		Health Rd, Hometown, PA	
Last name	**First name**	**Attending doctor**	**Patient ID #**
Elliot	Terry	Dr. Kyle Stevens	123456789

Date ordered	**Date discontinued**	**ORDERS**
07/10/19		Start cephalexin 500 mg BID P.O.
		Increase wound care to BID
		Increase SN visits to daily X 2 wks per Dr. M.
		Goodman's order. Read back and verified by Dr.
		Goodman.

Signature of nurse receiving order	**Date/time**	**Signature of doctor**	**Date/Time**
Jane Smith, RN	7/10/19 1400	M. Goodman, MD	07/11/19 1300

Keep the copy of the signed verbal order in the patient's record until the original copy with the physician's or nurse practitioner's signature is returned to the office. The original order must be signed within 48 hours.

Essential Documentation

The nurse should make sure the verbal order form includes the patient's complete name and identification number. Record the complete name, title, and signature of the person who received the order and the complete name of the physician or nurse practitioner who gave the order. Include a place for the physician's or nurse practitioner's signature. Document the complete contents of the order as it was given and that the order was read back and verified.

In addition to writing up the verbal order, document in the patient's record the reason it was initiated. Describe the circumstances that prompted the conversation with the patient's physician or nurse practitioner as well as the reason for giving the order. Be sure to communicate the order to everyone on the patient's health care team who needs to know it and document the communication.

See *Home care telephone order form*, page 179, for sample documentation.

Home Care Telephone Order

4/10/2019	1400	**NURSING ASSESSMENT:** Called Dr. M. Goodman to report increase in yellow drainage from leg wound, no odor. Skin around wound red, warm, and tender. P 88, BP 138/74, oral T 100.6°F. ______
		NURSING ORDERS: Dr. Goodman gave telephone order to start cephalexin 500 mg BID P.O., increase skilled nurse visits to daily × 14 days, and to call doctor in 2 weeks for follow-up orders. Orders read back and verified with Dr. Goodman and transcribed on telephone order sheet. ______
		PATIENT TEACHING: Explained to pt. and caregiver the indications for antibiotic, frequency, dosage, and possible adverse effects. Also explained the need for more frequent wound care. Instructed them on signs and symptoms to report to doctor and home care agency, including increase in drainage, dressing saturation, odor from wound, and increase in temperature. Pt. and caregiver verbalized understanding of antibiotic, signs and symptoms to report, and more frequent wound care. Written instructions provided. ______
		______ **Jane Smith, RN**

HYPERGLYCEMIA

Defined as an elevated blood glucose level, hyperglycemia results from not enough insulin or the body's inability to effectively use insulin. Extremely high blood glucose levels can lead to ketoacidosis, a potentially life-threatening condition.

Diabetes mellitus is the most common cause of hyperglycemia, but it may also be attributable to Cushing's syndrome; stresses, such as trauma, infections, burns, and surgery; and drugs such as corticosteroids. Patients with diabetes may develop hyperglycemia as a result of not enough insulin, poor compliance with diet, and illness.

If the patient develops hyperglycemia, the physician or nurse practitioner should be notified, and the nurse should anticipate orders for regular insulin therapy and fluid and electrolyte replacement. Prompt interventions are necessary to prevent ketoacidosis and a potentially fatal outcome.

Essential Documentation

Caring for a patient with hyperglycemia requires frequent assessments and interventions. The nurse should document on a timely basis and avoid block charting.

The nurse should record the date and time of the entry. The patient's blood glucose level and nurse's assessment findings, such as polyuria, polydipsia, polyphagia, glycosuria, ketonuria, blurry vision, flushed cheeks, dry skin and mucous membranes, poor skin turgor, weak and rapid pulse, hypotension, Kussmaul's respirations, acetone breath odor, weakness, fatigue, and altered level of consciousness, should be recorded. The nurse should document the name of the physician or nurse practitioner notified, the time of notification, and the orders given. Record interventions, such as subcutaneous or IV administration of regular insulin, frequent blood glucose monitoring, and IV fluid and electrolyte replacement. Include the patient's response to these interventions. Use the appropriate flow sheets to record intake and output, IV fluids, drugs, and frequent vital signs and blood glucose level. Document any patient education, such as proper nutrition, proper use of insulin, and disease management, that is provided.

Hyperglycemia		
9/27/2019	1800	**NURSING ASSESSMENT:** Pt. states, "I vomited and feel weak and dizzy." Face flushed, skin and mucous membranes dry, skin tents when pinched, breath has acetone odor, BP 100/50, P 98 and weak, RR 28 and deep, oral T 98.8°F, blood glucose 398 mg/dl by fingerstick. ______ **NURSING INTERVENTION:** Dr. P. Kelly notified at 1740 and orders given. I.V. infusion of 1000 mL NSS started in left forearm with 22G catheter at 100 mL/hr. Regular insulin 15 units I.V. given in left upper arm. Lab called to draw blood for electrolytes and blood glucose levels. ______ **PATIENT TEACHING:** Explained rationales for therapy to pt. See flow sheets for frequent documentation of VS, I/O, I.V. fluids, and blood glucose levels. ______ ______ **Cass McGuigan, RN**
9/27/2019	1800	**NURSING ASSESSMENT:** BP 122/60, P 90 and strong, RR 18. Pt. denies nausea, vomiting, and dizziness. Lab called to report blood glucose of 375 mg/dl, potassium 3.0 mEq/L. **NURSING INTERVENTION:** Dr. R. Kelly notified of results and ordered 40 mcg KCL rider I.V. ______ **Cass McGuigan, RN**

HYPEROSMOLAR HYPERGLYCEMIC NONKETOTIC SYNDROME

A complication of type 2 (non-insulin-dependent) diabetes mellitus, hyperosmolar hyperglycemic nonketotic syndrome (HHNS) is a condition marked by blood glucose levels as high as 1,000 mg/dL but without ketosis. Although the patient with HHNS produces enough insulin to prevent diabetic ketoacidosis, it isn't enough insulin to prevent dangerously high hyperglycemia, vast diuresis, and extracellular fluid losses. The incidence of HHNS is increasing with the increase in diabetes. Underlying infection is the most common cause. If left untreated, HHNS can lead to dehydration, seizures, coma, and death.

If the patient with type 2 diabetes mellitus develops hyperglycemia, the nurse should call the physician or nurse practitioner and anticipate orders for administering large amounts of IV fluids and, possibly, a transfer to the intensive care unit.

Essential Documentation

The nurse should record the date and time of the entry. The patient's glucose level and nursing assessment findings, such as dry skin and mucous membranes, poor skin turgor, extreme polyuria, hypotension, tachycardia, seizures, aphasia, somnolence, and coma, should be recorded. The interventions, such as cardiac monitoring; seizure precautions; maintaining a patent airway; and IV fluid, insulin, and electrolyte administration, should be recorded. The nurse should document the patient's responses to the interventions. Cardiopulmonary, renal, and neurologic assessments should be recorded frequently.

Hyperosmolar Hyperglycemic Nonketotic Syndrome		
9/15/2019	1900	**NURSING ASSESSMENT:** Blood glucose level 950 mg/dl at 1830. P 104, BP 88/64, RR 18, oral T 99.4°F. Pt. drowsy, but arousable, oriented to person but not place and time. Skin and mucous membranes dry, skin tents when pinched. Foley catheter drained 35 mL over last hour. Breath sounds clear. Placed on portable cardiac monitor showing sinus tachycardia. Side rails padded, bed in low position, airway taped to headboard of bed, suction equipment placed in room. ________
		NURSING INTERVENTION: Dr. T. Ramirez notified of assessment findings and elevated blood glucose level at 1835. Came to see pt. at 1840 and orders given. O_2 started at 2 L/min via NC. I.V. infusion of 1000 mL NSS in left antecubital increased to 1 L/hr. ________
		NURSING INTERVENTION: Infusion of 100 units regular insulin/100 mL of NSS started at 5 units/hr. Respiratory therapy called to obtain blood sample for ABG. Lab notified for stat CBC, BUN, creatinine, electrolytes, and blood glucose levels. Pt. being transferred to ICU, report called to Rose D'Amato, RN. Nursing supervisor, Marie Stone, RN, notified. Called pt.'s husband and notified him of wife's condition and transferred to ICU.
		________ **Tom Woods, RN**

HYPERTENSIVE CRISIS

A hypertensive crisis is a medical emergency in which the patient's diastolic blood pressure suddenly rises above 120 mm Hg. Precipitating factors include abrupt discontinuation of antihypertensive drugs; increased salt consumption; increased production of renin, epinephrine, and norepinephrine; and added stress.

Prompt recognition of a hypertensive crisis and appropriate nursing interventions to lower blood pressure are vital for preventing stroke, blindness, renal failure, hypertensive encephalopathy, left-sided heart failure, pulmonary edema, and even death. Anticipate assisting with the insertion of an arterial catheter for continuous blood pressure monitoring, administering IV antihypertensive drugs, and preparing the patient for transfer to the intensive care unit.

Essential Documentation

The nurse should record the date and time of the entry. Also, the patient's blood pressure and the assessment findings, including any cardiopulmonary, neurologic, and renal system findings, such as headache, nausea, vomiting, seizures, blurred vision, transient blindness, confusion, drowsiness, heart failure, pulmonary edema, chest pain, and oliguria, should be recorded. The nurse should document the measures taken to ensure a patent airway. The name of the physician or nurse practitioner notified; time of notification; and orders given, such as continuous blood pressure and cardiac monitoring, IV antihypertensive drugs, blood work, supplemental oxygen, and seizure precautions, should be recorded. See "Arterial line insertion," pages 22 and 23, for documenting the insertion of an arterial line. The patient's response to nursing interventions should be documented. The appropriate flow sheets for intake and output, IV fluids, drugs, and frequent vital signs should be used. Document patient education and emotional support given.

Hypertensive Crisis

3/2/2019	1500	**NURSING ASSESSMENT:** Pt. arrived in ED with c/o headache, blurred vision, and vomiting. BP 220/120, P 104 bounding, RR 16 unlabored, oral T 97.4° F. Pt. states, "I stopped taking my blood pressure pills 2 days ago when I ran out." Drowsy, but oriented to place and person, knew year but not day of week or time of day. No c/o chest pain, neck veins not distended, lungs clear. Cardiac monitor shows sinus tachycardia, no arrhythmias noted. ___
		NURSING INTERVENTION: Dr. P. Kelly notified and in to see pt. at 1045, orders written. O_2 at 4 L/min administered via NC. Dr. Kelly explained need for arterial line for BP monitoring. Pt. understands procedure and signed consent. ___
		___ **Alan Walker, RN**

Hypertensive Crisis (*continued*)

3/2/2019	1530	**NURSING INTERVENTION:** Assisted Dr. Kelly with insertion of arterial line in right radial artery using 20G 21/2" arterial catheter, after a positive Allen's test. Catheter secured with 1 suture. Right hand and wrist secured to arm board. Transducer leveled and zeroed. Initial BP reading 238/124, mean arterial pressure 162 mm Hg with pt.'s head at 30°. Readings accurate to cuff pressures. Line flushes easily. I.V. line inserted in right forearm with 18G catheter. ________ ________ **Alan Walker, RN**
3/2/2019	1600	**NURSING INTERVENTION:** Nitroprusside sodium 50 mg in 250 mL D5W started at 0.30 mcg/kg/min. See frequent vital signs flow sheet for frequent vital signs. Blood sent to lab for stat CBC, ABG, electrolytes, BUN, creatinine, blood glucose level. Stat ECG and portable CXR done, results pending. Foley catheter inserted, urine sent for UA. Side rails padded, bed in low position, airway taped to headboard of bed, suction equipment placed in room. ________ **PATIENT TEACHING:** All procedures explained to pt. and wife. ________ ________ **Alan Walker, RN**
3/2/2019	1600	**NURSING ASSESSMENT:** Pt. resting comfortably in bed, with HOB at 30°. B/P 190/106. Pt. states he's no longer nauseated and headache "is much better." ________ ________ **Alan Walker, RN**

HYPERTHERMIA-HYPOTHERMIA BLANKET

A hyperthermia-hypothermia blanket raises, lowers, or maintains body temperature through conductive heat or cold transfer between the blanket and the patient. It can be operated manually or automatically.

The blanket is used most commonly to reduce high fever when more conservative measures, such as baths, ice packs, and antipyretics, are unsuccessful. Its other uses include maintaining normal temperature during surgery or shock; inducing hypothermia during surgery to decrease metabolic activity and thereby reduce oxygen requirements; reducing intracranial pressure; controlling bleeding and intractable pain in patients with amputations, burns, or cancer; and providing warmth in cases of severe hypothermia.

Essential Documentation

The nurse should record the date and time of the entry. It should also be documented that the procedure was explained to the patient. The patient's vital signs, neurologic signs, fluid intake and output, skin condition, and position changes should be recorded. Vital signs should be documented every 30 minutes until the desired body temperature is reached, then every 15 minutes until the temperature is stable as ordered. These measurements may be documented on a frequent vital signs assessment sheet. (See *Vital signs, frequent,* page 430.) The nurse should document the type of hyperthermia-hypothermia unit used, control settings, and whether a rectal probe was used. The duration of the procedure and patient tolerance should be documented. The measures taken to prevent skin injury should be recorded. Signs of complications, such as shivering, marked changes in vital signs, signs of increased intracranial pressure, respiratory distress or arrest, cardiac arrest, oliguria, and anuria, should be recorded. Document the physician or nurse practitioner notified, time of notification, orders given, nursing actions, and patient's response.

Hyperthermia-Hypothermia Blanket		
1/19/2019	1000	**NURSING ASSESSMENT:** Need for hypothermia blanket explained to pt.'s wife by Dr. S. Albright. Preprocedure VS: Rectal T 104.3°F, P 112 and regular, RR 28, BP 138/88. ________ **Jane Walters, RN**
1/19/2019	1030	**NURSING INTERVENTION:** Automatic hypothermia blanket, set at 99°F, placed under pt. at 0945. Rectal probe inserted. Sheet placed between pt. and hypothermia blanket. ________ **NURSING ASSESSMENT:** Skin intact, flushed, warm to the touch. Pt. drowsy, but easily arousable and oriented to place and person but not time, able to feel light touch in all extremities, moving all extremities on own, no c/o numbness or tingling, PERRL. See I/O and frequent vital signs flow sheets for hourly intake and output, and VS. No shivering noted, Foley catheter intact draining clear amber urine, no dyspnea. ________ **Jane Walters, RN**

HYPOGLYCEMIA

Occurring when the blood glucose level drops below 60 mg/dL, hypoglycemia is a potentially fatal metabolic disorder. Hypoglycemia may occur as a complication of diabetes mellitus, but it may also occur as a result of adrenal insufficiency, myxedema, poor nutrition, hepatic disease, alcoholism, vigorous exercise, and certain drugs (e.g., pentamidine). If signs and symptoms of hypoglycemia are recognized, the nurse should obtain a blood glucose level; immediately notify the physician and nurse practitioner; and administer a carbohydrate or glucagon, as ordered, to increase the blood glucose level quickly.

Essential Documentation

The nurse should record the date and time of entry. The patient's signs and symptoms of hypoglycemia, such as hunger, weakness, shakiness, paresthesia, nervousness, palpitations, tachycardia, diaphoresis, and pallor, should be documented. With more severe hypoglycemia, the nurse may assess drowsiness, reduced level of consciousness, slurred speech, behavior changes, incoordination, seizures, and coma. Document the results of the blood glucose level determined by fingerstick. Note the name of the health care provider notified, the time of notification, and the orders given. For a conscious patient, record the type, amount, and route of carbohydrate given and the patient's response. If the patient is unconscious, record whether IV carbohydrates or subcutaneous glucagon was administered. Again, record the amount given, the route, and the patient's response.

Record all repeat blood glucose determinations and the measurement method used. If repeat doses are necessary, write a separate note for each administration, including the patient's response. Avoid block charting. Document other nursing interventions that may be necessary, such as maintaining a patent airway and seizure precautions, and the patient's response. Use the appropriate flow sheets to record intake and output, IV fluids, drugs, and frequent vital signs and blood glucose levels. Document any patient education, such as signs and symptoms of hypoglycemia, treating hypoglycemic episodes, preventive measures to avoid hypoglycemia, and disease management.

Hypoglycemia		
7/19/2019	1845	**NURSING ASSESSMENT:** While performing p.m. care at 1840, noted pt. had slurred speech and shaky hands. When questioned, pt. stated, "I feel OK, just a little headache." Pt. stated she wasn't very hungry at dinner. P 108, RR 14, BP 110/60, oral T 97.4°F. Skin pale and diaphoretic. Denies paresthesia. Received glyburide 5 mg at 1700. Blood glucose level by fingerstick 50 mg/dl. ______
		NURSING INTERVENTION: Dr. A. Luu notified at 1845 and ordered 1/2 amp of 50% Dextrose I.V. Gave 1/2 cup of orange juice. ______
		______ **Mary Kelly, RN**

Hypoglycemia (*continued*)		
7/19/2019	1900	**NURSING ASSESSMENT:** Blood glucose level 71 mg/dl by fingerstick. Speech clear, skin pale and dry, denies paresthesia, still c/o headache. P 104, RR16, BP 118/70. ________ **NURSING INTERVENTION:** Gave pt. an additional 1/2 cup orange juice. ________ **Mary Kelly, RN**
7/19/2019	1915	**NURSING ASSESSMENT:** Blood glucose level by fingerstick 98 mg/dl. P 88, RR 16, BP 118/68. Speech clear, skin pink, sl. diaphoresis noted, reports headache gone. Pt. states, "I feel much better." ________ **PATIENT TEACHING:** Explained relationship between oral hypoglycemic and timing of meals, reviewed s/s of hypoglycemia and its treatment. ________ **Mary Kelly, RN**

HYPOTENSION

Defined as blood pressure below 90/60 mm Hg, hypotension reduces perfusion to the tissues and organs of the body. Severe hypotension is a medical emergency that may progress to shock and death if left untreated.

Various disorders of the cardiopulmonary, neurologic, and metabolic systems may cause hypotension. It may also result from the use of certain drugs, stress, and position changes. Moreover, changes in heart rate or rhythm, the pumping action of the heart, and fluid loss may result in hypotension.

Because hypotension can be fatal, prompt recognition and interventions are necessary to save the patient's life. The nurse should notify the physician or nurse practitioner immediately, insert an IV line to administer fluids, begin cardiac monitoring, and administer oxygen. Anticipate administering vasopressor drugs and hemodynamic monitoring. Follow Advanced Cardiac Life Support (ACLS) protocols, as necessary.

Essential Documentation

The nurse should record the date and time of entry. Blood pressure and other vital signs should be recorded. Assessment findings, such as cardiac rhythm; weak pulses; cool, clammy skin; oliguria; reduced bowel sounds; dizziness; syncope; and reduced level of consciousness, should be recorded. Note the name of the physician and nurse practitioner notified, the time of notification, and any orders given, such as continuous blood pressure and cardiac monitoring; obtaining a 12-lead ECG; and administering supplemental oxygen, fluids, and vasopressor drugs.

Describe other interventions, such as lowering the head of the bed, inserting an indwelling urinary catheter, and assisting with insertion of hemodynamic monitoring lines. Document adherence to ACLS protocols, using a code sheet to record interventions if necessary. (See "Cardiopulmonary arrest and resuscitation," pages 61 to 63.) Use the appropriate flow sheets to record intake and output, IV fluids, drugs, and frequent vital signs. Record the patient's responses to these interventions. Include any emotional support and patient education.

Hypotension		
8/1/2019	1000	**NURSING ASSESSMENT:** Pt. c/o dizziness. BP 78/40, P 120, RR 20, oral T 99.6°F. Large amount of bloody drainage noted on abdominal dressing. **NURSING INTERVENTION:** Dr. M. Short notified NSS bolus of 1 L to be given. STAT ECG ordered. ________ **Jane George, RN**
8/1/2019	1000	**NURSING ASSESSMENT:** ECG shows ST rate 22. BP 86/46. See frequent VS sheet. STAT CBC drawn. HOB flat. ________ **Jane George, RN**
8/1/2019	1030	**NURSING INTERVENTION:** BP 90/50. CBC results called to Dr. Short. Pt. to receive 2 units PRBCs. ________ **Jane George, RN**

HYPOVOLEMIA

When a patient is hypovolemic, reduced intravascular blood volume causes circulatory dysfunction and inadequate tissue perfusion. Without sufficient blood or fluid replacement, the patient develops hypovolemic shock, which can progress to irreversible cerebral and renal damage, cardiac arrest, and ultimately, death.

The most common cause of hypovolemic shock is acute blood loss. Other causes include severe burns; intestinal obstruction; peritonitis; acute pancreatitis; ascites; dehydration from excessive perspiration, severe diarrhea, or protracted vomiting; diabetes insipidus; diuresis; and inadequate fluid intake.

When the patient is hypovolemic, the nurse should assess for and maintain a patent airway, breathing, and circulation. The nurse should expect to administer blood or fluid replacement. Inotropic and vasopressor drugs may also be administered. Other nursing interventions focus on identifying and treating the underlying cause.

Essential Documentation

The nurse should record the date and time of the entry. Record the assessment findings, such as decreased blood pressure; increased heart rate; abnormal cardiac rhythm; rapid, shallow respirations; reduced urine output; cold, pale, clammy skin; weight loss; poor skin turgor; weak, diminished, or absent pulses; and reduced level of consciousness. Document the measures taken to ensure a patent airway, breathing, and circulation and the patient's responses to the interventions.

Record the name of the health care provider notified; the time of notification; the orders given; and nursing actions, such as continuous blood pressure and cardiac monitoring, IV inotropic and vasopressor drugs, IV blood and fluid replacement, laboratory tests, supplemental oxygen, and assisting with insertion of hemodynamic monitoring lines. Chart the patient's response to these interventions. Refer to "Arterial line insertion", pages 22 and 23, and *Hemodynamic monitoring*, page 158, for instruction on documenting the insertion of these lines. Use the appropriate flow sheets to record intake and output, IV fluids, drugs, and frequent vital signs. Include patient education and emotional support given.

Hypovolemia		
10/17/2019	1435	**NURSING ASSESSMENT:** Pt. restless and confused to time and place. P 120 reg, BP 88/58, RR 28 shallow, rectal T 96.8°F. Lungs clear, neck veins flat, skin cold and clammy, skin tents when pinched, peripheral pulses weak. Urine output last hour 25 mL via Foley catheter. ______ **NURSING INTERVENTION:** Placed pt. flat in bed, on left side. Notified Dr. R. Diegidio at 1410, came to see pt., and orders written. Continuous cardiac monitoring shows sinus tachycardia. Automated cuff placed for continuous BP monitoring. Dr. Diegidio explained need for hemodynamic monitoring to pt.'s husband who signed consent. ______ ______ **Andrew Miller, RN**
10/17/2019	1500	**NURSING INTERVENTION:** Assisted Dr. Diegidio with insertion of Swan-Ganz catheter into right subclavian vein. Pressures on insertion: CVP 2 mm Hg, PAD 4 mm Hg, PAWP 5 mm Hg. Wedge tracing obtained with 1.5 mL balloon inflation. Using flush solution of 500 units heparin in 500 mL NSS. Catheter sutured in place and site covered with transparent semipermeable dressing. Portable CXR confirmed line placement. ______ ______ **Andrew Miller, RN**
10/17/2019	1600	Lab in to draw blood for CBC, electrolytes, BUN, creatinine, serum lactate, and coagulation studies at 1420. ABG drawn by Thomas Reilly, RPT, NSS infusing at 500 mL/hr × 2 hr. O_2 at 4L via NC w/pulse oximetry of 95%. See flow sheets for frequent VS, I/O, and hemodynamic readings. **PATIENT TEACHING:** All procedures explained to pt. and husband. Pt. lying comfortably in bed, oriented to time, place, and person. ______ ______ **Andrew Miller, RN**

HYPOXEMIA

Defined as a low concentration of oxygen in the arterial blood, hypoxemia occurs when the partial pressure of arterial oxygen (PaO_2) falls below 60 mm Hg. Hypoxemia causes poor tissue perfusion and may lead to respiratory failure. Hypoxemia may be caused by any condition that results in hypoventilation abnormalities (e.g., head trauma, stroke, or drugs that depress the central nervous system), diffusion abnormalities (including pulmonary edema, pulmonary fibrosis, and emphysema), ventilation/perfusion mismatches (e.g., chronic obstructive pulmonary disease or restrictive lung disorders), and shunting of blood (e.g., pneumonia, atelectasis, acute respiratory distress syndrome, pulmonary edema, and pulmonary embolism).

If the patient is suspected to be hypoxemic, the pulse oximetry reading should be obtained, if possible; the physician and nurse practitioner should be notified; and the nurse should anticipate interventions to prevent and treat respiratory failure.

Essential Documentation

The nurse should record the date and time of the entry. Record the patient's vital signs and pulse oximetry reading; PaO_2 level; and cardiopulmonary assessment findings, such as a change in level of consciousness, tachycardia, increased blood pressure, tachypnea, dyspnea, mottled skin, cyanosis, and in patients with severe hypoxemia, bradycardia, and hypotension. Chart the name of the health care provider notified, the time of notification, and any orders given. Record the nursing interventions, such as measuring oxygen saturation continuously by pulse oximetry, obtaining arterial blood gas values, providing supplemental oxygen, positioning the patient in a high Fowler's position, assisting with endotracheal intubation, monitoring mechanical ventilation, and providing continuous cardiac monitoring. Document any chest x-ray findings or other testing results. Also document any respiratory treatments given. Document the patient's responses to these interventions. Use the appropriate flow sheets to record intake and output, IV fluids, drugs, and frequent vital signs. Include any emotional support and patient education.

Hypoxemia

7/19/2019	1400	**NURSING ASSESSMENT:** Pt. restless and confused, SOB, skin mottled. P 112, BP 148/78, RR 32 labored, axillary T 97.4°F. ______ **NURSING INTERVENTION:** Dr. J. Bouchard notified and came to see pt.'s ABGs drawn by doctor and sent to lab. ______ **NURSING ASSESSMENT:** Pulse oximetry 86% on O_2 3 L/min by NC. ______ **NURSING INTERVENTION:** Placed on O_2 100% via nonrebreather mask with pulse oximetry 92%. Pt. positioned in high Fowler's position. Continuous cardiac monitoring shows sinus tachycardia at 116, no arrhythmias noted. Radiology called for stat portable CXR. Respiratory treatment given. ______ ______ **Donna Damico, RN**

SELECTED READINGS

Adeyinka, A., & Kondamudi, N. P. (2018). *Hyperosmolar hyperglycemic nonketotic coma (HHNC, hyperosmolar hyperglycemic nonketotic syndrome)*. Retrieved from https://www.ncbi.nlm.nih.gov/books/NBK482142/

Alliance for Home Health Quality and Innovation. (2019). *What is home health care?* Retrieved from http://www.ahhqi.org/home-health/what-is

Aronow, W. S. (2017). Treatment of hypertensive emergencies. *Annals of Translational Medicine, 5*(Suppl, 1), S5. doi:10.21037/atm.2017.03.34

Barber, C. (2018). Working with informal caregivers: Advice for nurses. *British Journal of Nursing, 27*(19), 1104–1105.

Buckley, L. F., Cooper, I. M., Navarro-Velez, K., Shea, E. L., Joly, J. M., Mehra, M. R., ... Desai, A. S. (2018). Burden of nursing activities during hemodynamic monitoring of heart failure patients. *Heart & Lung, 47*(4), 304–307.

Chiumello, D., & Brioni, M. (2016). Severe hypoxemia: Which strategy to choose. *Critical Care, 20*(1), 132. doi:10.1186/s13054-016-1304-1307

Cousins, J. L., Wark, P. A., & McDonald, V. M. (2016). Acute oxygen therapy: A review of prescribing and delivery practices. *International Journal of Chronic Obstructive Pulmonary Disease, 11*, 1067–1075. doi:10.2147/COPD.S103607.

Freeland, B. (2016). Hyperglycemia in the hospital setting. *Medsurg Nursing, 25*(6), 393–396.

Fritz, D. (2015). Cardiac assessment. *Home Healthcare Now, 33*(9), 466–472.

Funk, A., & Garcia, C. (2018). Understanding the hospital experience of older adults with hearing impairment. *American Journal of Nursing, 118*(6), 28–35.

Ingraham, P. (2016). *Heat for pain.* Retrieved from https://www.painscience.com/articles/heating.php

Klinkner, G. (2016). The importance of glycemic control in the hospital and the role of the infusion nurse. *Journal of Infusion Nursing, 39*(2), 87–91.

Landers, S., Madigan, E., Leff, B., Rosati, R. J., McCann, B. A., Hornbake, R., ... Breese, E. (2016). The future of home health care. *Home Health Care Management and Practice, 28*(4), 262–278.

Malanga, G. A., Yan, N., & Stark, J. (2015). Mechanisms and efficacy of heat and cold therapies for musculoskeletal injury. *Postgraduate Medical Journal, 127*(1), 57–65.

Mayer, S., Commichau, C., Scarmeas, N., Presciutti, M., Bates, J., & Copeland, D. (2001). Clinical trial of an air-circulating cooling blanket for fever control in critically ill neurologic patients. *Neurology, 56*(3), 292–298.

Mills, P. B., Fung, C. K., Travlos, A., & Krassioukov, A. (2015). Nonpharmacologic management of orthostatic hypotension: A systematic review. *Archives of Physical Medicine & Rehabilitation, 96*(2), 366–375.

O'Connor, M., & Davitt, J. K. (2012). The Outcome and Assessment Information Set (OASIS): A review of validity and reliability. *Home Health Care Services Quarterly, 31*(4), 267–301.

Saari, M., Xiao, S., Rowe, A., Patterson, E., Killackey, T., Raffaghello, J., & Tourangeau, A. E. (2018). The role of unregulated care providers in home care: A scoping review. *Journal of Nursing Management, 26*(7), 782–794.

Strachan, P. H., Kaasalainen, S., Horton, A., Jarman, H., D'Elia, T., Van Der Horst, M. L., ... Heckman, G. A. (2014). Managing heart failure in the long-term care setting. *Nursing Research, 63*(5), 357–365.

Torossian, A., Van Gerven, E., Geertsen, K., Horn, B., Van de Velde, M., & Raeder, J. (2016). Active perioperative patient warming using a self-warming blanket (BARRIER EasyWarm) is superior to passive thermal insulation: A multinational, multicenter, randomized trial. *Journal of Clinical Anesthesia, 34,* 547–554. doi:10.1016/j.jclinane.2016.06.030.

Trilla, F., DeCastro, T., Harrison, N., Mowry, D., Croke, A., Bicket, M., & Buechner, J. (2018). Nurse practitioner home-based primary care program improves patient outcomes. *Journal for Nurse Practitioners, 14*(9), e185–e188.

U.S. Department of Health and Human Services. (2013a). *Summary of the HIPAA privacy rule.* Retrieved from https://www.hhs.gov/hipaa/for-professionals/privacy/laws-regulations/index.html

U.S. Department of Health and Human Services. (2013b). *What does the HIPAA privacy rule do?* Retrieved from https://www.hhs.gov/hipaa/for-individuals/faq/187/what-does-the-hipaa-privacy-rule-do/index.html.

Van der Mullen, J., Wise, R., Vermeulen, G., Moonen, P. M., & Jalbrain, M. L. (2018). Assessment of hypovolemia in the critically ill. *Anaesthesiology Intensive Therapy, 50*(2), 150–159.

Varounis, C., Katsi, V., Nihoyannopoulos, P., Lekakis, J., & Tousoulis, D. (2016). Cardiovascular hypertensive crisis: Recent evidence and review of the literature. *Frontiers in Cardiovascular Medication, 3,* 51. doi:10.3389/fcvm.2016.00051

Watts, S. A. (2018). Diabetes basics for the inpatient nurse. *Medsurg Nursing, 27*(3), 161–185.

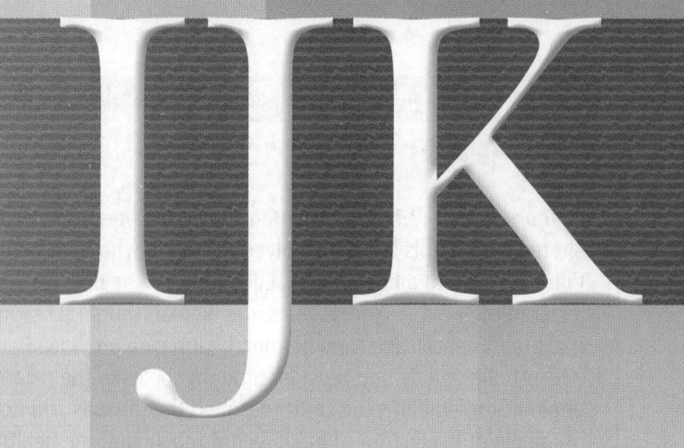

ILLEGAL ALTERATION OF A MEDICAL RECORD

As a general rule, the medical record is presumed to be accurate if there is no evidence of fraud or tampering. Tampering or illegal alteration of a medical record includes adding to someone else's note, destroying the patient's chart, not recording important details, recording false information, writing an incorrect date or time, adding to previous notes without marking the entry as being late, and rewriting notes. Evidence of tampering can cause the medical record to be ruled inadmissible as evidence in court.

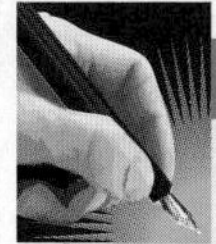

AccuChart

DOCUMENTING AN ALTERED MEDICAL RECORD ON THE INCIDENT REPORT

If the nurse discovers that a medical record has been altered, the nurse should document the findings in an incident report.

INCIDENT REPORT

DATE OF INCIDENT	TIME OF INCIDENT
4/9/19	0400

Name Greta Manning
Address 7 Worth Way, Boston, MA
Phone (617) 555-1122

EXACT LOCATION OF INCIDENT (Bldg, Floor, Room No, Area)
4-Main, Rm. 447

Addressograph if patient

TYPE OF INCIDENT
(CHECK ONE ONLY) ☑ PATIENT ☐ EMPLOYEE ☐ VISITOR ☐ VOLUNTEER ☐ OTHER (specify)

DESCRIPTION OF THE INCIDENT (WHO, WHAT, WHEN, WHERE, HOW, WHY)
(Use back of form if necessary) Called Dr. James at 0400 on 4/9/19 to report pt. had chest pain, radiating to jaw. Doctor said to give pt. Mylanta 30 ml × 1. 0430 called doctor to report continuing chest pain despite Mylanta 30 ml. × 1 dose. Doctor said to put nitroglycerin patch on now, rather than 6 a.m. When asked, doctor stated pt. didn't need nitro SL. Tonight, 4/8/19, when I came in, found doctor's order timed for 0400, 4/9/19, for nitro 1/150 gr SL q5min × 3 for chest pain.

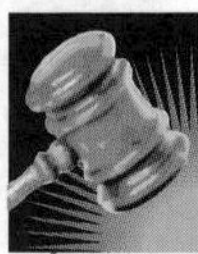

Legal Casebook

REWRITING RECORDS

In *Thor v. Boska (1974)*, a rewritten copy of a patient's record was suspected of being an altered record. This lawsuit involved a woman who had seen her health care provider several times because of a breast lump. Each time, the health care provider examined her and made a record of her visit. After 2 years, the woman sought a second opinion and learned that she had breast cancer. She sued her first health care provider. Rather than producing his records in court, the health care provider brought copies of the records and said he had copied the originals for legibility. The court reasoned that he was withholding evidence and held in favor of the plaintiff. Electronic health records document the health care provider's entered data at the time of patient care in a permanent manner. EHR documents are permanently stored in a digital format by the institution and readily retrievable by subpoena.

Electronic health records (EHRs) track the date and time of data entry and the identity of the user who is logged in. To prevent use by another party that would be recorded under the health care provider's log-in identifiers, the provider should be sure to keep all usernames and passwords private and log out of the computer whenever it is left unattended. See *Rewriting records* above.

Essential Documentation

The nurse should record the date and time that the incident report was completed. Write a factual account of what was observed in the medical record or the conversations with the colleague asking for alterations in the record. Include the names and titles of persons notified.

See *Documenting an altered medical record on the incident report,* page 193, for how to report an altered medical record.

IMPLANTED PORT, ACCESSING

Surgically implanted under local anesthesia by a health care provider, an implanted port consists of a silicone catheter attached to a reservoir, which is covered with a self-sealing silicone rubber septum. It is used most commonly when an external central venous access device is not desirable for long-term intravenous (IV) therapy. Typically, implanted ports deliver intermittent infusions. They are used to deliver chemotherapy and other drugs, IV fluids, and blood. They can also be used to obtain blood.

To access an implanted port, a noncoring or Huber needle is attached to an extension set, flushed with normal saline solution, and inserted into the reservoir. After checking for blood return, the implanted port is flushed with normal saline solution, according to the facility's policy. Consider adding a heparin flush to maintain line patency.

While the patient is hospitalized, a Luer-lock injection cap may be attached to the end of an extension set to provide ready access for intermittent infusions. In addition to saving time, a Luer-lock cap reduces the discomfort of accessing the implanted port and prolongs the life of the implanted port septum by decreasing the number of needle punctures.

Essential Documentation

An EHR or flow sheet should note the date and time that the implanted port was accessed. Within the EHR or flow sheet, the nurse should note whether signs or symptoms of infection or skin breakdown are present. Describe any pain or discomfort that the patient experienced when the implanted port was accessed. If nursing interventions included ice or local anesthetic, make sure to chart it. Describe how the area was cleaned before accessing the implanted port. Note whether resistance was met when inserting the needle and whether a blood return was obtained. Include the number of attempts made to access the implanted port. Record any problems with the normal saline flush, such as swelling or pain. Chart the time that the health care provider was notified of any problems, any orders given, nursing interventions, and the patient's response. Also, document the patient education provided.

Accessing an Implanted Port		
10/20/2019	1200	**NURSING ASSESSMENT:** No breakdown, redness, warmth, or drainage noted at implanted port site in left chest. ______ **NURSING INTERVENTION:** Site cleaned with chlorhexidine, per protocol, and anchored by hand while noncoring needle was inserted perpendicular to port septum on first attempt. No resistance noted. Blood return observed and implanted port flushed with NSS, per protocol. Antibiotic infusing without problem. ______ **PATIENT TEACHING:** Pt. has been using implanted port at home for 3 months and verbalized understanding of its use. Pt. will access implanted port with next drug infusion, with nurse watching to evaluate his technique. ______ ______ **Chelsea Burton, RN**

IMPLANTED PORT, CARE OF

After insertion of an implanted port, the nurse should monitor the site for signs of hematoma and bleeding. Edema and tenderness may persist for about 72 hours. The incision site requires routine postoperative care for 7 to 10 days. The nurse should assess the implantation site for signs of infection, port rotation, and skin erosion. Depending on the health care facility's policy, a dressing may or may not be necessary except during infusions or to maintain an intermittent infusion port.

Patients receiving continuous or prolonged infusions require a dressing and needle change every 7 days. The nurse will also change the tubing and IV solution for long-term central venous infusion according to facility policy. After a bolus injection or at the end of an infusion, flush the implanted port with normal saline solution followed by heparin, according to the facility's policy. For a patient receiving an intermittent infusion, the implanted port should be flushed periodically with heparin solution. When the implanted port isn't being used, it should be flushed every 4 weeks. During the course of therapy, the nurse may need to clear a clotted implanted port with a fibrinolytic drug, as ordered.

Essential Documentation

Within the EHR, the nurse should enter the date and time. Also note the appearance of the site, bleeding, edema, or hematoma. Document any sign of skin infection or device rotation. Indicate the type of therapy that the patient is receiving, such as continuous infusion or intermittent therapy. Document normal saline solution and heparin flushes as well as measures taken to maintain a patent infusion. Record all dressing, needle, and tubing changes.

Care of Implanted Port		
11/30/2019	0930	**NURSING ASSESSMENT:** Implanted port site clean, dry, and intact. No redness, warmth, drainage, bleeding, swelling, or discoloration noted. **NURSING INTERVENTION:** Non-coring needle, extension set, transparent dressing, tubing, and solution replaced. Implanted port flushed with heparin solution, per protocol. ________ ________ **Mae Robinson, RN**

IMPLANTED PORT, WITHDRAWING ACCESS

When the nurse is caring for a patient with an implanted port, the nurse will need to remove the noncoring Huber needle every 7 days (according to facility policy) or at the end of therapy. After the dressing is removed, attach a 10-mL syringe containing normal saline solution (according to facility policy), aspirate for blood, then flush the catheter. Follow this with a heparin flush according to facility policy. The extension tubing should then be reclamped to maintain positive forward flow. The nurse should stabilize the implanted port with the nondominant thumb and forefinger while gently pulling the needle upward. Protective devices are available to prevent a rebound needlestick. Discard the needle in the appropriate container. Apply adhesive dressing to the site according to facility policy.

Essential Documentation

The EHR will enter the date and time that access is withdrawn from the implanted port. The nurse should note that the procedure was explained to the patient. Document the solutions, amounts, and size of the syringes used to flush the extension tubing. The solutions and their volumes are typically recorded in the medication administration record (MAR) of the EHR; A flow sheet should also note whether blood was aspirated or resistance was met. Record that the needle was removed, noting any clots on the needle tip. Describe the condition of the site and the type of dressing applied.

Withdrawing Access to Implanted Port		
12/19/2019	1930	**PATIENT TEACHING:** Explained procedure for deaccessing implanted port to pt. Pt. was concerned about pain. Reassured her that removing needle shouldn't cause her any pain. ________
		NURSING INTERVENTION: Blood easily aspirated from extension tubing. Flushed tubing with 5 mL NSS, followed by 5 mL of 100 unit/mL heparin, using 10-mL syringes. While stabilizing implanted port, needle was easily withdrawn. ________
		NURSING ASSESSMENT: Except for needle puncture wound, skin at access site is intact and without redness, drainage, swelling, bleeding, or hematoma. ________
		NURSING INTERVENTION: Adhesive bandage placed over site. Told pt. bandage may be removed in 30 to 60 minutes. ________
		________ **Danielle Ford, RN**

INAPPROPRIATE COMMENT IN THE MEDICAL RECORD

Negative language and inappropriate information should not be included in a medical record. Such comments are unprofessional and can also trigger difficulties in legal cases. A lawyer may use negative or inappropriate comments to show that a patient received poor care. (See *Unprofessional documentation* below.)

Essential Documentation

Documentation in the medical record should contain descriptive, objective information: what the nurse sees, hears, feels, smells, measures, and counts. The nurse should not suppose, infer, conclude, or assume. Describe events or behaviors objectively, and avoid labeling them with such expressions as "bizarre," "spaced out," or "obnoxious." (See *Charting objectively*, page 199.)

The following note is an example of a nurse using inappropriate words with negative connotations:

1/19/2019	1400	**PATIENT TEACHING:** Pt. was obnoxious when I went to give him his medications and threw me out of his room. ______
		______ **Anne Curry, RN**

The next note concerns the same situation, but it is written objectively:

1/19/2019	1400	**PATIENT TEACHING:** Attempted to give pt. his medication, but he said, "I've had enough pills. Now leave me alone." Explained the importance of the medication and attempted to determine why he wouldn't take it. Pt. refused to talk. Dr. Ellis notified that medication was refused. ______
		______ **Anne Curry, RN**

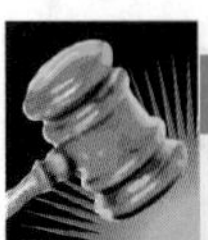

LEGAL CASEBOOK

UNPROFESSIONAL DOCUMENTATION

Negative language and inappropriate information should not be included in a medical record and can be used against the nurse in a lawsuit. For example, one elderly patient's family became upset after the patient developed pressure ulcers. They complained that the patient wasn't receiving adequate care. The patient later died of natural causes.

However, because the patient's family was dissatisfied with the care that the patient received, they sued. In the patient's chart, under prognosis, the health care provider had written "PBBB." After learning that this stood for "pine box by bedside," the insurance company was only too happy to settle for a significant sum.

CHARTING OBJECTIVELY

What the nurse says and how that message is relayed are of utmost importance in documentation. Keeping the patient's chart free from negative, inappropriate information can be quite a challenge when writing detailed narrative notes. Here are some guidelines to help the nurse sidestep charting pitfalls and record an accurate account of the patient's care and status.

Avoid Reporting Staffing Problems

Even though staff shortages may affect patient care or contribute to an incident, staffing problems should not be included in a patient's chart. Instead, discuss them in a forum that can help resolve the problem. In a confidential memo or an incident report, call the situation to the attention of the appropriate personnel, such as the nurse manager. Also review the facility's policy and procedure manuals to determine how employees are expected to handle this situation.

Keep Staff Conflicts and Rivalries out of the Record

Entries about disputes with nursing colleagues (including characterization and criticism of care provided), questions about a health care provider's treatment decisions, or reports of a colleague's rude or abusive behavior reflect personality clashes and do not belong in the medical record. They aren't legitimate concerns about patient care.

As with staffing problems, address concerns about a colleague's judgment or competence in the appropriate setting. Discuss all facts with the nurse manager. Consult with the health care provider directly if an order is concerning. Share opinions, observations, or reservations about colleagues with the nurse manager only; avoid mentioning them in a patient's chart.

If personal accusations or charges of incompetence are discovered in a chart, discuss this with the nurse supervisor.

Steer Clear of Words Associated with Errors

Terms such as *by mistake, accidentally, somehow, unintentionally, miscalculated,* and *confusing* can be interpreted as admissions of wrongdoing. Instead, let the facts speak for themselves—for example, "Pt. was given Demerol 100 mg I.M. at 1300 hours for abdominal pain. Dr. Jones was notified at 1305 and is on his way here. Pt.'s vital signs are BP 120/82, P 80, RR 20, T 98.4°F."

If the ordered drug dose was 50 mg, this entry will let other health care providers know that the patient was overmedicated.

Avoid Bias

Don't use words that suggest a negative attitude toward the patient. For example, do not use unflattering or unprofessional adjectives, such as *obstinate, drunk, obnoxious, bizarre*, or *abusive*, to describe the patient's behavior. If a patient is difficult or uncooperative, document the behavior objectively. Negative words could cause a plaintiff's attorney to attack the nurse's professionalism with an argument such as this: "Look at how this nurse felt about my client—the nurse called the patient 'rude, difficult, and uncooperative.' No wonder the nurse didn't take good care of the patient; the nurse didn't like the patient."

Don't Assume

The nurse should always aim to record the facts about a situation, not assumptions or conclusions. The nurse should only record only what is seen and heard. For example, the nurse should not record that a patient pulled out an IV line if it was not witnessed. The nurse should, however, describe findings—for example, "Found pt., arm board, and bed linens covered with blood. IV line and IV catheter were untaped and hanging free."

INCIDENT REPORT

An incident is an event that's inconsistent with the facility's ordinary routine, regardless of whether injury occurs. In most health care facilities, any injury to a patient requires an incident report (also known as an event report or occurrence report). Patient's complaints, medication errors, and injuries to employees and visitors require incident reports as well.

An incident report serves two main purposes:

- to inform hospital administration of the incident so that it can monitor patterns and trends, thereby helping to prevent future similar incidents (risk management)
- to alert the administration and the hospital's insurance company to the possibility of liability claims and the need for further investigation (claims management)

Essential Documentation

When filing an incident report, the nurse should include only the following information:

- the exact time and place of the incident

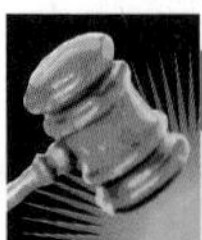

LEGAL CASEBOOK

REPORTING AN INCIDENT

Nurses have a duty to report any incident witnessed firsthand. Failure to report an incident has many consequences, including termination and exposure to personal liability for malpractice—especially if failure to report the incident causes injury to a patient.

Failure to document the incident, treatment, follow-up care, and patient's response may result in the interpretation that the nurse is withholding information. If the case goes to court, the jury may be asked to determine if the patient received appropriate care after the incident.

In the incident report and progress note, the nurse should include any statements made by the patient or the patient's family concerning their role in the incident. For example, "Patient stated, 'The nurse told me to ask for help before I went to the bathroom, but I decided to go on my own.'" This kind of statement helps the defense attorney prove that the patient was entirely or partially at fault. If the jury finds that the patient was partially at fault, the concept of contributory negligence may be used to reduce or even eliminate the patient's recovery of damages.

- the names of the persons involved and any witnesses
- factual information about what happened and the consequences to the person involved (supply enough information so that the administration can decide whether the matter needs further investigation)
- any relevant facts (such as immediate actions in response to the incident—e.g., notifying the patient's health care provider)

After completing the incident report, the nurse should sign and date it. (See *Tips for writing an incident report* below.)

See *Completing an incident report*, page 202, for how to document a patient incident.

TIPS FOR WRITING AN INCIDENT REPORT

When a malpractice lawsuit reached the courtroom in years past, the plaintiff's attorney wasn't allowed to see incident reports. Today, in many states, the plaintiff is legally entitled to a record of the incident if he or she requests it through the proper channels.

When writing an incident report, keep in mind the people who may read it, and follow the guidelines given here.

Write Objectively

The nurse should record the details of the incident in objective terms, describing exactly what was seen and heard. For example, unless the nurse actually saw a patient fall, the nurse should document: "Found patient lying on the floor." Then the nurse should only describe the actions taken to provide care at the scene, such as helping the patient back into bed, assessing the patient for injuries, and calling the health care provider.

Avoid Opinions

Don't commit opinions to writing in the incident report. Rather, verbally share suggestions or opinions on how an incident may be avoided with the nursing supervisor and risk manager.

Assign No Blame

Do not admit to liability, and do not blame or point the finger at colleagues or administrators. Steer clear of such statements as "Better staffing would have prevented this incident." State only what happened.

Avoid Hearsay and Assumptions

Each staff member who knows about the incident should write a separate incident report. If one patient is injured in another department, the staff members in that department are responsible for documenting the details of the incident.

File the Report Properly

Consult the facility risk manager or nursing supervisor in writing and filing an incident report.

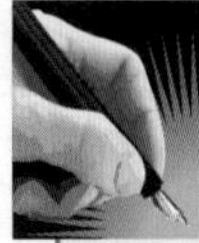

AccuChart

COMPLETING AN INCIDENT REPORT

When a reportable event is discovered, the nurse must fill out an incident report. Forms vary, but most include the following information.

INCIDENT REPORT

Name: Greta Manning
Address: 7 Worth Way, Boston, MA
Phone: (617) 555-1122
Addressograph if patient ____

DATE OF INCIDENT	TIME OF INCIDENT
4/05/19	1300

EXACT LOCATION OF INCIDENT (Bldg, Floor, Room No, Area): 3B-Room 310

TYPE OF INCIDENT (CHECK ONE ONLY) ☑ PATIENT ❑ EMPLOYEE ❑ VISITOR ❑ VOLUNTEER ❑ OTHER (specify)

DESCRIPTION OF THE INCIDENT (WHO, WHAT, WHEN, WHERE, HOW, WHY)
(Use back of form if necessary) Pt. found on floor next to bed. States she was trying to reach her slippers, which were under the bed, and lost her balance.

Patient fall incidents

FLOOR CONDITIONS ❑ OTHER ____ ☑ CLEAN & SMOOTH ❑ SLIPPERY (WET)

FRAME OF BED ☑ LOW ❑ HIGH

NIGHT LIGHT ❑ YES ☑ NO

WERE BED RAILS PRESENT? ❑ NO ☑ 1 UP ❑ 2 UP ❑ 3 UP ❑ 4 UP

OTHER RESTRAINTS (TYPE AND EXTENT): N/A

AMBULATION PRIVILEGE ☑ UNLIMITED ❑ LIMITED WITH ASSISTANCE ❑ COMPLETE BEDREST ❑ OTHER

WERE OPIOIDS, ANALGESICS, HYPNOTICS, SEDATIVES, DIURETICS, ANTIHYPERTENSIVES, OR ANTICONVULSANTS GIVEN DURING LAST 4 HOURS?
❑ YES ☑ NO DRUG ____ AMOUNT ____ TIME ____

Patient incidents

PHYSICIAN NOTIFIED — Name of Physician: J. Reynolds, MD — DATE: 4/05/19 — TIME: 1310 — COMPLETE IF APPLICABLE

Employee incidents

DEPARTMENT ____ JOB TITLE ____ SOCIAL SECURITY # ____

MARITAL STATUS ____

All incidents

NOTIFIED	DATE	TIME	LOCATION WHERE TREATMENT WAS RENDERED
C. Smith, RN	4/05/19	1310	

NAME, ADDRESS AND TELEPHONE NUMBERS OF WITNESS(ES) OR PERSONS FAMILIAR WITH INCIDENT - WITNESS OR NOT
Janet Adams (617) 555-0912 1 Main St., Boston, MA

SIGNATURE OF PERSON PREPARING REPORT	TITLE	DATE OF REPORT
Connie Smith	RN	4/05/19

PHYSICIAN'S REPORT — To be completed for all cases involving injury or illness (do not use abbreviations) (Use back if necessary)

DIAGNOSIS AND TREATMENT

DISPOSITION

PERSON NOTIFIED OTHER THAN HOSPITAL PERSONNEL — DATE — TIME
NAME AND ADDRESS

PHYSICIAN'S SIGNATURE — DATE

INCREASED INTRACRANIAL PRESSURE

The skull is a rigid compartment filled to capacity with three components: brain tissue, blood, and cerebrospinal fluid (CSF). Intracranial pressure (ICP) is the pressure exerted by these three components against the skull. When the volume of one or more of these components increases, the volume of the other two must decrease, or ICP will rise. If increased ICP goes untreated, it can lead to brain herniation and death.

Causes of increased ICP include tumors, abscesses, hemorrhage, head injuries, brain surgery, infection, cerebral infarct, conditions that obstruct venous outflow and cerebral edema.

If increased ICP is suspected, immediately notify the health care provider and ensure adequate airway, breathing, and circulation. Anticipate endotracheal intubation and mechanical ventilation, monitor for changes in level of consciousness (LOC), prepare for ICP monitoring, and anticipate orders for osmotic diuretics.

Essential Documentation

The EHR documents the date and time of the entry. A flow sheet should record the patient's ICP when on continuous ICP monitoring. The nurse should record assessment findings such as reduced LOC (e.g., confused, restless, agitated, lethargic, or comatose), pupillary changes (including unequal size and sluggish or absent response to light), headache, seizures, focal neurologic signs, increased blood pressure, widened pulse pressure, bradycardia, decorticate or decerebrate posturing, and vomiting. Record the name of the health care provider notified, the time of notification, and the orders given. Document actions taken, such as maintaining a patent airway and ventilation, administering oxygen, administering osmotic diuretics, proper head positioning, and monitoring ICP. Use the appropriate flow sheets to record ICP readings, Glasgow Coma Scale (GCS) scores, intake and output, IV fluids given, drugs administered, and frequent vital signs. Monitor the patient frequently, as ordered, and time and record each assessment. Chart all patient education and emotional support provided.

Increased Intracranial Pressure

12/28/2019	1300	**NURSING ASSESSMENT:** Pt. fell 10 feet and hit head at 0900. Now c/o headache, pupils equal with sluggish response on right. P 66, BP 146/50, RR 12. Rectal T 97.2°F. No evidence of seizures, hand grasp on right sl. weaker than left, opens eyes to verbal command, localizes and pushes away painful stimulus, oriented to name but not time and place. Glasgow Coma score 10. ______ **NURSING INTERVENTION:** Dr. Harper notified at 1250 and came to examine pt., orders given. O_2 at 2 L/min via NC started. HOB elevated and maintained at 15-degree angle, head maintained in straight alignment. Lights low, noise level to a minimum. CT scan ordered STAT by physician. Doctor Harper will contact pt.'s wife to discuss ICP monitoring and obtain consent for insertion of ICP monitor. See flow sheets for frequent VS, I/O, and Glasgow Coma scores. ______ **PATIENT TEACHING:** Reorienting pt. to time and place. Explaining all procedures to pt. ______ ______ **Erin O'Leary, RN**

INFECTION CONTROL

Meticulous record keeping is an important contributor to effective infection control. Various federal agencies require documentation of infections so that the data can be assessed and used to help prevent and control future infections. In addition, the data recorded will assist the health care facility in meeting national and local accreditation standards.

The nurse should report any culture result that shows a positive infection and any surgery, drug, elevated temperature, x-ray finding, or specific treatment related to infection.

Essential Documentation

The EHR documents the date and time. The nurse should document the health care provider who was notified of the signs and symptoms of suspected infection, instructions received, and treatments initiated. It is important to record the proper precautions (contact, high-level contact, droplet, airborne, etc.) for the suspected infection. Record that the patient and family have been educated regarding these precautions; include this information in the patient education portion of the EHR. Record the dates and times of nursing interventions in the patient's chart.

Note the name of the health care provider notified of the results of any culture and sensitivity studies, and record the time of notification. If the health care provider prescribes a drug to treat the infection, this information will be recorded in the MAR of the EHR.

Infection Control		
11/28/2019	1300	**NURSING ASSESSMENT:** Standard precautions maintained. P 96, BP 132/82, rectal T 102.3°F. Large amount of purulent yellow-green, foul-smelling drainage from incision soaked through (6) 4 inch × 4 inch gauze pads in 2 hours. ______ **NURSING INTERVENTION:** Dr. L. Levin notified. Ordered Tylenol 650 mg P.O. q 4hr prn for temp greater than 101.7°F, given at 1250. Repeat C&S obtained and sent to lab. Wound cleaned w/NSS and covered with 6 sterile 4 inch × 4 inch gauze pads using sterile technique. Reinforced standard precautions to pt. and wife. ______
		______ **Lynne Kasoff, RN**

INFORMED CONSENT, INABILITY TO GIVE

Informed consent relies on the patient's capacity or ability to make decisions at a particular time under specific circumstances. To make medical decisions, a person must possess not only the capacity but also the competence to make such decisions.

If there is reason to believe that a patient is incompetent to participate in giving consent because of a medical condition, sedation, language barrier, or cognitive impairment, the nurse has an obligation to bring it to the health care provider's attention immediately.

Along with discussing the matter with the health care provider and the nursing supervisor, the nurse must assess the patient's understanding of the information provided by the health care provider. If the patient can't provide consent, follow facility policy on contacting legal guardians or family members or interpreters for consent before the procedure. (See *When a patient can't give consent,* page 206.)

Essential Documentation

Document conversations with the patient, including the patient's mental status and understanding of the procedure, complications, and expected outcomes. If the patient is confused or medicated, does not comprehend the information conveyed, does not understand the procedure, or is incompetent to provide consent then the patient cannot give consent. Record the names of the health care provider and nursing supervisor notified, and note the time of notification.

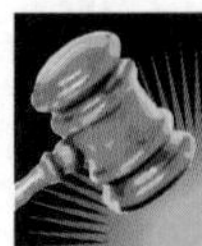

Legal Casebook

WHEN A PATIENT CAN'T GIVE CONSENT

If the nurse believes a patient is incompetent to participate in giving consent and the patient undergoes the procedure without giving proper consent, the nurse may be a co-defendant in a battery lawsuit. Lawyers, judges, and juries will look closely at the medication records to see when, in relation to the signing of the consent form, the patient was last medicated and the patient's response to the medication as documented in the record. The nurse could be held jointly responsible for the patient undergoing a procedure that the patient didn't consent to if:

- The nurse took part in the battery by assisting with the treatment.
- The nurse knew it was taking place and didn't try to stop it.

If the health care provider fails to provide adequate information for consent because of the patient's status, the patient may sue the health care provider for lack of informed consent due to temporary incapacitation. The courts might hold the nurse responsible if the nurse, knowing the health care provider has not provided adequate information to a patient, fails to try to stop the procedure until proper consent can be obtained.

Inability to Give Informed Consent

6/19/2019	0700	**NURSING INTERVENTION:** Pt. given morphine 4 mg IV push at 0630 for chest pain. Dr. K. James in to see pt. at 0645 to explain cardiac cath procedure and obtain informed consent. ______ **NURSING ASSESSMENT:** Pt. keeps asking, "Where am I? What's happening?" Dr. James explained that she was in CCU with chest pain and was scheduled for a cardiac catheterization this a.m. Pt. keeps asking, "What is this test and why do I need it?" Cardiac cath. canceled for this a.m. Doctor will come back to see pt. later today. ______ **Mary Higgins, RN**

INFORMED CONSENT IN EMERGENCY SITUATION

A patient must sign a consent form before most treatments and procedures. Informed consent means that the patient understands the proposed therapy, alternative therapies, the risks of the therapy, and the hazards of not undergoing any treatment at all.

However, in specific circumstances, emergency treatment (to save a patient's life or to prevent loss of organ, limb, or a function) may be done without first obtaining consent. If the patient is unconscious or a minor who can't give consent, emergency treatment may be performed without first obtaining consent. The presumption is that the patient would have consented if able, unless there's a reason to believe otherwise. For example, to sustain the life of unconscious patients in the emergency department, intubation has been held to be appropriate even if no one is available to consent to the procedure.

Courts will uphold emergency medical treatment as long as reasonable effort was made to obtain consent and no alternative treatments were available to save life or limb.

Essential Documentation

The nurse should record the date and time of the entry. Document the emergency and the reason the patient cannot give informed consent, such as being unconscious. Describe efforts to reach family members to obtain consent. List the names, addresses, telephone numbers, and relationships of the people who were attempted to reach. Record that no alternative treatment was available to save life or limb.

Informed Consent in Emergency		
5/26/2019	1000	**NURSING ASSESSMENT:** Pt. arrived in ED at 0940 via ambulance following motor vehicle accident. Pt. not responding to verbal commands, opens eyes and pushes at stimulus in response to pain, making no verbal responses. Pt. has bruising across upper chest, labored breathing, skin pale and cool, normal S_1 and S_2 heart sounds, diminished breath sounds throughout left lung, normal breath sounds left lung, no tracheal deviation. P 112, BP 88/52, RR 26. ________ **NURSING INTERVENTION:** Dr. Mallory called at 0945 and came to see pt. IV line inserted in left antecubital with 20G catheter. 1000 mL NSS infusing at 125 mL/hr. 100% oxygen given via nonrebreather mask. Stat CXR ordered to confirm pneumothorax. Pt. identified by driver's license and credit cards as Michael Brown of 123 Maple St., Valley View. Dr. Mallory called house to speak with family about need for immediate chest tube and treatment, no answer, left message on voicemail. ________ **Sandy Becker, RN**
5/26/2019	1000	**NURSING ASSESSMENT:** Tracheal deviation to left side, difficulty breathing, cyanosis of lips, and mucous membranes, distended neck veins, absent breath sounds in right lung, muffled heart sounds. P 120, BP 88/58, RR 32. Neurologic status unchanged. See neuro flow sheet. Dr. Mallory called pt.'s home and wife's place of business but was unable to speak with her. Again, left messages. Because of pt.'s deteriorating condition, pt.'s inability to give consent, and inability to reach wife, Dr. Mallory has ordered chest tube to be inserted on right side to relieve tension pneumothorax. ________ **Sandy Becker, RN**

INFORMED CONSENT, LACK OF UNDERSTANDING OF

Informed consent means that the patient has consented to a procedure after receiving a full explanation and understanding of it, its risks and complications, and the risk if the procedure isn't performed at this time. As a patient's advocate, it's the nurse's responsibility to help ensure that the patient is truly making an informed choice. If the patient does not understand English, a language interpreter should be provided by the facility. If the nurse determines that the patient did not understand the informed-consent discussion with the health care provider, treatment should not proceed. Notify the health care provider that the patient can't give informed consent without further information from the health care provider or an interpreter. After the health care provider or interpreter clarifies the procedure or treatment, have the patient explain their understanding in their own words.

Essential Documentation

The nurse should document the date and time of the discussion with the patient. Note whether the patient signed the consent form. Record the name of the health care provider interpreter or interpretation modality used, the time of notification, and what was communicated. Record whether the patient could explain the procedure and the patient's ability to answer questions.

Lack of Understanding of Informed Consent		
7/16/2019	0945	**NURSING ASSESSMENT:** While performing morning care, pt. asked, "Will I have periods after my tubal ligation?" and "How will I know if I am pregnant?" Tubal ligation is scheduled for tomorrow morning and signed consent is in chart. ________
		NURSING INTERVENTION: Notified Dr. Newcomb at 0915 that, because pt. is asking questions about getting pregnant, she doesn't understand the full implications of the procedure and that her consent wasn't informed. Dr. Newcomb came to see pt. and husband at 0930 and explained the procedure and consequences of tubal ligation. When asked to repeat back what the doctor said, pt. replied, "I understand now. I'll still get periods. This surgery will prevent eggs from reaching my uterus so they won't be able to be fertilized by sperm. I won't be able to have any more children. But, that's OK since we don't want any more. Four is enough."
		________ **Fran Cervone, RN**

INFORMED CONSENT WHEN PATIENT IS A MINOR

Informed consent involves ensuring that the patient or someone acting on the patient's behalf has enough information to know the risks and consequences of a treatment, procedure, drug, or surgery. When the patient is a minor, it's essential that the health care provider give a full explanation of care to the parent or designated adult responsible for signing the consent. (See *When a minor can give consent* below.) Ethically, there's certainly a duty to inform a minor of the procedure and risks regardless of whether the minor can consent to care. Wherever and whenever possible, children should at least be given the opportunity to participate in the decision making for their care. Parents ultimately have the responsibility for making health care decisions, but children benefit greatly by involvement in their care and treatment. Generally, when controversies arise and a court hearing ensues, the older the minor is, the more likely the minor's wishes will be followed.

Essential Documentation

The nurse should record the date and time that the patient or health care proxy gave consent. Describe the involvement of the child, where

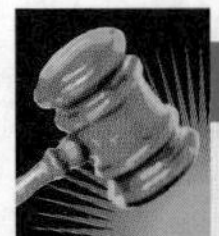

LEGAL CASEBOOK

WHEN A MINOR CAN GIVE CONSENT

The ability of a minor to give consent varies with the condition being treated, the age of the minor, and the state where the condition is being treated. Because privacy issues are involved, the nurse must understand the specific circumstances in which a minor can give consent and when to contact the parent or legal guardian.

A teenage mother must give consent before her baby can receive treatment but generally isn't permitted to determine the course of her own health care. Under federal law, adolescents can be tested and treated for human immunodeficiency virus without parental involvement. However, parental consent is required to set an adolescent's fractured arm in most cases.

Every state will allow an emancipated minor to consent to his or her own medical care and treatment. State definitions of emancipation vary, but it is generally recognized that to be emancipated, the individual must be a minor by state definition and must have obtained a legal declaration of freedom from the custody, care, and control of his or her parents.

Most states will allow teenagers to consent to treatment in cases involving pregnancy and sexually transmitted diseases.

An unemancipated minor in his or her mid- to late teens who shows signs of intellectual and emotional maturity is considered a "mature minor" and, in some cases, is allowed to exercise some of the rights regarding health care that are generally reserved for adults.

possible. Include information on other persons present. Record any questions or comments that the child, parents, or significant others had. Witness the signature of the responsible adult per facility policy. Ask the responsible adult to restate the purpose of the procedure, medication, or surgery in his or her own words. Record the responsible adult's responses. Also, ask the child to do the same, and chart the response.

Informed Consent When Patient Is a Minor		
11/12/2019	1420	**NURSING ASSESSMENT:** Consent obtained by Dr. W. Mason for Scott Jones' tonsillectomy from Mr. and Mrs. Jones, parents of Scott, at 1400 at the preop clinic appt. Parents were able to state the purpose of the surgery and the risks involved. Scott agreed to the operation and stated that he understood that he "needs it to get well." ________ ________ **Richard Lyons, RN**

INTAKE AND OUTPUT

Many patients require 24-hour intake and output monitoring. They include surgical patients; patients on IV therapy; patients with fluid and electrolyte imbalances; and patients with burns heart or renal failure, hemorrhage, or edema.

For easy reference, list the volumes of specific containers. Infusion devices make documenting enteral and IV intake more accurate. However, keeping track of intake that isn't premeasured—for example, food such as gelatin that's normally fluid at room temperature—requires the cooperation of the patient, family members (who may bring the patient snacks and soft drinks or help the patient to eat at the health care facility), and other caregivers. Therefore, the nurse must make sure that everyone understands how to record or report all foods and fluids that the patient consumes orally.

IV infusions, drugs given by IV push, patient-controlled analgesics, any irrigation solutions that are not withdrawn, IV heparin flushes, and saline flushes should also be accounted for. The nurse will need to know whether the patient receives any fluids orally or IV while off the unit.

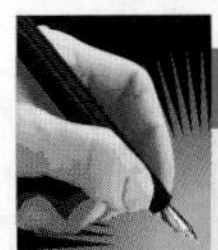

AccuChart

INTAKE AND OUTPUT

As the sample shows, the nurse can monitor the patient's fluid balance by using an intake and output record.

Name: Josephine Klein

Medical record #: 49731

Admission date: 8/13/19

INTAKE AND OUTPUT RECORD

	INTAKE						OUTPUT				
	Oral	Tube feeding	Instilled	I.V. and IVPB	TPN	Total	Urine	Emesis Tubes	NG	Other	Total
Date 8/15/19											
0700-1500	250	320	H_2O 50	1100		1720	1355				1355
1500-2300	200	320	H_2O 50	1100		1670	1200				1200
2300-0700		320	H_2O 50	1100		1470	1500				1500
24hr total	450	960	H_2O 150	3300		4860	4055				4055
Date											
24hr total											
Date											
24hr total											
Date											
24hr total											

Key: IVPB = I.V. piggyback TPN = total parenteral nutrition NG = nasogastric

Standard measures

Styrofoam cup	240 ml	Water (large)	600 ml	Milk (large)	600 ml	Ice cream, sherbet, or gelatin	120 ml
Juice	120 ml	Water pitcher	750 ml	Coffee	240 ml		
Water (small)	120 ml	Milk (small)	120 ml	Soup	180 ml		

Recording fluid output accurately requires the cooperation of the patient and staff members in any other departments the patient goes to. If the patient is ambulatory, remind the patient to use a urinal or a commode.

The amount of fluid lost through the GI tract is normally 100 mL or less daily. However, if the patient's stools become excessive or watery, they must be counted as output. The nurse should follow the facility standards and orders for the patient (e.g., strict intake and output or every 4 hour intake and output). Vomiting, drainage from suction devices and wound drains, and bleeding are other measurable sources of fluid loss. This fluid should be accounted for if possible If the patient is incontinent, document this as well as tube drainage and irrigation volumes.

Essential Documentation

The nurse should make sure the patient's name is on the intake and output record. Record the date and time of the shift on the appropriate line. EHR documentation will automatically populate and record the date and time under the user's name. Record the total intake and output for each category of fluid for the nursing shift, then total these categories and provide a shift total for intake and output. At the end of 24 hours, a daily total is calculated.

See *Intake and output,* page 211, for an example of proper documentation.

INTESTINAL OBSTRUCTION

An intestinal obstruction is a partial or complete blockage of the lumen in the small or large bowel. A small-bowel obstruction is far more common and usually more serious. A complete obstruction can cause death within hours from shock and vascular collapse. Intestinal obstructions are most likely to occur from adhesions caused by previous abdominal surgery, external hernias, volvulus, radiation enteritis, intestinal wall hematomas (after trauma or anticoagulant therapy), and neoplasms.

When the patient has an intestinal obstruction, the nurse should assess and treat the patient for peritonitis and shock, which are life-threatening conditions. Anticipate administering IV fluids, electrolytes, blood, and antibiotics. Assist with the insertion of a nasogastric or intestinal tube for decompression of the bowel. Prepare the patient for surgery, if necessary.

Essential Documentation

Record the results of the GI assessment, such as colicky pain, abdominal tenderness, rebound tenderness, nausea, vomiting, constipation, liquid stools, bowel sounds or absent bowel sounds, and abdominal distention. Also, record the results of the cardiopulmonary, renal, and neurologic assessments. Document the name of the health care provider notified, the time of notification, the orders given, nursing actions, and the patient's response. Use the appropriate flow sheets to record intake and output, IV fluids given, drugs administered, and frequent vital signs. Record the type of decompression tube inserted; the name of the health care provider inserting the tube (typically recorded as a "tube" in the flow sheet of the EHR for continued documentation); the suction type and amount; the color, amount, and consistency of drainage; and mouth and nose care provided. Note the patient's tolerance of the procedure. Document the patient's level of pain on a scale of 0 to 10, with 10 being the worst pain; nursing interventions; and the patient's response. Include patient education and emotional support given.

Intestinal Obstruction		
9/1/2019	1810	**NURSING ASSESSMENT:** Pt. c/o nausea and cramping abdominal pain. Vomited 150 mL green liquid. States he hasn't had BM × 5 days. P 112, BP 128/72, RR 28, oral T 99.0°F. Abdominal exam shows rebound tenderness, distention, and high-pitched hyperactive bowel sounds. Pt. is alert and oriented to time, place, and person. Normal heart sounds. Breath sounds clear. Skin pale, cool, peripheral pulses palpable. Voiding approx. 400 mL q4hr. ________
		NURSING INTERVENTION: Notified Dr. Brunell at 1745 of pt.'s condition. Orders given. Pt. NPO. ________
		PATIENT TEACHING: Explained NPO to pt. and wife, answered their questions, and explained treatments being done. Stat abdominal X-ray done at 1755. Lab in to draw blood for electrolytes, BUN, creatinine, CBC w/diff. at 1800, I.V. infusion started in right forearm with 18G catheter. 1000 mL of D5NSS w/KCL 20 mEq/L infusing at 75 mL/hr. Dr. Brunell in at 1805 to explain possible bowel obstruction to pt. and wife. Told them that depending on the results of X-ray, pt. may need decompression tube, and explained to them the reasons for this treatment. See I.V., I/O, and VS flow sheets. ________
		________ **Mary Wagner, RN**

INTRA-AORTIC BALLOON COUNTERPULSATION CARE

The patient receiving intra-aortic balloon counterpulsation (IABC) therapy requires continuous monitoring and care to ensure proper IABC function, patient comfort, and early detection and treatment of complications. Refer to *Intra-aortic balloon insertion,* pages 216 to 217, for a discussion of common uses of IABC therapy.

Essential Documentation

The nurse should record the patient's arm (brachial or radial) and foot (dorsalis pedis or posterior tibial) pulses, sensation and movement, color, and temperature every 15 minutes for 1 hour, then reassess the arms every 2 hours and the legs every hour while the balloon is in place, or per facility policy.

Document hourly intake and output. Monitor and record bowel sounds or absence of bowel sounds, abdominal distention, tenderness, and elimination patterns every 4 hours, or per facility policy. Record vital signs, pulmonary artery pressure, and pulmonary capillary wedge wedge pressure frequently, as ordered. Monitor and record laboratory values, such as arterial blood gases, blood urea nitrogen, creatinine, complete blood count with differential, partial thromboplastin time, and electrolytes. Place a waveform strip in the chart to document balloon function. In EHR documentation, there may be a box to document waveform appearance (normal, dampened, etc.). Check the insertion site for redness, swelling, bleeding, hematoma, and drainage, and record all site care according to facility policy. Record the name of the health care provider notified of any changes in the patient's condition or complications, the time of notification, the orders given, nursing actions, and the patient's response. Use the appropriate flow sheets to record intake and output, IV fluids given, drugs administered, and frequent hemodynamic measurements and vital signs. A critical care flow sheet or the EHR may also be used to document frequent assessments. Include any teaching and emotional support given. Record routine checks of equipment, problems, and troubleshooting.

Intra-Aortic Balloon Counterpulsation Care

9/24/2019	0900	**NURSING ASSESSMENT:** Monitor shows normal inflation-deflation timing and augmentation, NSR, no arrhythmias noted. Radial pulses strong, hands pink and warm, able to move fingers and feel light touch bilaterally. Pedal pulse palpable and strong, feet warm to touch, able to move toes and ankles and feel light touch bilaterally + bowel sounds in all 4 quadrants, medium-sized BM this a.m. No abdominal tenderness or distention. P 94, BP 122/72, RR 18, oral T 98.8°F, PAP 15/5, PCWP 4. Normal heart sounds. Breath sounds clear. ________
		NURSING INTERVENTION: Blood drawn and sent to lab at 0845 for BUN, creatinine, CBC w/diff., PT/PTT. Results pending. ________
		NURSING ASSESSMENT: IABC insertion site without redness, warmth, bleeding, hematoma, or drainage. See critical care flow sheet for I/O, I.V. fluids, frequent assessments. ________
		PATIENT TEACHING: Reminded pt. to keep affected leg straight, HOB not more than 30 degrees, and to call for help to move in bed. Call bell placed within reach. ________
		________ **Darcy Stone, RN**

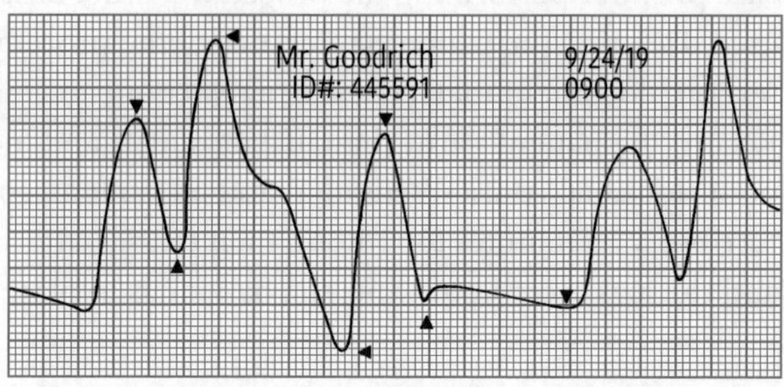

INTRA-AORTIC BALLOON INSERTION

Providing temporary support for the heart's left ventricle, IABC mechanically displaces blood within the aorta by means of an intra-aortic balloon (IAB) attached to an external pump console. The IAB is inserted inserted through the femoral artery and threaded into the aorta. It monitors myocardial perfusion and the effects of drugs on myocardial function and perfusion. IABC improves two key aspects of myocardial physiology: it increases the supply of oxygen-rich blood to the myocardium, and it decreases myocardial oxygen demand.

IABC is indicated for patients with low-cardiac-output disorders or cardiac instability, including refractory angina, ventricular arrhythmias associated with ischemia, and pump failure caused by cardiogenic shock, intraoperative myocardial infarction (MI), or low cardiac output after bypass surgery. IABC is also indicated for patients with low cardiac output secondary to acute mechanical defects after MI, such as ventricular septal defect, papillary muscle rupture, or left ventricular aneurysm.

Essential Documentation

Record the date and time of IAB insertion. Note that the patient or family understands the procedure and that a signed consent form is in the chart. Before insertion, document vital signs as well as the pulses, sensation, movement, color, and temperature of all extremities. If a sedative was ordered, chart it on the MAR. Record the name of the health care provider performing the procedure, other assistants, and the leg used. Describe the patient's tolerance of the procedure. After IAB insertion, document that a chest x-ray was done to confirm placement. Record the patient's arm (brachial or radial) and foot (dorsalis pedis or posterior tibial) pulses, sensation and movement, color, and temperature every 15 minutes for 1 hour, then reassess the arms every 2 hours and the legs every hour while the balloon is in place.

Intra-Aortic Balloon Insertion		
5/30/2019	1300	**PATIENT TEACHING:** Pt. and wife verbalize understanding of IAB procedure, signed consent form is in chart. ____ **NURSING ASSESSMENT:** P 98, BP 102/68, RR 18, oral T 98.4°F. Dorsalis pedis, posterior tibial, and radial pulses palpable bilaterally. Pt. able to feel light touch and move all extremities bilaterally. Hands pink and warm, feet pink and cool to touch bilaterally. Transported to cardiac cath lab via stretcher for IAB insertion. ____ **Barry Moore, RN**
5/30/2019	1400	**NURSING ASSESSMENT:** Returned from cath lab. P 92, BP 114/88, RR 16, oral T 98.67°F. IAB inserted into right femoral artery. Hands warm to touch, skin pink, radial pulse 2/4 bilaterally, able to feel light touch and move hands and fingers bilaterally. Feet cool, dorsalis pedis and posterior tibial pulses 2/4 bilaterally, able to move right leg, foot, and toes without

Intra-Aortic Balloon Insertion (*continued*)

difficulty, moving left foot and toes without problem. + bowel sounds active in all 4 quadrants, no abdominal tenderness or distention. Monitor shows normal waveform. No bleeding, hematoma, drainage, redness, or swelling at insertion site. Reminded pt. to keep right leg straight and to call nurse with complaints of pain in leg, numbness or tingling. Call bell placed within reach. No c/o discomfort at insertion site. ________________ **Barry Moore, RN**

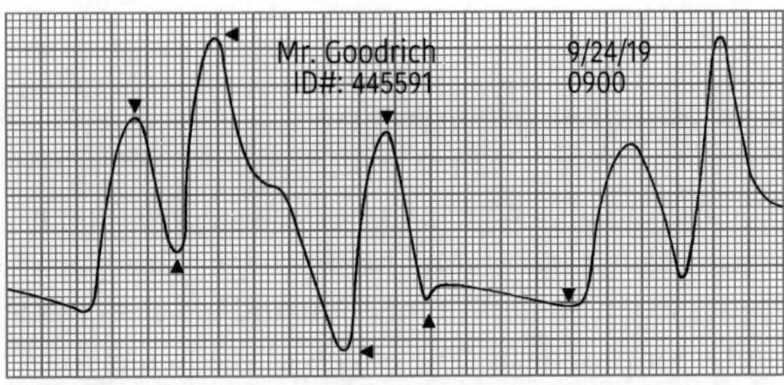

INTRA-AORTIC BALLOON REMOVAL

The IAB may be removed when the patient's hemodynamic status remains stable after the frequency of balloon augmentation is decreased. The control system should be turned off and the connective tubing disconnected from the catheter to ensure balloon deflation. After the balloon and introducer sheath are removed, pressure is applied manually, then by pressure dressing. Provide wound care according to the facility's policy.

Essential Documentation

Record the time and date of balloon removal. Chart the name of the health care provider removing the balloon. Indicate how pressure is applied and for how long. Record the patient's pedal pulses and the color, temperature, and sensation of the affected limb. Describe the type of dressing applied. Record any bleeding and hematoma formation. Document frequent assessments of the insertion site and circulation to the affected leg according to the facility's policy. Include any patient education.

Intra-Aortic Balloon Removal		
1/30/2019	1015	**NURSING INTERVENTION:** IAB in right groin removed by Dr. Johnson. Pressure applied for 30 minutes by Dr. Johnson followed by application of a pressure dressing. Pt. instructed to keep right leg straight. Right foot warm and pink, dorsalis pedis and posterior tibial pulses 2/4 bilaterally, able to feel light touch in lower extremities bilaterally. No bleeding or hematoma noted at right groin site. ________
		________ **Pat Schuler, RN**

INTRACEREBRAL HEMORRHAGE

The rupture of a cerebral vessel causes bleeding into the brain tissue, resulting in intracerebral hemorrhage. This type of hemorrhage usually causes extensive loss of function and has a very slow recovery period and poor prognosis. The effects of the hemorrhage depend on the site and extent of the bleeding. Intracerebral hemorrhage may occur in patients with hypertension or atherosclerosis. Other causes include aneurysm, arteriovenous malformation, tumors, trauma, or bleeding disorders.

If intracerebral hemorrhage or stroke is suspected, ensure a patent airway, breathing, and circulation (ABC). Perform a neurologic examination, and alert the health care provider of the findings.

Essential Documentation

Evaluate the patient's airway, breathing, and circulation, and document the findings, actions taken, and the patient's response. Record the neurologic assessment (e.g., reduced LOC, confused, restless, agitated, lethargic, or comatose), pupillary changes (including unequal size and sluggish or absent response to light), headache, seizures, focal neurologic signs, increased blood pressure, widened pulse pressure, bradycardia, decorticate or decerebrate posturing, and vomiting. Document the name of the health care provider notified, the time of notification, and the orders given. Record nursing actions, such as drug and fluid administration, assisting with ICP monitoring, administering oxygen, assisting intubation, and maintaining mechanical ventilation. Chart the patient's responses to these interventions. Record any patient and family education and support given.

Assess the patient frequently, and record the specific time and results of the assessments. Use the appropriate flow sheets to record intake and output, IV fluids given, drugs administered, and frequent hemodynamic measurements and vital signs. A neurologic flow sheet, such as the GCS or the National Institutes of Health Stroke Scale, may be used to record frequent neurologic assessments.

Intracerebral Hemorrhage

10/28/2019	0810	**NURSING ASSESSMENT:** Pt. found in bed at 0735 unresponsive to verbal stimuli but grimaces and opens eyes with painful stimuli. PERRL. Moving right side of body but not left. Airway is patent, with unlabored breathing. BP 100/60, P 72 and regular, RR 16, rectal T 98°F. Breath sounds clear, normal heart sounds. Skin cool, dry. Peripheral pulses palpable.
		NURSING INTERVENTION: Dr. Martinez notified at 0740 and orders given. Administering O_2 at 2 L/min by NC. I.V. infusion started in right forearm with 18G catheter. NSS infusing at 30 mL/hr. #16 Fr. Foley catheter inserted. MRI scheduled for 0900. Dr. Martinez in to see pt. at 0750. Dr. called wife, Patricia Newman, to notify her of change in pt.'s condition. Wife consented to MRI. Glasgow Coma score of 7. See Glasgow Coma Scale, I.V., I/O, and VS flow sheets for frequent assessments.
		Juanita Perez, RN

INTRACRANIAL PRESSURE MONITORING

ICP monitoring measures pressure exerted by the brain, blood, and CSF. Indications for monitoring ICP include head trauma with bleeding or edema, overproduction or insufficient absorption of CSF, cerebral hemorrhage, and space-occupying brain lesions. ICP monitoring can detect elevated ICP early, before clinical danger signs develop. Prompt interventions can then help avert or diminish neurologic damage caused by cerebral hypoxia and shifts of brain mass. The procedure for placement of a device to measure ICP is always performed by a neurosurgeon in the operating room, emergency department, or critical care unit.

Essential Documentation

The nurse should document that the procedure has been explained to the patient or his or her family and that the patient or a responsible family member has signed the consent form. Record the time and date of the insertion procedure, the name of the health care provider performing the procedure, and the patient's response. Note the insertion site and the type of monitoring system used. Record ICP digital readings and waveforms and cerebral perfusion pressure hourly. Document any factors that may affect ICP (e.g., drug administration, stressful procedures, or sleep).

Record neurologic assessment results and vital signs hourly (including temperature, pulse, respirations, blood pressure, LOC, pupillary activity, and orientation to time, place, person, and date, GCS score), and describe the patient's clinical status. Note the amount, character, and frequency of any CSF drainage (e.g., "between 1800 and 1900, 15 mL of blood-tinged CSF") and record it in the flow sheet. Describe the insertion site and any site care and dressing changes performed. Describe any patient and family education and support given.

Intracranial Pressure Monitoring

05/6/2019	1100	**PATIENT TEACHING:** ICP insertion and monitoring procedures explained to pt.'s wife by Dr. M. Norton. Wife verbalized understanding of procedure and signed consent form. ______
		NURSING ASSESSMENT: Subarachnoid bolt placed by Dr. Norton on left side of skull behind hairline. Initial ICP 16 mm Hg, MAP 110 mm. Site clean, no drainage or redness, covered with sterile dressing. See flow sheets for hourly ICP, VS, neuro. checks. BP 154/88, P 98 and regular, RR 16 and regular, rectal T 99.4°F. Opens eyes and moves right extremities to painful stimuli, makes incomprehensible sounds. PERRL. No purposeful movement on left side. Breath sounds clear, normal heart sounds, peripheral pulses palpable. Skin pale, cool. Foley catheter drained 100 mL of clear amber urine last hr. ______
		______ **Mary Steward, RN**

Mr. Paul
05/6/19

1100
ID#: 563421

INTRAVENOUS CATHETER COMPLICATION: CANNULA DISLODGMENT

A common IV catheter complication, cannula dislodgment occurs when the cannula becomes partially shifted out of the vein. The infusing solution can also infiltrate into the surrounding tissue.

Cannula dislodgment can be caused by loosened tape or tubing that becomes snagged in bed lines, resulting in partial retraction of the cannula. The cannula can also be pulled out by a confused patient.

Essential Documentation

In the nursing notes or on the appropriate IV flow sheet, the nurse should record the date and time of entry. Record the signs and symptoms of the catheter dislodgment, such as swelling, burning, discomfort, changes in skin temperature, or pain. Document the nursing actions (e.g., stopping the infusion and applying ice or warm compresses). Restart the infusion when new IV access is established, and note the new insertion site, catheter size, number of IV attempts, the name of the provider who placed the IV, and any complications during insertion (e.g., bleeding). Document all fluids that are infusing. Document any patient education or emotional support provided.

IV Cannula Dislodgment		
1/4/2019	0800	**NURSING ASSESSMENT:** Assessed IV site inserted 1/2/2019 in right forearm. D5W infusing at 100 mL/hr. Insertion site without redness, warmth, or tenderness but distal site is cool to touch and swollen. IV fluids run sluggishly off pump and no blood return is noted. Pt. states that arm “looks puffy.” ______ **NURSING INTERVENTION:** IV discontinued and warm compresses applied. New site started in left forearm with #20 catheter after site cleaned and prepped with 2% chlorhexidine solution. Catheter secured and positive blood return noted. D5W resumed at 100 mL/hr with new tubing. ______ ______ **Jane Worth, RN**

INTRAVENOUS CATHETER COMPLICATION: PHLEBITIS

Phlebitis is another IV catheter complication. It most commonly occurs after the third or fourth day following insertion. It can be due to poor blood flow around the venous access device, friction from the cannula movement in the vein, a venous access device that is left in too long, a drug solution with high or low pH or high osmolarity, or clotting at the cannula tip.

Signs and symptoms of possible phlebitis include tenderness at the tip of and proximal to the venous access device, redness at the tip of the cannula along the vein, puffy area over the vein, vein hardness on palpation, or elevated skin temperature around the vein.

Essential Documentation

Record any signs and symptoms, including tenderness or pain at the insertion site, puffiness, elevated skin temperature, or vein hardness on palpation. Document the nursing actions (e.g., stopping the infusion and applying ice or warm compresses). Record the name of the health care provider notified and the time of the notification. Restart the infusion when new IV access is established, and note the new insertion site, catheter size, number of IV attempts, the name of the provider who placed the IV, and any complications during insertion (e.g., bleeding). Document all fluids that are infusing. Document any patient education or emotional support provided.

Complication Phlebitis		
1/4/2019	0800	**NURSING ASSESSMENT:** IV site in right forearm observed. Insertion date 1/1/19. D5W infusing at 50 mL/hr via infusion pump. Redness and warmth noted at insertion site. Pt. states site is painful to touch and pain has increased over the past hour. ______ **NURSING INTERVENTION:** IV discontinued and new IV site started in left forearm with #20 catheter after site cleaned and prepped with 2% chlorhexidine solution. Catheter secured and positive blood return noted. D5W resumed at 50 mL/hr with new tubing. Cool compress applied to former IV site and Dr. J. Cross notified of events at 0830. ______ ______ **Jill Miller, RN**

INTRAVENOUS CATHETER INSERTION

Peripheral IV line insertion involves the selection of a venipuncture device and an insertion site, application of a tourniquet, preparation of the site, and venipuncture. Selection of a venipuncture device and site depends on the type of solution to be used; the frequency and duration of infusion; the patency and location of accessible veins; the patient's age, size, and condition.

IV catheters are inserted to administer medications, blood, or blood products or to correct fluid and electrolyte imbalances.

Essential Documentation

In the nursing notes or on the appropriate IV flow sheets, record the date and time of the venipuncture; the type, gauge, and length of the needle or catheter; and the anatomic location of the insertion site. Also, document the number of attempts at venipuncture (if more than one attempt was made); the type and flow rate of the IV solution; the name and amount of medication in the solution, if any (this should be documented in the MAR of the EHR); and any adverse reactions and actions taken to correct them. If the IV site was changed, document the reason for the change. Document patient teaching and evidence of patient understanding.

IV Catheter Insertion

10/3/2019	1100	**NURSING INTERVENTION:** 20G 11/29 catheter inserted in right forearm without difficulty on the first attempt. Site dressed with transparent dressing and tape. I.V. infusion of 1000 mL D5W started at 100 mL/hr. I.V. infusing without difficulty. ________
		PATIENT TEACHING: Pt. instructed to notify nurse if the site becomes swollen or painful, or catheter becomes dislodged or leaks. No c/o pain after insertion. ________
		________ **David Stevens, RN**

INTRAVENOUS CATHETER REMOVAL

A peripheral IV line is removed on completion of therapy, for cannula site changes, and for suspected infection or infiltration.

Essential Documentation

After removing an IV line, the nurse should document the date and time of removal. Describe the condition of the site. Note any excess bleeding or drainage from the site. If necessary, document that the tip of the device was sent to the laboratory for culture, according to the facility's policy. It may also be necessary to send a sample of unusual drainage from the IV site for culture as well, according to the facility's policy. Record any site care administered and the type of dressing applied. Include any patient education.

IV Catheter Removal		
10/15/2019	1000	**NURSING INTERVENTION:** IV catheter removed from right forearm vein. Pressure held for 2 min until bleeding stopped. **NURSING ASSESSMENT:** Site clean and dry, no redness, drainage, warmth, or pain noted. **NURSING INTERVENTION:** Dry sterile dressing applied to site. **PATIENT TEACHING:** Pt. instructed to call nurse if bleeding, swelling, redness, or pain occurs at the removal site. **Jane Newport, RN**

INTRAVENOUS SITE CARE

Proper IV site care is the single most important intervention for prevention of infection and other complications. The site should be assessed every 2 hours—assess every hour if there is a continuous infusion running or if a transparent semipermeable dressing is used, or with every dressing change otherwise. Check the facility's policy for the frequency of IV dressing changes and the type of site care to be performed.

Essential Documentation

In the nursing notes or on the appropriate IV flow sheet, the nurse should record the date and time of the dressing change. Chart the condition of the insertion site, noting whether there are signs of infection (redness and pain), infiltration (coolness, blanching, and edema), or thrombophlebitis (redness, firmness, pain along the path of the vein, and edema). If complications are present, note the name of the health care provider notified, the time of notification, the orders given, nursing interventions, and the patient's response. Record site care given and the type of dressing applied. Document patient education. For a central IV line, the catheter length should be noted and compared to the last dressing change noted in the chart to ensure that the IV line has not become displaced.

IV Site Care		
12/3/2019	0910	**NURSING ASSESSMENT:** Transparent IV dressing wet and curling at edges. **NURSING INTERVENTION:** Dressing removed. Skin cleaned with alcohol, air dried. **NURSING ASSESSMENT:** No redness, blanching, warmth, coolness, edema, drainage, or induration noted, No c/o pain at site. **NURSING INTERVENTION:** New transparent dressing applied and secured with tape. Pt. told to report any pain at site. **Gina Antenucci, RN**

INTRAVENOUS SITE CHANGE

Routine maintenance of an IV site and rotation of the site help prevent complications, such as thrombophlebitis and infection. The IV site is changed, according to the facility's policy. An IV site that shows signs of infection, infiltration, or thrombophlebitis should be changed immediately.

Essential Documentation

In the nursing notes or on the appropriate IV flow sheet, the nurse records the date and time that the IV line was removed. Note whether the site change is routine or due to a complication. Describe the condition of the site. Record any site care given and the type of dressing applied.

Document the new IV insertion site. Record the type, gauge, and length of the needle or catheter. Include the type and flow rate of the IV solution; the name and amount of medication in the solution, if any (this documentation will be included in the MAR of an EHR); and any adverse effects and actions taken to correct them. Describe any patient education.

IV Site Care		
9/2/2019	0900	**NURSING ASSESSMENT:** IV line in place for 72 hours and removed from right forearm according to facility policy. Site without redness, warmth, swelling, or pain. 2" × 2" gauze dressing applied. **NURSING INTERVENTION:** IV infusion restarted in left forearm using 20G 11/2" catheter on first attempt. Site dressed with transparent dressing. I.V. infusion of 500 mL of NSS at 50 mL/hr without difficulty. Pt. instructed to call nurse immediately for any pain at I.V. site. **Leigh Adams, RN**

INTRAVENOUS SITE INFILTRATION

Infiltration of an IV site occurs when an IV solution enters the surrounding tissue as a result of a punctured vein or leakage around a venipuncture site. If vesicant drugs or fluids infiltrate, severe local tissue damage may result. Because infiltration can occur without pain or in unresponsive patients, the IV site must be monitored frequently.

Document assessments of the IV site and the site care provided. Such documentation is important in the prevention and early detection of infiltration and other complications.

Essential Documentation

The nurse should record the date and time of entry. Record signs and symptoms of infiltration at the IV site, such as swelling, burning, discomfort, or pain; tight feeling; decreased skin temperature; and blanching. Chart an assessment of circulation to the affected and unaffected limbs, such as skin color, capillary refill, pulses, and circumference. Document nursing actions, such as stopping the infusion. Estimate the amount of fluid infiltrated. Restart the infusion, and note the new location in the unaffected limb. Record any emotional support and patient education.

IV Infiltration		
10/31/2019	1900	**NURSING ASSESSMENT:** IV site in right forearm swollen and cool at 1820. Pt. c/o of some discomfort at the site. Hands warm with capillary refill less than 3 seconds, radial pulses 2/4 bilaterally. ___ **NURSING INTERVENTION:** IV line removed and sterile gauze dressing applied. Approx. 30 mL of NSS infiltrated. Dr. Horning notified at 1830, and orders given that IV therapy may be discontinued. Right arm elevated on 2 pillows and ice applied in wrapped towel for 20 min. ___ **NURSING ASSESSMENT:** After ice application, skin cool, intact. No c/o burning or numbness. ___ **PATIENT TEACHING:** Explained importance of keeping arm elevated and to call nurse immediately for any pain, burning, numbness in right forearm. ___ **Betsy Rothman, RN**

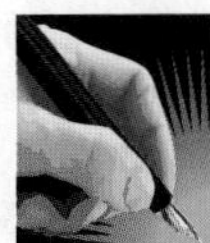

ACCUCHART

INTRAVENOUS FLOW SHEET

This sample shows the typical features of an IV flow sheet.

INTRAVENOUS CARE RECORD

INTRAVENOUS CARE COMMENT CODES C = CAP F = FILTER T= TUBING D = DRESSING
RFA = RIGHT FORERM LFA = LEFT FOREARM

START DATE/ TIME	INITIALS	I.V. VOLUME & SOLUTION	ADDITIVES	FLOW RATE	SITE	STOP DATE/ TIME	TUBING CHANGE	COMMENTS/ASSESSMENT OF SITE
11/30/19 1100	DS	1000 cc D_5W	20 mEq KCL	100/hr	RFA	11/30/19 2100	T	
11/30/19 2100	JM	1000 cc D_5W	20 mEq KCL	100/hr	RFA	12/1/19 0700		
12/1/19 0700	DS	1000 cc D_5W	20 mEq KCL	100/hr	12/2/19 LFA		TD	

INTRAVENOUS THERAPY, CONTINUOUS

More than 89% of hospitalized patients receive some form of IV therapy. Whether providing fluid or electrolyte replacement, total parenteral nutrition, drugs, or blood products, the nurse will need to carefully document all facets of IV therapy—including administration and any subsequent complications of IV therapy.

Keep in mind that an accurate description of care provides a clear record of treatments and drugs received by the patient. This record provides legal protection for the nurse and the facility and furnishes health care insurers with the data they need to approve and provide reimbursement for equipment and supplies.

Depending on the facility's policy, document IV therapy on a special IV therapy sheet, nursing flow sheet, or in another format (EHR).

Essential Documentation

On each shift, the nurse should document the type, amount, and flow rate of IV fluid, along with the condition of the IV site. The nurse should chart each time he or she flushes the IV line, and identify any drug used to flush the line (saline or heparin). Any change in routine care should be documented, along with follow-up assessments. Record any patient teaching provided for the patient and family.

See *Intravenous flow sheet,* page 227, for documentation of routine care during continuous IV administration.

SELECTED READINGS

Azagury, D., Liu, R. C., Morgan, A., & Spain, D. A. (2015). Small bowel obstruction: A practical step-by-step evidence-based approach to evaluation, decision making, and management. *Journal of Trauma & Acute Care Surgery, 79*(4), 661–668.

Carr, P. J., Rippey, J. C. R., Cooke, M. L., Higgins, N. S., Trevenen, M., Foale, A., & Rickard, C. M. (2018). From insertion to removal: A multicenter survival analysis of an admitted cohort with peripheral intravenous catheters inserted in the emergency department. *Infection Control & Hospital Epidemiology, 39*(10), 1216–1221.

Conley, S. B., Buckley, P., Magarace, L., Hsieh, C., & Vitale Pedulla, L. (2017). Standardizing best nursing practice for implanted ports: Applying evidence-based professional guidelines to prevent central line-associated bloodstream infections. *Journal of Infusion Nursing, 40*(3), 165–174.

Fowler, S. B., Penoyer, D. A., & Bourgault, A. M. (2018). Insertion and removal of PIVCs: Exploring best practices. *Nursing, 48*(7), 65–67.

Harth, I. (2007). Critical incident reporting: Learning from errors to improve patient safety. *CONNECT: The World of Critical Care Nursing, 5*(4), 101–103.

Hemphill, J. C., Greenberg, S. M., Anderson, C. S., Becker, K., Bendok, B. R., Cushman, M., ... Council on Clinical Cardiology. (2015). Guidelines for the management of spontaneous intracerebral hemorrhage: A guideline for healthcare professionals from the American Heart Association/American Stroke Association. *Stroke, 46*(7), 2032–2060.

Johnson Hall, S. (2018). Considering the "informed" in informed consent. *Dimensions of Critical Care Nursing,* 37(5), 237–238.

Jones, A. (2018). Infection prevention and control at a glance. *Journal of Perioperative Practice, 28*(10), 250.

Kear, T. (2017). Fluid and electrolyte management across the continuum. *Nephrology Nursing Journal, 44*(6), 491–497.

Laham, R. J., Aroesty, J. M., & Pinto, D. S. (2018). *Intraaortic balloon pump counterpulsation.* Retrieved from UpToDate website: http://www.uptodate.com

McNett, M. M., & Olson, D. M. (2013). Evidence to guide nursing interventions for critically ill neurologically impaired patients with ICP monitoring. *Journal of Neuroscience Nursing, 45*(3), 120–123.

Mihala, G., Ray-Barruel, G., Chopra, V., Webster, J., Wallis, M., Marsh, N., ... Rickard, C. M. (2018). Phlebitis signs and symptoms with peripheral intravenous catheters: Incidence and correlation study. *Journal of Infusion Nursing, 41*(4), 260–263.

Patient safety: Incident reports reflect ongoing blame games. (2017). *Nursing, 47*(11), 25.

Perez-Barcena, J., Llompart-Pou, J. A., & O'Phelan, K. H. (2014). Intracranial pressure monitoring and management of intracranial hypertension. *Critical Care Clinics, 30*(4), 735–750.

Schimpf, M. M. (2012). Diagnosing increased intracranial pressure. *Journal of Trauma Nursing, 19*(3), 160–167.

Schuster, C., Stahl, B., Murray, C., Keleekai, N. L., and Glover, K. (2016). Development and testing of a short peripheral intravenous catheter insertion skills checklist. *Journal of the Association for Vascular Access, 21*(4), 196–204.

Silk, B. J. (2018). Infectious disease threats and opportunities for prevention. *Journal of Public Health Management & Practice, 24*(6), 503–505.

Xu, L., Hu, Y., Huang, X., Fu, J., & Zhang, J. (2017). Clinically indicated replacement versus routine replacement of peripheral venous catheters in adults: A nonblinded, cluster-randomized trial in China. *International Journal of Nursing Practice, 23*(6).

L

LANGUAGE DIFFICULTIES

Entering a health care facility or using a health care service can be a daunting experience for a person who does not speak English. Nurses and other health care workers face similar obstacles to communication. A patient may be unable to communicate questions, concerns, needs, and fears, and the nurse may be unable to perform a health history, ask about symptoms, or provide education. In fact, every part of the nurse–patient relationship may be compromised.

When a patient does not speak English, the nurse will need to find an interpreter. Interpreters should not be family members, interpreters should be objective translators hired by the facility or through a translator service. Telephone interpretation services are also available. It is best to use an objective translator because family members can be biased and not accurately reflect the patient's words, or patients may be reluctant to be truthful with family member as translator. The facility should supply an objective interpreter or employ a service. Health care providers need to obtain truthful history information from the patient and in some cultures this may not be possible if you use a family member as a translator. This is a patient safety issue.

Children and adolescents should never be put in a situation in which they are expected to interpret for parents and other adult family members unless it is an emergency situation.

For informed consent or end-of-life care conversations, finding a neutral third party who also speaks the patient's language is a prudent idea when possible. Health care institutions are supposed to provide interpreters or interpretation devices for patients who cannot speak English. A spouse or family member or a staff member should not be used for interpretation in order to maintain confidentiality for the patient. Failure to have a reliable translator can result in a lack of informed consent and liability for the health care facility.

Essential Documentation

The nurse needs to:

- Document the primary language spoken by the patient.
- Include the names, addresses, and telephone numbers of interpreters.
- Place in the patient's chart a list of staff members approved by the facility to act as interpreters. When a translator is used for an event, such as patient education, discharge instructions, or informed consent, record the name of the translator on the appropriate form or in the nurse's notes. If a telephone interpretation service is used, record the call number assigned by the service for future reference.
- Describe alternative forms of communication used, such as a picture board or flash cards.

Because narrative notes are often permitted but rarely used in electronic health records (EHRs), a narrative note should be inserted. The nurse needs to describe why the interpreter was called, particularly if the conversation is a preoperative or preprocedural informed-consent discussion. Interpreters are absolutely required in the creation of vital documents such as a health care power of attorney (HPOA) or guardian for surrogate decision-making, durable power of attorney (DPOA), or creation of last will and testament. These are legal documents that have requirements in order to be considered valid. If there is concern about how these conversations are being conducted, it is necessary to notify the nursing supervisor and the agency's on-call administrator. It is important to document the names of all present during conversations and their relationships to the patient, as well as to document the patient's level of consciousness (LOC) and ability to participate in the discussion.

LAST WILL AND TESTAMENT, PATIENT REQUEST FOR WITNESS OF

Patients, especially those who believe or have been told that they are dying, may ask that the nurse witness a last will and testament. In many states, a nurse can witness a patient's signature on a will. However, the nurse does not have a legal or ethical responsibility to act as a witness. Before witnessing a will, a nurse should check the facility's policy or ask the facility's legal consultant. (See *Witnessing a will*, page 233.)

If patients ask the nurse to be a witness for either an informed-consent conversation or when they draw their last will and testament, the nurse should notify the health care provider and supervisor before acting as a witness. It is not appropriate to give any legal advice or offer assistance in the wording of the document. Equally inappropriate is commenting on the nature of the patient's choices. The nurse's note should document the nurse's actions. The nurse should avoid being involved in the creation of a last will and testament if the patient does not meet the four tests of legal competency: (1) that a choice has been made, (2) evidence of choice, (3) that the choice is one that a reasonably prudent person would also have made under similar circumstances, and (4) the patient's understanding.

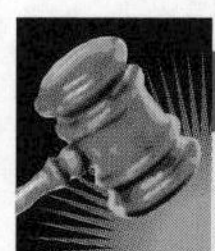

LEGAL CASEBOOK

WITNESSING A WILL

In many states, the nurse's signature on a will certifies that

- the nurse witnessed the signing of the will,
- the nurse heard the maker of the will declare it to be the patient's will, and
- all witnesses and the maker of the will were actually present during the signing.

By attesting to the last two facts, the nurse helps to ensure the authenticity of the will and the signatures. However, the nurse's signature does not certify the competency of the maker of the will.

Before signing any document, the nurse should read at least enough of it to make sure it is the type of document the maker represents it to be. Usually, it does not require reading all of the text, and legally, that is not necessary for the nurse's signature to be valid. However, the nurse should always examine the document's title and first page and give careful attention to what's written immediately above the place for the witness signature.

Because family members' judgment may be swayed according to whether or not they are beneficiaries of the will, a court-appointed guardian ad litem may be indicated in some cases. The American Nurses Association (ANA, 2015) *Code of Ethics for Nurses with Interpretive Statements* places the primacy of the patient as the nurse's first priority. If the nurse suspects coercion, inducement, or unfair persuasion of the patient, it is essential to notify the supervisor and the organization's legal counsel immediately.

Essential Documentation

When witnessing a written will, the nurse should:

- Document that it was signed and witnessed, who signed and witnessed it, who was present, what was done with it after signing, and what the patient's condition was at the time.
- Document the name of the health care provider, facility attorney, or any other person (e.g., nursing supervisor) who was notified, and record the time of notification.
- Record instructions that were given and the actions taken by the nurse.
- Record that the nurse heard the maker of the will declare it to be the will of the patient and that all witnesses and the maker of the will were actually present during the signing.
- Make sure to obtain and make copies of any documents, such as living wills, durable HPOAs, DPOAs, or other legal documents pertaining to provision of the nursing and other health care providers at hand, and include them in the patient's paper record or scan them into the patient's EHR.

Witnessing a Will		
7/17/2019	1300	**NURSING INTERVENTION:** Pt. asked me to witness his will. Dr. Pershing; Edward Ewing, hospital attorney; and Nancy Strom, RN, nursing supervisor, were contacted at 1245. Mr. Ewing; Ms. Strom; pt.'s daughter, Mrs. Pope; pt.; and I were present at the signing. The document was entitled "My last will and testament." Pt. signed the will. It was witnessed by the above people and me. Will was placed with pt.'s personal belongings in his closet after signing. At pt.'s request, a copy was given to Mrs. Pope. At the signing, pt. was alert and oriented to time, place, and person. Pt. is also aware of his poor prognosis and has had many discussions with me about "putting my affairs in order before I die." ________ **Sally Ball, RN**

LATE-DOCUMENTATION ENTRY

Late-documentation entries are appropriate in the situations noted in the following list. However, keep in mind that a late or altered chart entry can arouse suspicions and can be a significant problem in the event of a malpractice lawsuit. (See *Avoiding late entries*, below.)

- If the chart was unavailable when it was needed—for example, when the patient was away from the unit (e.g., for x-rays or physical therapy)
- If important information needs to be added after notes were completed
- If notes were forgotten to be written on a particular chart
- If the EHR goes offline, for example, in a power outage or a hacking incident. In that case, follow the organization's protocol for creating handwritten narrative notes, as well as maintaining all flow-sheet-style documentation, in the frequency that was ordered by the physician. If there is a handwritten note, scan that entry into the EHR.

Essential Documentation

If a nurse must make a late entry or alter an entry, it is necessary to find out if the facility has a protocol for doing so (many do). If not, the best approach is to add the entry to the first available line and label it "late entry" to indicate that it is out of sequence. Then, the nurse records the date and time of the entry and, in the body of the entry, records

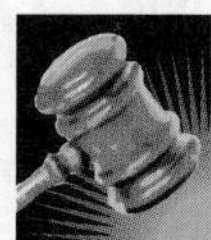

LEGAL CASEBOOK

AVOIDING LATE ENTRIES

If the court uncovers alterations in a patient's chart during the course of a trial, suspicions may be aroused. The court may logically infer that additional alterations were made. In such situations, the value of the entire medical record may be brought into question.

That happened in one case involving a nurse who failed to chart her observations of a patient for 7 hours after surgery, during which time the patient died. The patient's family later sued the hospital, charging the nurse with malpractice. The nurse insisted that she had observed the patient, but because her particular unit was understaffed and overpopulated, she was not able to record her observations. She explained that the assistant director of nursing later instructed her about the hospital's policy on charting late additions. The nurse subsequently added her observations to the patient's medical record.

However, the court was not convinced that the nurse had indeed observed the patient during the postoperative period. Suspicious of the altered record, it ruled that the nurse's failure to chart her observations at the proper time supported the plaintiff's claim that she had made no such observations.

the date and time it should have been made. EHRs generally allow for the creation of late entries that are placed in the correct sequence in the documentation, but the actual date and time the data entries were made are also recorded. Therefore, honest documentation not only adheres to the provisions of the ANA (2015) *Code of Ethics for Nurses with Interpretive Statements* but also protects patient safety.

Late Entry		
6/14/2019	0900 Late entry	**NURSING ASSESSMENT:** On 6/13/19 at 1300, pt. stated she felt faint when getting OOB on 6/13/19 at 1200 and she fell to the floor. Pt. states she didn't hurt herself at the time and didn't think she had to tell anyone about this until her husband encouraged her to report it. Right wrist bruised and slightly swollen. Pt. c/o some tenderness. ________ **NURSING INTERVENTION:** Dr. Muir notified at 1310 and came to see pt. at 1320 on 6/13/19. X-ray of wrist ordered. ________ ________ **Elaine Kasmer, RN**

LATEX HYPERSENSITIVITY

Latex, derived from the sap of the rubber tree, is used throughout the health care industry. The increased use of latex may be related to the increased hypersensitivity reactions experienced by health care workers and patients, with reactions ranging from local dermatitis to anaphylaxis. There are many health care organizations that have become latex-free zones and purchase only products with no latex components. Only when it is suspected that a patient may be hypersensitive to latex should the nurse advocate for the use of these products. The nurse might be the first health care professional in the patient's timeline who identifies this as an allergy concern for that individual.

If the patient has latex hypersensitivity, only nonlatex products should be used. The nurse needs to be prepared to treat life-threatening hypersensitivity with antihistamines, epinephrine, corticosteroids, intravenous (IV) fluids, oxygen, intubation, and mechanical ventilation, if necessary. The pharmacy and other departments need to be alerted that the patient has a latex allergy so that latex-free materials can be provided. The nurse should place a band on the patient's wrist and a note in the medical record to identify the hypersensitivity to latex.

Essential Documentation

The nurse needs to:

- Record the date and time of the entry.
- At admission, record all allergies, including reactions to latex.
- Document signs and symptoms that are observed or that the patient reports to the nurse, such as red skin, itching, itchy or runny eyes and nose, coughing, hives, shortness of breath, wheezing, bronchospasm, or laryngeal edema.
- Include information about diagnostic testing the patient may undergo to confirm latex hypersensitivity.
- Record that other departments have been notified of the patient's latex allergy and that identification of this allergy has been placed on the patient's wrist and on the front of the medical record.
- Describe measures taken to prevent latex exposure. Be sure to chart patient teaching about latex reactions.

Latex Hypersensitvitiy		
4/3/2019	1120	**NURSING ASSESSMENT:** Pt. reports that she has a latex allergy and has developed red skin and itching with past exposures to latex. ______ **NURSING INTERVENTION:** Latex allergy wristband placed on pt.'s left wrist. Latex precautions stickers placed on pt.'s medical record, MAR, nursing Kardex, and door to pt.'s room. Pharmacy, dietary, lab, and other departments notified of latex allergy by automated record-keeping system. Supply cart with latex-free products kept by pt.'s room. **PATIENT TEACHING:** Pt. very knowledgeable about her latex allergy and was able to describe s/s of reactions, products to avoid, and how to respond to a reaction with autoinjectable epinephrine, if necessary. Pt. already sent away for an ID bracelet to identify her latex allergy, but she hasn't yet received it. ______ ______ **Kate Wilson, RN**

LEVEL OF CONSCIOUSNESS, CHANGES IN

A patient's LOC provides information about the patient's respiratory, cardiovascular, and neurologic status. The Glasgow Coma Scale (GCS; see discussion later in this chapter) provides a standard reference for assessing or monitoring the LOC of a patient with a suspected or confirmed brain injury. This scale measures three responses to stimuli—eye-opening response, motor response, and verbal response—and

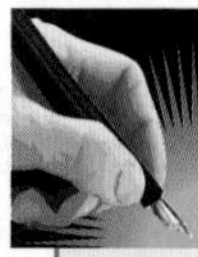

AccuChart

USING THE GLASGOW COMA SCALE

The GCS is a standard reference that is used to assess or monitor LOC in a patient with a suspected or confirmed brain injury. This scale measures three responses to stimuli—eye-opening response, motor response, and verbal response—and assigns a number to each of the possible responses within these categories.

The lowest possible score is 3; the highest is 15. A score of 7 or lower indicates coma. This scale is commonly used in the emergency department, at the scene of an accident, and for the evaluation of a hospitalized patient.

GLASGOW COMA SCALE

Characteristic	Response	Score
Eye opening response	▪ Spontaneous	4
	▪ To verbal command	(3)
	▪ To pain	2
	▪ No response	1
Best motor response	▪ Obeys commands	(6)
	▪ To painful stimulus:	
	– Localizes pain; pushes stimulus away	5
	– Flexes and withdraws	4
	– Abnormal flexion	3
	– Extension	2
	– No response	1
Best verbal response (arouse patient with painful stimulus, if necessary)	▪ Oriented and converses	5
	▪ Disoriented and converses	(4)
	▪ Uses inappropriate words	3
	▪ Makes incomprehensible sounds	2
	▪ No response	1
	Total:	13

assigns a number to each of the possible responses within these categories. The lowest possible score is 3; the highest is 15. A score of 7 or lower indicates a coma. It is also necessary to evaluate a patient's cranial nerves, pupil size, and reactivity to light and accommodation (PERRLA – pupils equally round and reactive to light and accommodation), and the absence or presence of a widening pulse pressure (the number of the diastolic blood pressure [BP] subtracted from the systolic BP pressure gets larger over time); if indicated, physicians may add assessment for cold caloric reflexes when assessing LOC. All of these assessments must be recorded and the status of the patient appreciated and evaluated for further assessment by the nurse. If the patient has invasive electronic monitoring lines, the values and interpretation of these values should also be recorded regularly as ordered and more often when unstable. Subtle changes and trends in the changes of these numbers may mean rapid neurologic deterioration. Notification by the nurse to the physician could save the patient from a life-threatening brainstem-herniation event. Visitors and their relationships to the patient should also be recorded.

Essential Documentation

The nurse needs to:

- Record the date and time of the assessment. (Depending on the facility's GCS flow sheet, the nurse will either circle the number that describes the patient's response to stimuli or will write in the number of the corresponding response. See *Using the Glasgow Coma Scale*, page 238, for an example of how to document a patient's LOC.)
- Record the *total* of the three responses.

LUMBAR PUNCTURE

A lumbar puncture involves the insertion of a sterile needle into the subarachnoid space of the spinal canal, usually between the third and fourth lumbar vertebrae. This process is used to detect increased intracranial pressure (ICP) or the presence of blood in the cerebrospinal fluid (CSF), obtain CSF specimens for laboratory analysis, and inject dyes or gases for contrast in radiologic studies. It is also used to administer drugs (including anesthetics) and to relieve ICP by removing CSF. This procedure should be used with caution in patients with increased ICP because the rapid reduction in pressure that follows the withdrawal of CSF can cause herniation of the brainstem and medullary compression, resulting in death.

Essential Documentation

The nurse needs to:

- Document that the patient understands the lumbar puncture (LP) procedure and has signed a consent form.
- Record the patient education provided regarding what to expect before, during, and after the procedure.
- Record the date of the procedure as well as the initiation and completion times.

- Take a baseline set of vital signs before the procedure and record the values. Include prior pupil checks (PERRLA). The pupil changes and emotional responses of the patient must be included in the documentation as well.
- Record circumstances for children and patients with special needs with limited capacity who must be restrained or sedated in some way, either physically or with sedatives.
- Document any physical restraints that were applied, and if necessary, get a physician's order for them. Include the timing of their application and release.
- Document adverse reactions, such as changes in LOC or vital signs or dizziness. Chart that these responses were reported to the health care provider, and note his or her response, the nurse's actions, and the patient's response.
- Record the number of test tube specimens of CSF that were collected and the time they were transported to the laboratory.
- Describe the color, consistency, and other characteristics of the collected specimens.
- Document the patient's tolerance of the procedure.
- After the procedure, document nursing interventions, such as keeping the patient flat in bed for 6 to 12 hours, encouraging fluid intake, assessing for headache, and checking the puncture site for leakage of CSF.
- Record the patient's responses to these interventions.

Lumbar Puncture		
3/4/2019	0900	**PATIENT TEACHING:** Lumbar puncture explained to pt. by Dr. Wells. Pt. verbalized understanding of the procedure and signed consent form. Explained what to expect before, during, and after the procedure and answered his questions. ______
		NURSING INTERVENTION: Pt. positioned on left side for lumbar puncture. Pt. draped and prepped by Dr. Wells. Specimen obtained on first attempt. One test tube obtained and sent to lab. Specimen clear and straw colored. ______
		NURSING ASSESSMENT: Preprocedure, 0815, P 88, BP 126/82, RR 18, oral T 98.2°F. During procedure, 0830, P 92, BP 128/80, RR 18. After procedure, 0845, P 86, BP 132/82, RR 20, oral T 98.0°F. ______
		NURSING INTERVENTION: Pt. maintained in supine position as instructed. I.V. of NSS infusing at 100 mL/hr in right forearm. Puncture site dressed by Dr. Wells. ______
		NURSING ASSESSMENT: Site clean, dry, and intact. No leakage. Pt. has no c/o of headache or dizziness. Pt. reports no pain after procedure. Pt. lying flat in bed without difficulty. Pt. drank 240 mL ginger ale. ______
		______ **Jeanette Kane, RN**

SELECTED READINGS

American Nurses Association. (2015). *Code of ethics for nurses with interpretive statements.* Silver Spring, MD: Author. Retrieved from https://www.nursingworld.org/coe-view-only

Chae, D., & Park, Y. (2019). Organisational cultural competence needed to care for foreign patients: A focus on nursing management. *Journal of Nursing Management, 27*(1), 197–206.

Liberatore, K. (2018). Protecting patients with latex allergies. *The American Journal of Nursing, 119*(1), 60–63.

Pechak, C., Summers, C., & Velasco, J. (2018). Improved knowledge following an interpreter-use training. *Journal of Allied Health, 47*(3), 159–166.

Perry, S., Barnes, J., & Allan, A. (2018). Performing and interpreting a lumbar puncture. *British Journal of Hospital Medicine, 79*(12), C183–C187.

Reith, F., Brande, R., Synnot, A., Gruen, R.; Maas, A., Van den Brande, R., & Maas, A. (2016). The reliability of the Glasgow Coma Scale: A systematic review. *Intensive Care Medicine, 42*(1), 3–15.

Ratwani, R. M., Moscovitch, B., & Rising, J. P. (2018). Improving pediatric electronic health record usability and safety through certification. *JAMA Pediatrics, 172*(11), 1007–1008. doi:10.1001/jamapediatrics.2018.2784

Showstack, R. E, Guzman, K., Chesser, A. K, & Woods, N. K. (2019). Improving Latino health equity through Spanish language interpreter advocacy in Kansas. *Hispanic Health Care International, 17*(1), 18–22.

Turnbull, J., Arenth, J., Payne, K., Lantos, J. D., & Fanning, J. (2019). When only family is available to interpret. *Pediatrics, 143*(4), 1–4.

SELECTED READINGS

M

MECHANICAL VENTILATION

A mechanical ventilator moves air in and out of a patient's lungs. Although the equipment ventilates a patient, it doesn't ensure adequate gas exchange. Mechanical ventilation may use either positive or negative pressure to ventilate a patient.

Positive-pressure ventilators exert a positive pressure on the airway, which causes inspiration while increasing tidal volume. The inspiratory cycles of these ventilators may vary in volume, pressure, or time. A high-frequency ventilator uses high respiratory rates and low tidal volume to maintain alveolar ventilation.

Negative-pressure ventilators create negative pressure, which pulls the thorax outward and allows air to flow into the lungs. Examples of such ventilators are the iron lung, the cuirass (chest shell), and the body wrap. Negative-pressure ventilators are mainly used to treat neuromuscular disorders, such as Guillain–Barré syndrome, myasthenia gravis, and poliomyelitis.

Other indications for ventilator use include central nervous system disorders, such as cerebral hemorrhage and spinal cord transection; acute respiratory distress syndrome; pulmonary edema; chronic obstructive pulmonary disease; flail chest, and acute hypoventilation.

Essential Documentation

The nurse should document the date and time that mechanical ventilation began. Note the type of ventilator used as well as its settings, such as ventilatory mode, tidal volume, rate, fraction of inspired oxygen, positive end-expiratory pressure (PEEP), and peak inspiratory flow. Record the size of the endotracheal (ET) tube, centimeter mark of the ET tube, and cuff pressure or if the patient has a tracheostomy. Describe the patient's subjective and objective responses to mechanical ventilation, including vital signs, pulse oximetry reading, arterial blood gas (ABG) results, breath sounds, use of accessory muscles, comfort level, and physical appearance.

Throughout mechanical ventilation, list any complications and subsequent interventions. Record pertinent laboratory data, including ABG analyses and oxygen saturation findings. Also record tracheal suctioning and the character of secretions.

If the patient is receiving pressure-support ventilation or is using a T-piece or tracheostomy collar, note the duration of spontaneous breathing and the patient's ability to maintain the weaning schedule. If the patient is receiving intermittent mandatory ventilation, with or without pressure-support ventilation, record the control breath rate, the time of each breath reduction, and the rate of spontaneous respirations.

Record adjustments made in ventilator settings as a result of ABG levels, and document adjustments of ventilator components, such as changing, cleaning, or discarding the tubing. Also, record teaching efforts and emotional support given.

Mechanical Ventilation		
3/16/2019	1015	**NURSING ASSESSMENT:** Pt. on Servo ventilator set at TV 750, Fio_2 45%, 5 cm PEEP, AC 12. RR 20 and nonlabored; no SOB noted. #8 ETT in right corner of mouth taped securely at 22-cm mark. ______
		NURSING INTERVENTION: Suctioned via ETT for large amt. of thick white secretions. ______
		NURSING ASSESSMENT: Pulse oximetry reading 98%. Left lung clear. Right lung with basilar crackles and expiratory wheezes. ______
		NURSING INTERVENTION: Dr. M. Short notified at 1000; no treatment at this time. ______
		PATIENT TEACHING: Explained all procedures including suctioning to pt. Pt. nodded head "yes" when asked if he understood explanations.
		______ **Janice Del Vecchia, RN**

MEDICAL ADVICE, PATIENT OR FAMILY REQUEST FOR

A patient or family member may seek the nurse's advice about a particular treatment the patient is receiving. The nurse should be careful to provide objective information and not advice about the treatment.

Giving medical advice can be looked upon as providing medical treatment without a license and could subject the nurse to legal concerns. Instead of offering advice, offer rationales for the treatment rather than recommending alternative treatment options or comparing one treatment to another.

Evaluate what patients know and understand about their treatment and what they understand about what the health care provider has told them about their treatment. Then, explain how the treatment works to alleviate or cure the patient's condition. Suggest that the patient should speak to his or her health care provider if the patient still does not understand the explanation or has questions or doubts. Inform the health care provider of the patient's or family member's concerns and the information or teaching that has been provided, and suggest that the health care provider speak to the patient or family member.

If the patient or family member is asking for the nurse's opinion about the abilities of a particular health care provider, the nurse must be careful to avoid negative comments because he or she could be charged with defamation of character. Ask if a friend or family member has had previous experience with the health care provider. If the patient or family member is questioning the care that the patient is receiving, the nurse can suggest that the patient seek a second opinion. In fact, most health care providers will suggest that the patient should ask for a second opinion before treatment is performed. If the patient or family member is asking about the skill of the health care provider, the nurse should ask what concerns are causing these questions to identify any underlying issues.

Essential Documentation

The nurse's progress notes should document the patient's or family member's questions or concerns as well as the response provided. The nurse should also document any teaching that was provided and the response to that teaching. If the nurse told the patient or family member that the nurse would speak to the health care provider document when the health care provider was called and whom the nurse spoke to.

Patient or Family Request for Medical Advice

4/29/2019	0045	**PATIENT TEACHING:** Called to pt.'s room because pt. says he's worried about his medications. Pt. asked me if I thought the doctor prescribed the correct medications for his condition. He states that his brother had the "same thing" and he was on a different heart medication and feels wonderful now. I explained the purpose of lisinopril and metoprolol to pt. Pt. verbalized his understanding of his medications and their purpose but still had questions as to why his doctor chose these medications and not the ones his brother is on. I suggested he clarify his medications with his doctor. ______ **NURSING INTERVENTION:** Told pt. I would leave a message for Dr. C. Ward to speak to him. ______ ______ **Callie Burns, RN**
4/29/2019	0630	**NURSING INTERVENTION:** Reported to morning shift nurse Jill Spillane, RN, that pt. has a concern about his cardiac medications and that they're not the same as his brother takes for his heart condition. Pt. still wishes to speak to Dr. Ward. Jill Spillane states she would contact Dr. Ward's nurse, Barb Lawson, who accompanies him on morning rounds, that the patient wishes to discuss his medications with him. ______ **Callie Burns, RN**

MEDICATION ERROR

Medication errors are the most common, and potentially the most dangerous, errors. Mistakes in dosage, patient identification, or drug selection by nurses have led to vision loss, brain damage, cardiac arrest, and death. (See *Lawsuits and medication errors,* page 246.)

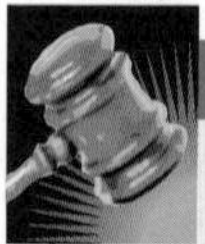

LEGAL CASEBOOK

LAWSUITS AND MEDICATION ERRORS

Unfortunately, lawsuits involving nurses' drug errors are common. The court determines liability based on the standards of care required of nurses who administer drugs. In many instances, if the nurse had known more about the proper dosage, administration route, or procedure connected with a drug's use, the nurse might have avoided the mistake.

In *Norton v. Argonaut Insurance Co.* (1962), an infant died after a nurse administered injectable digoxin at a dosage level appropriate for an elixir of Lanoxin, an oral drug. The nurse was unaware that digoxin was available in an oral form. The nurse questioned two health care providers who were not treating the infant about the order but failed to mention to them that the order was written for elixir of Lanoxin. She also failed to clarify the order with the health care provider who wrote it.

The nurse, the health care provider who ordered the drug, and the hospital were found liable.

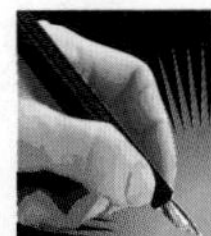

ACCUCHART

MEDICATION EVENT QUALITY REVIEW FORM

When a medication error occurs, most facilities require the nurse to complete a medication event report. The information is used to investigate the incident and develop an action plan to avoid future incidents.

QUALITY REVIEW FORM

Confidential — This is a peer review document and may be protected by applicable law. Not for distribution.

Patient information

Event data

Date and time of event: 10/8/19 1300

Date and time reported: 10/8/19 1315

Primary event type (check one only):
- ❑ Wrong drug
- ❑ Wrong dose
- ❑ Omitted dose
- ❑ Wrong route
- ☑ Wrong time
- ❑ Wrong patient
- ❑ Other ______

For wrong dose or omitted doses, # doses involved: ______

Event severity (check only one):
- ❑ 0 - potential error only
- ❑ 1 - error occurred, no harm to the patient
- ☑ 2 - error occurred, increased monitoring only
- ❑ 3 - error occurred, change in VS, additional labs, no permanent harm
- ❑ 4 - error occurred, required additional treatment, increased LOS
- ❑ 5 - error occurred, permanent harm to patient
- ❑ 6 - error resulted in patient's death

Contributing causes of event

Order related (check all that apply):

Type of order: ❑ Written ❑ Oral ❑ Telephone

- ❑ Order incomplete:
  - ❑ Not dated
  - ❑ No frequency
  - ❑ Not timed
  - ❑ No route
  - ❑ No dose
  - ❑ No drug parameters indicated
  - ❑ No signature
  - ❑ Signature illegible
- ❑ Order illegible
- ❑ Unacceptable abbreviation used: ______
- ❑ Decimal misplaced
- ❑ Inappropriate use of leading or trailing zeros
- ❑ Order not flagged correctly
- ❑ Order written on wrong patient's chart
- ❑ Inappropriate drug selection
- ❑ Inappropriate route selection
- ❑ Patient drug allergies not identified or documented
- ❑ Drug not renewed
- ❑ Drug not discontinued
- ❑ Drug not reordered postop
- ❑ Nonformulary request

Transcription related (check all that apply):
- ❑ Order not faxed
- ❑ Order not transcribed
- ❑ Pharmacy clarification of order not transcribed
- ❑ Incomplete order not clarified
- ❑ Order not completely signed off
- ❑ Incorrect transcription onto:
  - ❑ MAR ❑ Recopied MAR
- ❑ Transcription illegible on:
  - ❑ MAR ❑ Recopied MAR
- ❑ Incomplete allergy documentation
- ❑ Allergies not transcribed onto:
  - ❑ Order sheets ❑ MAR ❑ Recopied MAR
- ❑ Unacceptable abbreviations

Patient related (check all that apply):
- ❑ Took own meds
- ❑ Altered infusion rate
- ❑ Loss of venous access
- ❑ Medication refused

Dispensing related (check all that apply):
- ❑ Drug incompatibility
- ❑ Outdated product dispensed
- ❑ Patient allergies not identified
- ❑ Incorrect product chosen
- ❑ Product incorrectly labeled
- ❑ Product not delivered to nursing unit
- ❑ Delay in delivery due to:
  - ❑ Nonformulary request
  - ❑ Illegible order
  - ❑ Out of stock
  - ❑ Illegible fax
  - ❑ Further investigation required
  - ❑ Pneumatic tube problem
  - ❑ Other: ______
- ❑ Product incorrectly prepared in:
  - ❑ Pharmacy ❑ Nursing unit ❑ Other: ______
- ❑ Miscalculation
- ❑ No physician order

MEDICATION EVENT QUALITY REVIEW FORM *(continued)*

Dispensing related (continued)
- ❑ Incomplete physician order not clarified
- ❑ Unacceptable abbreviation used: ________
- ❑ Computer entry errors (pharmacy only):
  - ❑ Duplicate ❑ Wrong patient ❑ Wrong drug
  - ❑ Missed order ❑ Other
- ❑ Pharmacy clarification of order not documented

Administration related (check all that apply):
- ❑ Incorrect drug storage method
- ❑ Patient allergies not correctly checked against:
  - ❑ Allergy band ❑ MAR
- ❑ Patient allergy band not intact
- ❑ Patient not correctly identified
- ❑ No physician order
- ❑ Drug incompatibility
- ❑ Available product incorrectly prepared
- ❑ Miscalculation
- ❑ Incorrectly labeled
- ❑ Medication or I.V. not checked with MAR, order, I.V. record
- ☑ Time of last p.r.n. medication administration not checked
- ❑ Patient not observed taking medication
- ❑ Med. or I.V. not charted at time of administration
- ❑ Med. or I.V. not charted correctly
- ❑ Incorrect I.V. line used
- ❑ Incorrect setting on infusion pump
- ❑ Lock-out on infusion pump not used
- ❑ Outdated product given
- ❑ Forgotten or overlooked
- ❑ Product not available
- ❑ Extra or duplicated dose
- ❑ Monitoring, insufficient or not done

Event analysis

(Include additional information, such as staffing patterns, activity level, patient outcome, action plan, and conclusion)

Susan Jones, RN, had administered and documented giving p.r.n. Demerol 100 mg I.M. to the pt. at 1215. I did not review the p.r.n. MAR and administered the dose again at 1300. Pt. monitored q 15 min. for 2 hours. No adverse effects. Pt. alert and oriented to time, place, and person. Dr. G. Miller notified at 1305 and came to see pt.

Completed by: Aleisha Adams, RN Date completed: 10/8/19

A medication event report or incident report should be completed when a medication error is discovered. The nurse who discovers the medication error is responsible for completing the medication error report or incident report and for communicating the error to the patient's health care provider and the nursing practitioner. It is essential for the nurse to be aware of the agency's policy and procedure for medication error reporting.

Essential Documentation

The nurse's note should describe the situation objectively and include the name of the health care provider notified, the time of notification, and the provider's response. Avoid the use of such terms as "by mistake," "somehow," "unintentionally," "miscalculated," and "confusing," which can be interpreted as admissions of wrongdoing. Document the medication error on an incident report or medication event report. (See *Medication event quality review form,* pages 247 and 248.)

MEDICATIONS, RECONCILING

Reconciling medications is a process that develops an accurate, up-to-date medication list for patients at admission and then compares that list against the health care provider's admission orders. Any discrepancies in the patient's medications will be brought to the attention of the health care provider, and changes will be made to the orders as necessary. The process is designed to promote communication and information transfer during patient transfer and prevent errors, such as omissions, duplications, dosing errors, or drug interactions.

The ordering health care provider, the registered nurse, and the pharmacist all share accountability for accurate medication reconciliation. Reconciliation of medications should occur within 24 hours of patient admission and at every transition of care, such as a change in setting, service, practitioner, or level of care. The process of medication reconciliation includes five steps:

- developing a list of the patient's current medications
- developing a list of medications to be prescribed for the patient
- comparing the medications on the two lists
- making clinical decisions based on a comparison of the two lists
- communicating the new list to the patient and appropriate caregivers

Essential Documentation

The documentation should include the dosage, dosing frequency, date and time of last dose, and the purpose of each medication. It should also include the source of this information (patient, family member, caregiver, or medication bottle) and any patient allergies.

Reconciling medications is assisted by the completion of the facility's standardized documentation process for admission, transfer, and discharge of the patient. For accurate medication reconciliation after completion of the admission process, the nurse should obtain information from the patient, the patient's family, and the facility pharmacy as necessary. The nurse should take particular care when filling out the patient's discharge instructions.

MEDICATION RECONCILIATION

The following is an example of a completed medical reconciliation form.

Name: Benjamin Henry **Medical record #:** 13011976 **Admission date:** 1/19/19

Information Source:
- ☑ Patient
- ❑ Family
- ❑ Caregiver
- ❑ Medication bottle
- ❑ Other: ____

Allergies:
NKDA

❑ Unable to obtain Medication History – Reason:

Reconciliation
(Check yes if drug is ordered, no if drug is not ordered or the dose/frequency/route has been changed. Complete the comment section using the comment codes provided)

Medications on Admission							Admission Reconciliation (must be completed within 24 hours)			
Medication	**Dose**	**Route**	**Frequency**	**Date/time of last dose**	**Date & initials**	**Reason for medication**	**Yes**	**No**	**Comment***	**Date & initials**
Zetia	10 mg	P.O.	daily	1/18/19 2100	1/19/19 MG	high cholesterol	✓			1/19/19 MG
lisinopril	5 mg	P.O.	daily	1/18/19 2100	1/19/19 MG	hypertension	✓			1/19/19 MG
aspirin	81 mg	P.O.	daily	1/18/19 2100	1/19/19 MG	prophylactic	✓			1/19/19 MG

Signature & initials: Millie Gondek, RN MG Signature & initials: ____

Signature & initials: ____ Signature & initials: ____

NOTE:
- Place form on top of the current practitioner order sheet until admission reconciliation is complete.
- Place form with discharge instructions once admission reconciliation is completed.

*Comment Codes:
- DFR: Dose/frequency/route changes (see practitioner order)
- N/A: Not applicable based on diagnosis
- NPO: Patient status is NPO and an alternate route is not indicated
- TS: Therapeutic substitution
- PA: Practitioner aware
- Other: Note reason and continue on flowsheet or progress note as needed

THIS IS NOT A PRACTITIONER ORDER SHEET

MISUSE OF EQUIPMENT

At times, a patient may manipulate equipment or misuse supplies (e.g., pressing keys on a pump or monitor, detaching tubing, or playing with switches) without understanding the consequences. If a patient misuses equipment, the nurse should explain that such misuse can cause harm. Advise the patient to call for the nurse if the patient feels the equipment is not working properly, is causing discomfort, or for other concerns. The nurse should notify the patient's health care provider or nurse practitioner of any misuse that has resulted in injury or affected the patient's health status.

Essential Documentation

The nurse should record the date and time that the patient misused the equipment. Describe the patient's actions, and record the patient's response to safety education. Use the patient's own words in quotes. Document how the problem was corrected.

The nurse should document an assessment of the patient's condition. Chart the name of the health care provider notified, the time of notification, the orders given, the nurse's actions, and the patient's response. Include any patient teaching that is provided.

Misuse of Equipment by Patient		
2/6/2019	0930	**NURSING INTERVENTION:** I.V. of 1000 mL D5W hung at 0915 infusing at rate of 60 mL/hr via infusion pump. ______ **Kate Comerford, RN**
2/6/2019	1015	**NURSING ASSESSMENT:** Assessed I.V. infusion; 840 mL left in bag and pump infusing at 250 mL/hr. Pt. stated, "I flicked the switch because I didn't see anything happening. Then I pressed the green button and the arrow." I.V. pump reset to 60 mL/hr. ______ **NURSING ASSESSMENT:** P 80, BP 110/82, RR 18, oral T 98.4°F. Breath sounds clear; normal heart sounds; no peripheral edema. ______ **PATIENT TEACHING:** Instructed pt. not to touch the pump or I.V. line. I.V. pump placed on lock setting. Informed pt. he was not to change settings on pump. Pt. verbalized understanding and agreed not to touch equipment. ______ **NURSING INTERVENTION:** Dr. I. Huang notified at 1030. No new orders. ______ **Kate Comerford, RN**

MIXED VENOUS OXYGEN SATURATION MONITORING

This procedure uses a fiber-optic thermodilution pulmonary artery catheter to continuously monitor oxygen delivery to tissues and oxygen consumption by tissues. Monitoring of mixed venous oxygen saturation (So_2) allows rapid detection of impaired oxygen delivery, such as that from decreased cardiac output, hemoglobin level, or arterial oxygen saturation. It also helps evaluate a patient's response to drug therapy, ET tube suctioning, ventilator setting changes, PEEP, and fraction of inspired oxygen. The So_2 level usually ranges from 60% to 80%; the normal value is 75%.

Essential Documentation

The nurse should record the SvO_2 value on a flow chart and attach a tracing as ordered. Note significant changes in the patient's status and the results of any interventions. For comparison, note the SvO_2 value as measured by the fiber-optic catheter whenever a blood sample is obtained for laboratory analysis of SvO_2.

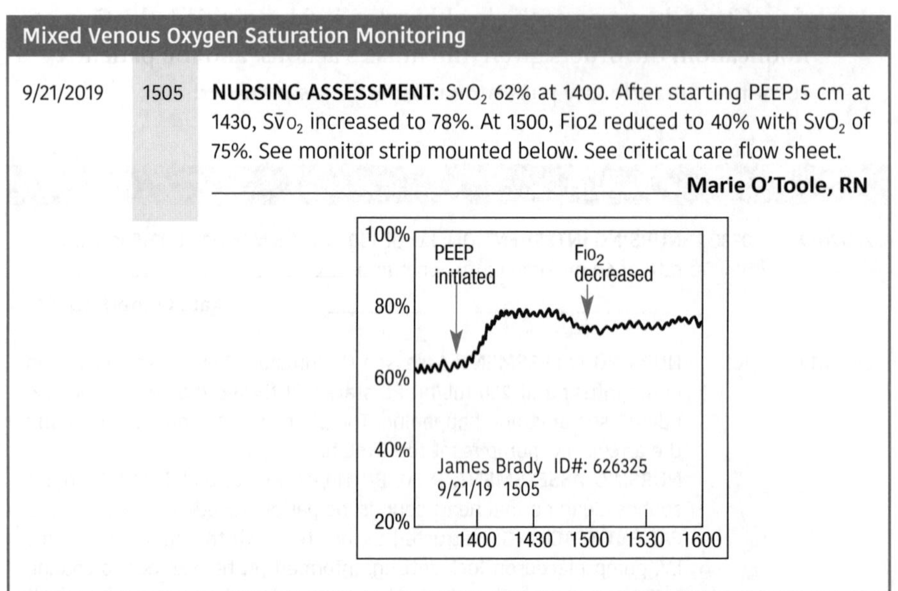

Mixed Venous Oxygen Saturation Monitoring
9/21/2019 1505 NURSING ASSESSMENT: SvO2 62% at 1400. After starting PEEP 5 cm at 1430, Sv̄o2 increased to 78%. At 1500, Fio2 reduced to 40% with SvO2 of 75%. See monitor strip mounted below. See critical care flow sheet.
Marie O'Toole, RN
100%
80%
60%
40%
20%
PEEP initiated
Fio2 decreased
James Brady ID#: 626325
9/21/19 1505
1400 1430 1500 1530 1600

MODERATE SEDATION

Moderate sedation, also called *conscious* or *procedural sedation*, produces a minimally depressed level of consciousness (LOC) in patients undergoing such tests and procedures as minor bone fracture reduction, breast biopsy, vasectomy, dental or plastic reconstructive surgery, or endoscopy. Moderate sedation allows the patient to respond to verbal or tactile commands during the procedure and helps maintain airway patency and protective reflexes while controlling anxiety and pain and producing amnesia. Following moderate sedation, the patient is able to return to daily activities within a short time.

Drugs, such as benzodiazepines (midazolam and diazepam) and opioids (morphine, hydromorphone, and fentanyl), may be used alone or in combination to produce moderate sedation. Emergency equipment, reversal drugs, and staff trained in advanced life support must be immediately available for the patient who slips into a deeper level of sedation.

Moderate sedation is administered by specially trained health care providers and nurses. Determine whether the state board of nursing and the facility allow the registered nurse to administer drugs that produce moderate sedation.

Essential Documentation

In the nurse's notes or on the appropriate flow sheet, the nurse should record the date and time of each entry. The frequency of nursing assessments depends on the facility's policy, the health care provider's orders, and the patient's condition. Charting should include the time the patient was received; assessment of the patient's airway and breathing, including breath sounds, respiratory rate and depth, pulse oximetry values, skin color, oxygen use, and positioning to maintain airway patency; vital signs; assessment of circulation, including heart rate and rhythm, pulses, skin temperature, and capillary refill; LOC; surgical- or procedural-site assessment, including drainage (amount, color, consistency), bleeding, swelling, condition of the skin around the site, and the presence and condition of any dressings or drains; and pain assessment, using a 0-to-10 scale (with 10 being the worst pain imaginable), analgesics or comfort measures given, and the patient's response.

Use the appropriate documentation to record frequent assessments, vital signs, intake and output, intravenous (IV) therapy, and neurologic assessments per the facility's policy. The nurse should document the name, dose, route, and frequency of any drugs given (e.g., analgesics, antiemetics, or reversal agents) on the medication administration record and note the patient's response. Record the name of the health care provider who was notified of any changes in the patient's condition, such as somnolence, confusion, reduced reflexes, respiratory depression or obstruction, apnea, coma, hypotension, and nausea and vomiting. Include the time the provider was notified, orders given, the nurse's actions, and the patient's response.

If the patient is being discharged, note that discharge criteria were met. For example, note that the patient's vital signs, LOC, and cardiopulmonary assessment were within an acceptable range; protective reflexes and motor and sensory control were present; pain was at an acceptable level; the wound or procedure site was stable; and the patient was without nausea and adequately hydrated.

Record patient and family teaching and any emotional support given. This may be documented on a separate patient education section of the patient's health record. Include verbal and written information given to the patient and family; verbalization of understanding of the instructions; a name and telephone number for the patient to call with questions; and the date, time, and name of the health care provider for follow-up. Note who was taking the patient home.

Moderate Sedation		
1/14/2019	1300	**NURSING ASSESSMENT:** Received pt. from endoscopy at 1230 via wheelchair following colonoscopy. P 82 regular, BP 128/72, RR 16 deep, oral T 98.8°F. Pt. awake, alert, and oriented to time, place, and person. Answering all questions appropriately. Breath sounds clear bilaterally, skin pink, pulse ox 98% on room air. Peripheral pulses strong, hands and feet warm to touch, Capillary refill less than 3 sec. Pt. moving all extremities and able to feel light touch. Cough and gag reflexes intact. Abdomen slightly distended, bowel sounds heard in all 4 quadrants. NSS infusing at 30 mL/hr in left hand via infusion pump. See flow sheets for frequent vital signs, I.V. therapy, I/O, and neuro assessments. **PATIENT TEACHING:** Explained to pt. that he may be discharged once he's able to urinate and drink fluids. ____ **NURSING INTERVENTION:** Brought pt. 120 mL of apple juice to sip. Pt. called wife to get him and requested that discharge instructions be given when she arrives. Pt. sitting up in bed drinking apple juice and watching the news. ____ ____ **Marcy Thayer, RN**

MULTIPLE TRAUMA

The patient with multiple trauma has injuries to more than one body system caused by such situations as a vehicular accident, violence, a fall, or a burn. The patient's injuries may involve penetrating wounds, blunt trauma, or both. The patient's chances of survival are improved when health care workers follow a systematic team approach of assessment, resuscitation, and treatment. The nurse will need to document assessments, interventions, and the patient's response. The nurse will also need to document emotional care given to the patient and the patient's family.

Essential Documentation

Immediately upon arrival at the health care facility, the patient will undergo a primary survey of airway, breathing, and circulation with resuscitation and treatment of life-threatening problems.

Documentation at this point in the patient's care must reflect:

- date and time that the patient is admitted to the facility
- assessment of airway, breathing, and circulation (including hemorrhage) and resuscitation and emergency treatment, such as cardiopulmonary resuscitation, ET tube intubation, mechanical ventilation, oxygen therapy, fluid or blood replacement, and direct pressure to control bleeding
- level of responsiveness

When the primary survey is complete, the nurse should document a more thorough secondary survey, including:

- cause and physical evidence of trauma
- vital signs
- head-to-toe assessment
- history
- diagnostic tests.

Record treatments provided, such as insertion of a nasogastric, urinary, or chest tube; neck and spine stabilization; drug therapy; splinting of fractures; and wound care. Include patient and family teaching and emotional support provided.

Continue to document ongoing frequent assessments and treatments until the patient's condition has stabilized.

Multiple Trauma		
8/15/2019	1330	**NURSING ASSESSMENT:** 18 y.o. male brought to ED after being struck by a car at 1245 while riding his bike. Pt. was wearing a helmet. Parents are present. Pt. is awake, alert, and oriented to person and place but not time. Pt. has trauma to face, airway is open, no stridor, RR 18 and nonlabored, Administering O_2 2 L/min by NC. Cervical collar in place. P 104, BP 90/62. Monitor shows sinus tachycardia, no arrhythmias. Bruising over abdomen. Pt. splinting abdomen and c/o abdominal pain and nausea. ________

Multiple Trauma (*continued*)

NURSING INTERVENTION: #16 Fr Foley catheter placed; no blood in urine. I.V. line started in right antecubital vein with 18G catheter. 1000 mL of lactated Ringer's infusing at 100 mL/hr. X-rays of neck, spine, and pelvis done at 1315; results pending. ________

NURSING ASSESSMENT: Moving upper extremities spontaneously and without pain. Moving left leg on own, without pain, right thigh has bruising and deformity, c/o of right thigh pain. Radial pulses 2/4 bilaterally. Dorsalis pedis and posterior tibial pulses palpable 2/4 bilaterally. Able to feel light touch to both legs. Dr. B. Moore discussing need for exploratory abdominal surgery and reduction of right thigh fracture with parents. See I.V., I/O, and VS flow sheets for frequent assessments.

PATIENT TEACHING: All procedures explained to pt. ________

________ **Carrie Burke, RN**

MYOCARDIAL INFARCTION, ACUTE

A myocardial infarction (MI) is due to an occlusion of a coronary artery that leads to oxygen deprivation, myocardial ischemia, and eventually, necrosis. The extent of functional impairment depends on the size and location of the infarct, the condition of the uninvolved myocardium, the potential for collateral circulation, and the effectiveness of compensatory mechanisms.

Mortality is high when treatment for an MI is delayed; however, the prognosis improves if vigorous treatment begins immediately. Therefore, prompt recognition of an MI and nursing interventions to relieve chest pain, stabilize heart rhythm, reduce cardiac workload, and reperfuse the coronary artery are essential to preserving myocardial tissue and preventing complications, including death. Expect to assist with thrombolytic therapy, administer oxygen, assist with the insertion of hemodynamic monitoring catheters, and prepare the patient for invasive procedures to improve coronary circulation. Also, anticipate administering drugs to relieve pain, inhibit platelet aggregation, treat arrhythmias, reduce myocardial oxygen demands, increase myocardial oxygen supply, and improve the patient's chance of survival.

Essential Documentation

All documentation should include the date and time. Describe the patient's chest pain and other symptoms of an MI, using the patient's own words whenever possible, as well as a pain scale rating. Assessment findings, such as feelings of impending doom, anxiety, restlessness, fatigue, nausea, vomiting, dyspnea, tachypnea, cool extremities, weak peripheral pulses, diaphoresis, third or fourth heart sounds, a new murmur, pericardial friction rub, low-grade fever, hypotension or hypertension, bradycardia or tachycardia, and crackles on lung auscultation, should all be documented.

The name of the health care provider who was notified; the time of notification; and the orders given, such as transfer to the coronary care unit, continuous cardiac monitoring, supplemental oxygen, 12-lead electrocardiogram, IV therapy, cardiac lab tests (including troponin and cardiac enzymes), nitroglycerin (sublingual or via an IV line), thrombolytic therapy, aspirin, morphine, bed rest, antiarrhythmics, beta-adrenergic blockers, angiotensin-converting enzyme inhibitors, and heparin, need to be documented.

Documentation of the nurse's actions and the patient's response to these therapies should be thorough and timely. Appropriate documentation to record intake and output, hemodynamic parameters, IV fluids given, drugs administered, and frequent vital signs is essential. Patient teaching, such as details about the disease process, treatments, drugs, signs and symptoms to report, exercise, sexual activity, proper nutrition, smoking cessation, support groups, and cardiac rehabilitation programs, should also be documented. Emotional support given to the patient and the patient's family should also be documented.

Acute Myocardial Infarction

12/30/2019	2310	**NURSING ASSESSMENT:** Pt. c/o severe crushing midsternal chest pain with radiation to left arm at 2240. Pt. pointed to center of chest and stated, "I feel like I have an elephant on my chest." Rates pain at 9 on a scale of 0 to 10. Pt. is restless in bed and diaphoretic, c/o nausea. P 84 and regular, BP 128/82, RR 24, oral T 98.8°F. Extremities cool, pedal pulses weak, normal heart sounds, breath sounds clear. ________
		NURSING INTERVENTION: Dr. D. Boone notified of pt.'s chest pain and physical findings at 2245 and came to see pt. and orders given. O_2 started at 2 L by NC. 12-lead ECG obtained; showed ST-segment elevation in anterior leads. Pt. placed on portable cardiac monitor. I.V. line started in left forearm with 18 G catheter with NSS at 30 mL/hr. Stat cardiac enzymes, troponin, and electrolytes sent to lab at 2255. Nitroglycerin 1/150 gr given SL, 5 minutes apart X 3 with no relief.
		PATIENT TEACHING: Explained all procedures to pt., who verbalized understanding. Assured him that he's being monitored closely and will be transferred to CCU for closer monitoring and treatment. ________
		NURSING INTERVENTION: Report called to CCU at 2255 and given to Laurie Feldman, RN. ________
		PATIENT/FAMILY TEACHING: Wife notified of events and pt.'s transfer.
		________ **Patricia Silver, RN**

SELECTED READINGS

American Nurses Association. (2015). *Code of ethics for nurses with interpretive statements.* Silver Spring, MD: Author.

Cattano, D. (2018). Questions about the practice management guidelines for moderate sedation and analgesia. *Anesthesiology, 129*(4), 855–855.

Cohen, M. R. (2019). *Medication errors. Nursing, 49*(4), 72–72.

De Jong, A., & Jaber, S. (2018). Focus on ventilation management. *Intensive Care Medicine, 44*(12), 2254–2256.

Dirik, H. F., Menevse, S., Seren Intepeler, S., & Hewison, A. (2019). Nurses' identification and reporting of medication errors. *Journal of Clinical Nursing, 28*(5/6), 931–938.

Edwards, S. L., & Axe, S. (2018). Medication management: Reducing drug errors, striving for safer practice. *Nurse Prescribing, 16*(8), 380–389.

Elliott, S., & Morrell-Scott, N. (2017). Care of patients undergoing weaning from mechanical ventilation in critical care. *Nursing Standard, 32*(13), 41–51.

Elliot, Z., & Elliot, S. (2018). An overview of mechanical ventilation in the intensive care unit. *Nursing Standard, 32*(28), 41–49.

Etchells, E., & Fernandes, O. (2018). Medication reconciliation: Ineffective or hard to implement? *BMJ Quality & Safety, 27*(12), 947–949.

Flanagan, N. (2018). Medication reconciliation: A necessary process for patient safety. *Caring for the Ages, 19*(8), 14–15.

Hartog, C., & Bloos, F. (2014). Venous oxygen saturation. *Best Practice & Research: Clinical Anaesthesiology, 28*(4), 419–428.

Ibrahim, A. W., Riddell, TC., & Devireddy, C. M. (2014). *Acute myocardial infarction. Critical Care Clinics, 30*(3), 341–364.

Koers, L., Eberl, S., Cappon, A., Bouwman, A., Schlack, W., Hermanides, J., & Preckel, B. (2018). Safety of moderate-to-deep sedation performed by sedation practitioners: A national prospective observational study. *European Journal of Anaesthesiology, 35*(9), 659–666.

Ladewig, E. L., & Lewis, P. A. (2014). Central venous oxygen saturation monitoring. *British Journal of Cardiac Nursing, 9*(2), 85–89.

Marshall, S. D., Chrimes, N. (2019). Medication handling: towards a practical, human-centred approach. *Anaesthesia, 74*(3), 280–284.

Mayer, K., Trzeciak, S., & Puri, N. K. (2016). Assessment of the adequacy of oxygen delivery. *Current Opinion in Critical Care, 22*(5), 437–443.

McDonald, K., Arndt, D., Myronuk, L. (2019). Uncovering the mysteries of electronic medication reconciliation. Studies in Health Technology & Informatics, 257, 303–309.

Mondor, E. (2017). Alveoli, airways, volumes and ventilators: Breathing easier about mechanical ventilation. *Canadian Journal of Critical Care Nursing, 28*(2), 43–43.

Mondor, E. (2018). Take a deep breath and relax: 10 things you need to know about mechanical ventilation. *Canadian Journal of Critical Care Nursing, 29*(2), 39–40.

New guidelines for moderate procedural sedation and analgesia. *AACN Bold Voices, Nov 2018, 10*(11), 15.

Norton, C. (2017). Acute coronary syndrome: assessment and management. *Nursing Standard, 31*(29), 61–71.

Richards, J. E, Conti, B. M., & Grissom, T. E. (2018). Care of the severely injured orthopedic trauma patient: Considerations for initial management, operative timing, and ongoing resuscitation. *Advances in Anesthesia, 36*(1), 1–22.

Romanoski, M. (2018). Improving practice—Reconciliation of medications. *Geriatric Nursing, 39*(6), 723–724.

Tisherman, S. A., & Stein, D. M.(2018). ICU management of trauma patients. *Critical Care Medicine, 46*(12), 1991–1997.

Wrigglesworth, S. (2018). Acute coronary syndrome. *Nursing Standard, 32*(25), 64–65.

Yamashita, K., Takami, A., Wakayama, S., Makino, M., Takeyama, Y. (2017). Effectiveness of new sedation and rehabilitation methods for critically ill patients receiving mechanical ventilation. *Journal of Physical Therapy Science, 29*(1), 138–143.

N

NASOGASTRIC TUBE CARE

Providing effective nasogastric (NG) tube care requires meticulous monitoring of the patient and the equipment. Monitoring the patient involves checking drainage from the NG tube and assessing the patient's gastrointestinal (GI) function. Monitoring the equipment involves verifying correct tube placement and irrigating the tube to ensure patency to prevent mucosal damage.

Specific care measures vary only slightly for the most commonly used NG tubes: the single-lumen Levin tube and the double-lumen Salem sump tube.

Essential Documentation

The nurse needs to:

- Record the date and time that care was provided.
- Regularly record tube placement confirmation (usually every 4 to 8 hours).
- Record fluids instilled in the NG tube and any NG output. This may be recorded on an intake and output flow sheet.
- Describe the NG drainage, noting its color, consistency, and odor.
- Track the irrigation schedule and note the actual time of each irrigation.
- Describe the condition of the patient's skin, mouth, and nares as well as care provided.

- Record tape changes and skin care provided.
- Chart the assessment of bowel sounds.
- Note any patient teaching provided by the nurse.

Nasogastric Tube Care		
11/30/2019	1100	**NURSING ASSESSMENT:** NG tube placement verified by pH of aspirate. NG tube drained 100 mL of clear and colorless fluid over 4 hr. Active bowel sounds in all 4 quadrants. Skin around mouth and nose intact. Assisted with mouth care. ________ **PATIENT TEACHING:** Explained importance of good oral hygiene to pt. ________ **Clarissa Stone, RN**

NASOGASTRIC TUBE INSERTION

Usually inserted to decompress the stomach, an NG tube can prevent vomiting after major surgery. An NG tube is typically in place for 48 to 72 hours after surgery, by which time peristalsis usually resumes. However, the NG tube may remain in place for shorter or longer periods, depending on its use.

The NG tube has other diagnostic and therapeutic applications, especially in assessing and treating upper GI bleeding, collecting gastric contents for analysis, performing gastric lavage, aspirating gastric secretions, and administering drugs and nutrients. Insertion of an NG tube demands close observation of the patient and verification of proper tube placement.

Essential Documentation

The nurse needs to:

- Record the type and size of the NG tube inserted; the date, time, and route of insertion; and confirmation of proper placement.
- Describe the type and amount of suction, if applicable; the drainage characteristics, such as amount, color (e.g., green, or coffee-ground), character, consistency, and odor; and the patient's tolerance of the insertion procedure.
- Include signs and symptoms signaling complications, such as nausea, vomiting, and abdominal distention.
- Document subsequent irrigation procedures and continuing problems after irrigations.

Nasogastric Tube Insertion		
4/22/2019	1700	**PATIENT TEACHING/INTERVENTION:** Procedure explained to pt. and #12 Fr. NG tube inserted via left nostril. Placement verified by pH of aspirate. Tube attached to low intermittent suction as ordered. Tube taped in place to nose. Drainage pale green, Hematest negative. Irrigated with 30 mL NSS per order. Hypoactive bowel sounds in all 4 quadrants. Pt. resting comfortably in bed. No c/o nausea or pain. ______ **Carol Allen, RN**

NASOGASTRIC TUBE REMOVAL

An NG tube typically remains in place for 48 to 72 hours after surgery and is removed when peristalsis resumes. Depending on its use, it may remain in place for shorter or longer periods.

Essential Documentation

The nurse needs to:

- Record the date and time that the NG tube is removed.
- Chart that the procedure has been explained to the patient.
- Describe the color, consistency, and amount of gastric drainage.
- Note the patient's tolerance of the procedure.

Nasogastric Tube Removal		
4/24/2019	0900	**PATIENT TEACHING/INTERVENTION:** Explained the procedure of NG tube removal to pt. Active bowel sounds heard in all 4 quadrants. NG tube clamped × 4 hr. Tolerating ice chips without nausea, vomiting, discomfort, or abdominal distention. NG tube removed without difficulty. Pt. taking small sips of water without c/o nausea. ______ **Carol Allen, RN**

NEWBORN IDENTIFICATION

Newborn identification is the process by which a newborn infant is identified and an individual health record established for the infant immediately following delivery. The identification process includes obtaining the footprints, fingerprints, or handprints of the newborn, and often the fingerprints of the mother, so that the infant can be properly identified if necessary. Armbands and ankle bands are also placed on the infant, mother, and father or significant other. Identification bands usually share a common identification number or code so that the infant and parent can be matched.

Essential Documentation

On the appropriate flow sheet or newborn identification record, the nurse should record the time and date of the entry. The newborn should have the mother's first and last names and the newborn's gender, boy or girl, written as an identifier on signage. The mother and baby should have corresponding ID bracelets with the mother's first and last names and the baby's gender (e.g., Smith Kate Boy), identification number, and barcode on each. There should be two sites of banding on the newborn. In the case of multiple births, a number should be placed in front of the mother's name, or a letter can be placed after mother's name (e.g., 1 Kate Smith, 2 Kate Smith, 3 Kate Smith or Smith Kate A, Smith Kate B). Communication tools among staff should be established, particularly if there are newborns with similar names. The record should have the date and time of the infant's birth; physical characteristics of the infant, including gender, length, weight, head circumference, hair and eye color, and any unique anatomical features such as birthmarks; time prints were recorded; who was present when prints were recorded and identification bands were applied; whether prints were taken from right, left, or both feet or hands; which finger the print was taken from; whether or not the mother's fingerprint was also recorded and which finger was printed; time when identification bands were applied; who received identification bands (mother, father, or significant other); which limbs (e.g., right leg, right wrist) identification bands were placed on; and any patient education that was performed at the time of newborn identification. Whether or not an identification photo was taken and where it is located in the chart should be noted.

It is important to use the proper hospital form when obtaining prints, along with the appropriate ink transferal device or ink pad. The nurse should be sure to double-check identification numbers on all identification bands to ensure that they match and to have another nurse witness the recording of the numbers on all the bands after they have been applied to both infant, mother, and father or significant other.

Newborn Identification		
3/1/2019	1400	**NURSING ASSESSMENT:** Baby girl Brown was delivered vaginally at 1312 on 3/1/2019 in Rm 32E (see separate note for delivery information). Infant is female, length $19\frac{1}{2}$ inches, weight 7 lb 4 oz, head circumference 35 cm. Fine, dark brown hair covers head, eyes are brown, no unique birth marks noted. ________
		NURSING INTERVENTION: Left footprint was obtained at 1324 on hospital form 1400e—newborn identification. Mother's left index fingerprint was recorded on same form at 1325. ID band number 13200564 was applied to infant's left wrist and left ankle at 1328. ID bands numbered 13200564 were also applied to mother's left wrist and father's left wrist at 1328. Mother, father, bedside nurse, and nurse Sheila Johnson were present when print was obtained and ID bands were applied. Security sensor armband was placed on infant's left bicep at this time. ________
		PATIENT/FAMILY EDUCATION: Parents were informed that security sensor will cause unit alarm, lock-down, and security team activation if infant is carried or otherwise conveyed beyond double doors at nurses' station. Parents had no questions about ID band procedure or security sensor and alarm system. ________
		NURSING INTERVENTION: ID photo was taken using unit's digital camera and a copy was printed and placed in identification section of infant's paper chart. ________
		________ **Geneva Thiel, RN**

PATIENT NONADHERENCE TO RECOMMENDED MEDICAL CARE

Occasionally, a patient does something—or fails to do something—that may contribute to an injury or explain the reason for nonresponsiveness to nursing and medical care.

Essential Documentation

The nurse needs to:

- Record the date and time of the entry.
- Document the patient's nonadherence to recommended medical care and the outcome. Although patients have the right to refuse medical and nursing care, it is important to be sure to document in the nurse's notes any behavior that runs counter to medical

instructions as well as the fact that the nurse informed the patient of the possible consequences of nonadherent actions.

- Document notification of the health care provider regarding patient behavior.

Patient Nonadherence		
8/31/2019	0800	**NURSING ASSESSMENT:** Pt. up and walking in hall without antiembolism stockings on. ______
		PATIENT TEACHING: Reminded pt. that stockings need to be put on before getting out of bed, before edema develops, to be most effective.
		NURSING ASSESSMENT: Pt. stated, "It's too early. I'll put them on after breakfast." ______
		NURSING INTERVENTION: Dr. Somers notified and told of situation. No orders given. Dr. Somers will talk with pt. this afternoon. ______
		______ **Casey Adams, RN**

SELECTED READINGS

Adelman, J., Aschner, J., Schechter, C., Angert, R., Weiss, J., Rai, A., ... Southern, W. (2015). Use of temporary names for newborns and associated risks. *Pediatrics, 136,* 327–333.

Freeman, G. (2016). Patient ID a top source of error; newborns high risk. *Healthcare Risk Management, 38*(12), 133–144.

Gray, J. E., Suresh, G., Ursprung, R., Edwards, W. H., Nickerson, J., Shiono, P. H., ... Horbar, J. (2006). Patient misidentification in the neonatal intensive care unit: Quantification of risk. *Pediatrics, 117,* e43–e47.

Hurlburt, J. (2018). *Leading hospital improvement: Newborn identification changes recommended to avoid misidentification.* Retrieved from https://www.jointcommission.org/the_view_from_the_joint_commission/newborn_identification_changes_recommended_to_avoid_misidentification

Jones, S. (2016). *The non-compliant versus non-adherent patient.* Retrieved from https://www.capphysicians.com/articles/noncompliant-vs-non-adherent-patient

Lyman, B., Peyton, C., & Healey, F. (2018). Reducing nasogastric tube misplacement through evidence-based practice: Is your practice up-to-date? *American Nurse Today, 3*(11), 6–11.

Taylor, S. J., Allan, K., Clemente, R., Marsh, A., & Toher, D. (2018). Feeding tube securement in critical illness: implications for safety. *British Journal of Nursing, 27*(18), 1036–1041.

The Joint Commission. (2015). Temporary names put newborns at risk. *Quick Safety, 17,* 1–2.

The Joint Commission. (2018). Distinct newborn identification requirement. *R3 Report. Requirement, Rationale, Reference, 17.* Retrieved from https://www.jointcommission.org/assets/1/18/R3_17_Newborn_identification_6_22_18_FINAL.pdf

Wallace, S. C. (2016). Newborns pose unique identification challenges. *Pennsylvania Patient Safety Advisory, 13,* 42–49.

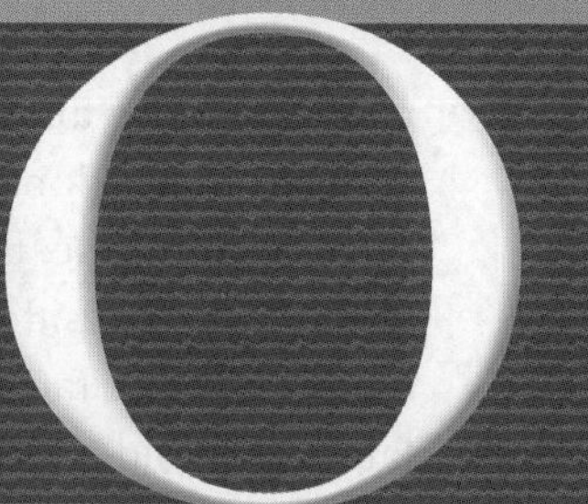

ORGAN DONATION

A federal requirement enacted in 1998 requires facilities to report deaths to the regional organ procurement organization (OPO). This regulation was enacted so that no potential donor would be missed. The regulation ensures that the family of every potential donor will understand the option to donate.

Collection of most organs, including the heart, liver, kidney, and pancreas, requires that the patient be pronounced brain dead but kept physically alive until the organs are harvested. Tissue, such as eyes, skin, bone, and heart valves, may be taken after death.

The nurse should follow the facility's policy for identifying and reporting a potential organ donor. Contact the local or regional OPO when a potential donor is identified. Typically, a specially trained person from the regional OPO will speak with the family about organ donation. The OPO coordinates the donation process after a family consents to donation.

Essential Documentation

Documentation will vary depending on the role of the nurse and the stage of the organ donation process. Separate documentation for each stage must be done. The date and time of each note must be recorded. The date and time that the patient is pronounced brain dead and the health care provider's discussions with the family about the prognosis must be included in the documentation. (See "Brain death", pages 49 to 51.) If the patient's driver's license or other documents indicate the patient's wish to donate organs, the nurse must place copies in the medical record and document that it was done. The individual who contacts the regional OPO must document the conversation, including the date and time, the name of the person contacted, and instructions given. If the bedside nurse was part of the discussion about organ donation with the family, the nurse documents who was present, what the family was told and by whom, and their response. Document the nursing care of the donor until the time of transfer to the operating room for organ procurement. Document teaching, explanations, and emotional support given to the family.

Organ Donation		
11/12/2019	0900	**PATIENT TEACHING:** At 0815. Dr. A. Silverstone explained to the family of Peter Hubbard that the patient was brain dead and the prognosis. Mary Hubbard, wife; Ron Hubbard, son; Mary Rundell, daughter; and Patty Fisher, RN, bedside nurse, were present. Family asked about organ donation. Wife stated, "My husband has spoken about donating his organs if this type of situation ever occurred." Patient's driver's license confirms patient's request for organ donation. Copy of license placed in Peter Hubbard's medical record. Dr. Silverstone explained the criteria for organ donation and the process to the family. Mrs. Hubbard stated "she would like more information from the regional organ procurement organization (OPO)." OPO was contacted by Patty Fisher, RN, at 0830, and the intake information was taken by Rhonda Tierney, RN. ______
		NURSING INTERVENTION: Appointment made for today at 1000 for OPO coordinator to meet with family in conference room on nursing unit.
		PATIENT/FAMILY TEACHING: All family questions were answered and emotional support provided. Chaplain paged per family request. ______
		______ **Patty Fisher, RN**

OSTOMY CARE

An ostomy is a surgically created opening used to replace a normal physiologic function. Ostomies are used to facilitate the elimination of solid or liquid waste or to support respirations if placed in the trachea. The type and amount of care an ostomy requires depend on the output and location of the stoma. The nurse is responsible for providing ostomy care and assessing the condition of the stoma. Provide patient and family teaching regarding ostomy and peristomal skin care. The nurse may also need to help the patient adapt to the care and wearing of an appliance while helping with acceptance of a change in body image.

Essential Documentation

Record the time of ostomy care. Describe the location of the ostomy and the condition of the stoma, including size, shape, and color. Chart the condition of the peristomal skin, noting any redness, irritation, breakdown, bleeding, or other unusual conditions. Note the character of drainage, including color, amount, type, and consistency. Record the type of appliance used, appliance size, and type of adhesive used. Document patient and family teaching, describing the teaching content. Record the patient's response to self-care, and evaluate learning progress. Some facilities use a patient-teaching record to document patient teaching.

Ostomy Care		
06/11/2019	1000	**NURSING ASSESSMENT:** Ostomy located in left upper abdomen. Appliance removed. Minimal amount of dark brown fecal material in appliance. Stoma is 4 cm in diameter, round, beefy red in color, no drainage or bleeding. Skin surrounding stoma is pink and intact. ______ **NURSING INTERVENTION:** Karaya ring applied to skin surrounding stoma after applying skin adhesive. New appliance snapped onto ring. Patient helped measure stoma and applied skin adhesive. ________ **PATIENT TEACHING:** Patient currently reading material on ostomy care. Discussed proper measurement of stoma and cutting hole in Karaya ring to proper size. Patient states understanding of teaching and agrees to cut skin barrier with next change. ________________ ______________________________ **Dawn March, RN**

OVERDOSE, DRUG

Consumption of drugs in an amount that produces a life-threatening response is a drug overdose, sometimes also called an *ingestional error*. The overdose can be intentional, such as a suicide gesture or attempt, or accidental, such as overmedicating with pain medicine. Either situation requires the nurse's prompt and skilled actions. If the nurse suspects that the patient has taken a drug overdose, the health care provider is immediately contacted, and measures are taken to ensure the patient's airway, breathing, and circulation are not compromised. Other interventions focus on identifying, removing, neutralizing, and enhancing excretion of the drug.

Essential Documentation

The date and time of the admission; a brief medical history, including allergies, current drugs, and history of substance abuse, if possible; the type and amount of drug taken and the route of ingestion; and signs and symptoms exhibited are documented. The nurse performs a comprehensive assessment of the patient and documents the findings. The physical assessment should include the patient's vital signs, noting the character of respirations and pulse oximetry reading; cardiac rhythm; and the patient's mental status, including level of consciousness (LOC), orientation, and ability to follow commands. The neurologic assessment includes pupillary reaction, cranial nerve assessment, fine and gross motor activity, sensory functioning, and reflexes.

Any interventions implemented before arrival to the health care facility should be noted in the clinical record. The nurse documents the name of the health care provider notified, time of notification, orders given, and nursing interventions performed, such as administering reversal agents (naloxone [Narcan] and flumazenil [Romazicon]) or gastrointestinal decontaminants (activated charcoal, gastric lavage, cathartics, and whole-bowel irrigation), as well as supportive therapies. It is important that the nurse include the patient's response to the nursing interventions. If gastric emptying is performed, the character and contents of the return should be documented. Flow sheets may be used to document frequent assessments, vital signs, intake and output, intravenous (IV) therapy, and laboratory values. The nurse should provide and document patient and family teaching, including strategies to prevent future drug overdose and emotional support.

Drug Overdose

09/17/2019	0200	Patient admitted to ED by ambulance with suspected opioid overdose. EMTs stated "friend of patient's at the scene indicated the patient may have taken 'painkillers' prescribed to treat his cancer pain." ______ **NURSING INTERVENTION:** Stat toxicology screen, CBC, BUN, creatinine, electrolytes, and ABG obtained. ______ **NURSING ASSESSMENT:** Patient unresponsive to painful stimulation. VS: P 56, BP 100/50, SpO_2 100%, tympanic T 96.8°F, pupils pinpoint and nonreactive to light. Extremities flaccid, deep tendon reflexes absent. Patient has a #7.0 ETT—on 100% O_2 via ambu. Bilateral breath expansion present and breath sounds clear. ______ **NURSING INTERVENTION:** IV access established in right antecubital vein with 18G catheter on second attempt. 1000 mL NS infusing at 100 mL/hr. Naloxone (Narcan) 1 ampule IV push administered. See MAR. Patient immediately began moving extremities and coughing. See flow sheets for frequent VS, I/O, IV therapy, and labs. ______ ______ **Anthony Gasso, RN**

OXYGEN ADMINISTRATION

A patient will need oxygen therapy when hypoxemia results from a respiratory or cardiac emergency or an increase in metabolic function. The adequacy of oxygen therapy is determined by arterial blood gas (ABG) analysis, pulse oximetry monitoring, and clinical assessments. The patient's disease, physical condition, and age will help determine the most appropriate method of administration.

Essential Documentation

Note the time that the oxygen was administered, oxygen delivery device used, and oxygen flow rate. The nurse performs a cardiopulmonary assessment and records findings, including vital signs, skin color and temperature, respiratory effort, use of accessory muscles, breath sounds, and LOC. Signs of hypoxia may include a decreased LOC, increased heart rate, arrhythmias, restlessness, dyspnea, use of accessory muscles, flared nostrils, cyanosis, and cool and clammy skin. The ABG or pulse oximetry values are recorded. If a health care provider was notified, the name of the health care provider, time notified, orders given, and whether the health care provider came to see the patient is recorded. The patient's response to oxygen therapy and patient and family teaching and emotional support given are documented.

Oxygen Administration		
02/06/2019	1152	**NURSING ASSESSMENT:** At 1130 noted patient sitting upright, pale, diaphoretic, taking deep, labored respirations using accessory muscles with nasal flaring. O_2 currently at 2 L by nasal cannula. Patient only able to speak 1 to 2 words at a time, stated his breathing has been "getting shorter" over the last hour. P 124 and regular, BP 134/88, RR 22 and labored. Tympanic temp. 97.2°F. Skin cool and pale. Circumoral cyanosis noted. Normal heart sounds, wheezes heard posteriorly on expiration. Patient alert and oriented to time, place, and person but appears anxious and restless. SaO_2 87%. ________ **NURSING INTERVENTION:** Dr. Desmond notified of findings at 1140 and examined patient at 1145. Orders given. O_2 increased to 4 L by nasal cannula. Albuterol 2 puffs administered by MDI. ________ **NURSING ASSESSMENT:** Patient stated "I am breathing easier". ____ ________ **Mindy Pressler, RN**

Oxygen Administration (*continued*)		
02/16/2019	1230	P 92 and regular, BP 128/72. RR 16 and unlabored. SaO_2 96%. No use of accessory muscles noted. Skin warm and pink, lungs clear. Patient states he "is comfortable." The importance of immediately reporting any signs of SOB to the nurse was explained. ______ **PATIENT TEACHING:** Patient verbalized understanding. Per orders O_2 to be titrated to keep O_2 sat greater than 95%. ______ ______ **Mindy Pressler, RN**

SELECTED READINGS

Budinger, G. S. R., & Mutlu, G. M. (2013). Balancing the risks and benefits of oxygen therapy in critically Ill adults. *Chest, 143*(4), 1151–1162.

Kirkland-Kyhn, H., Martin, S., Zaratkiewicz, S., Whitmore, M., & Young, H. M. (2018). Ostomy care at home. *American Journal of Nursing, 118*(4), 63–68.

Martin, D. S., & Grocott, M. P. (2013). Oxygen therapy in critical illness: Precise control of arterial oxygenation and permissive hypoxemia. *Critical Care Medicine, 41* (2). 423–432.

National Institute on Drug Abuse. (2018, April). *Opioid overdose reversal with naloxone (Narcan, Evzio).* Retrieved from https://www.drugabuse.gov/related-topics/opioid-overdose-reversal-naloxone-narcan-evzio

Shoar, N. S., & Saadabadi, A. (2018). Flumazenil. *Stat Pearls* [Internet]. Retrieved from https://www.ncbi.nlm.nih.gov/books/NBK470180/

Siela, D. (2017). Oxygen requirements for acute and critically ill patients. *Critical Care Nurse, 37*(4), 58–70.

The Joint Commission. (2017). *Facts about the official "Do Not Use" list of abbreviations.* Retrieved from https://www.jointcommission.org/facts_about_do_not_use_list/

P

PACEMAKER, CARE OF PERMANENT

A pacemaker is implanted when the heart's natural pacemaker fails to work properly. It provides electrical impulses to the cardiac muscle as a means to stimulate contraction and support cardiac output.

Many types of pacemakers are available for use; the majority can be programmed to perform various functions. When caring for a patient with a pacemaker, it's important to know the type of pacemaker, its rate, and how it works. This information will help the nurse ensure that the pacemaker is functioning properly and detect complications more quickly. The patient should have a manufacturer's card with pacemaker information; his medical records may also contain this information. The nurse can obtain this information from the patient or the patient's family.

Essential Documentation

Chart the date of insertion, type of pacemaker (demand or fixed rate), rate of pacing, chambers paced, chambers sensed, how the pulse generator responds, and whether it is rate-responsive. If the patient knows the three- or four-letter pacemaker code, record it. Document the patient's apical pulse rate, noting whether it is regular or irregular. If the patient is on a cardiac monitor, place a rhythm strip in the chart. Electronic health records may automatically demonstrate patient's rhythm. Note the presence of pacemaker spikes, P waves, and QRS complexes and their relationship to each other. Ask the patient about and record symptoms of pacemaker malfunction, such as dizziness, fainting, weakness, fatigue, chest pain, and prolonged hiccups. Check the pacemaker insertion site and describe its condition. Assess and document the patient's understanding of the pacemaker.

Nursing Care of Patient with Permanent Pacemaker		
11/24/2019	1500	**NURSING ASSESSMENT:** Pt. admitted to Rm 327A. Admission history and physical completed. Pt. reports having a permanent DDD pacemaker with low rate set at 60, high rate set at 125, and AV interval of 200 msec. Pacemaker inserted 2008. AP 72 and regular, BP 132/84, RR 18, oral T 97.0°F. Pacemaker site in right upper chest w/ healed incision. Pt. denies any dizziness, fainting spells, chest pain, or hiccups. Has been feeling weak and fatigued recently but states he feels this is due to a flare-up of his ulcerative colitis. ________
		PATIENT TEACHING/EDUCATION: Pt. able to explain pacemaker function, how to take his pulse, signs and symptoms to report, and need to avoid electromagnetic interference. ________
		________ **Thomas Harkin, RN**

PACEMAKER, CARE OF TRANSCUTANEOUS

Completely noninvasive and easily applied, a transcutaneous pacemaker proves especially useful in an emergency. Large skin electrodes are placed on the patient's anterior and posterior chest; then they are connected to a pulse generator to initiate pacing.

Nursing care of the patient receiving temporary transcutaneous pacing includes proper lead placement and attachment, assessment of the patient's response and cardiac rhythm, and monitoring for possible pacemaker malfunction. Because external pacing may be uncomfortable for the conscious patient, a sedative should be given.

Essential Documentation

Chart the patient's heart rate and rhythm. Note the pacemaker rate and the output, in milliamperes (mA), at which capture occurs. Describe whether or not all QRS complexes are captured; record as a percentage (such as 100% capture). Place a rhythm strip showing pacemaker function in the chart, if available. Electronic health records may automatically demonstrate patient's rhythm. Describe the condition of the skin at the electrode sites and any skin care performed. Record the assessment of the patient, including skin color and temperature, mental status, and urine output. Document measures to reduce anxiety and provide comfort as well as the patient's response to these measures. Record patient teaching and emotional support given.

Nursing Care of Patient with Transcutaneous Pacemaker		
8/25/2019	1800	**NURSING ASSESSMENT:** Transcutaneous pacing continues as 100% paced beats with pacemaker set at rate of 68 and output 50 mA. BP 88/50, RR 16. Pt. awaiting placement of transvenous pacemaker. Skin around electrodes slightly red and intact. Pt. c/o some burning at electrodes with each paced beat. ______
		NURSING INTERVENTION: Pt. given Valium 5 mg P.O. for anxiety and discomfort. Reassuring pt. that he's being monitored closely in CCU and that he'll be receiving transvenous pacemaker shortly. ______
		______ **Karen Forbes, RN**

PACEMAKER, CARE OF TRANSVENOUS

Transvenous pacing is accomplished by threading a pacing wire through a vein, such as the subclavian, antecubital, femoral, or jugular vein, to the right atrium (for atrial pacing), right ventricle (for ventricular pacing), or both (for dual-chamber pacing). Some pulmonary artery catheters also have a lumen for a transvenous pacing electrode. The pacing wire is then connected to a pulse generator outside the body.

If the patient has a transvenous pacemaker, the nurse should monitor the patient for complications such as pneumothorax, hemothorax, cardiac perforation and tamponade, diaphragmatic stimulation, pulmonary embolism, thrombophlebitis, and infection. Sometimes a patient may begin to hiccup from irritation of the diaphragm and phrenic nerve due to dislocation of the lead.

Also, if the health care provider threads the electrode through the antecubital or femoral vein, venous spasm, thrombophlebitis, or lead displacement may occur. Nursing interventions also focus on protecting the patient from microshock, preventing and detecting pacemaker malfunction, and providing patient education.

Pacemaker malfunction often begins with the patient experiencing bradycardia and signs of decreased cardiac output. Often the first symptoms may include diaphoresis, syncope, or postural hypotension. The occurrence of symptoms depends on how dependent the patient is on the pacemaker and on the degree that the pacemaker is actually malfunctioning.

Essential Documentation

Chart the pacemaker's settings. Document the patient's vital signs and include a rhythm strip in the note. Place a rhythm strip in the chart whenever pacemaker settings are changed or when the patient is treated for a complication caused by the pacemaker. Electronic health records may automatically demonstrate patient's rhythm. Document interventions to prevent shock and pacemaker malfunction. Chart the assessment of the pacemaker insertion site, noting drainage, redness, and edema. Describe site care and document dressing changes. Include signs and symptoms of other complications, the name of the health care provider notified, the time of notification, orders given, nursing interventions, and the patient's response. Record patient and family education and emotional support rendered.

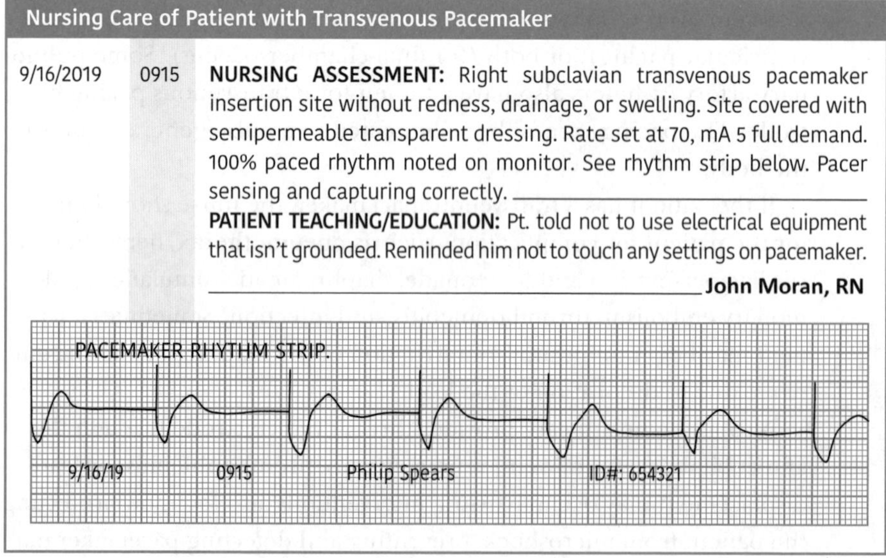

Nursing Care of Patient with Transvenous Pacemaker

9/16/2019	0915	**NURSING ASSESSMENT:** Right subclavian transvenous pacemaker insertion site without redness, drainage, or swelling. Site covered with semipermeable transparent dressing. Rate set at 70, mA 5 full demand. 100% paced rhythm noted on monitor. See rhythm strip below. Pacer sensing and capturing correctly. ______
		PATIENT TEACHING/EDUCATION: Pt. told not to use electrical equipment that isn't grounded. Reminded him not to touch any settings on pacemaker.
		______ **John Moran, RN**

PACEMAKER, INITIATION OF TRANSCUTANEOUS

A temporary pacemaker is usually inserted in an emergency. In a life-threatening situation, when time is critical, a transcutaneous pacemaker is the best choice. This device sends an electrical impulse from the pulse generator to the patient's heart by way of two electrodes, which are placed on the front and back of the patient's chest. Transcutaneous pacing is quick and effective, but it is only a temporary measure.

Essential Documentation

The nurse should chart the date and time transcutaneous pacing is initiated. Record the reason for transcutaneous pacing and the location of the electrodes. Chart the pacemaker settings. Note the patient's response to the procedure along with complications and interventions. If possible, obtain rhythm strips before, during, and after pacemaker use; whenever settings are changed; and when the patient is treated for a pacemaker-related complication. Electronic health records may automatically demonstrate patient's rhythm. Describe the frequency of paced or captured beats. During patient monitoring, record the patient's response to temporary pacing and note changes in the patient's condition. Record patient and family teaching, emotional support, and comfort measures provided.

Nursing Care in Initiation of Transcutaneous Pacemaker		
2/15/2019	1420	**NURSING ASSESSMENT:** Pt. with AP 48, BP 84/50, RR 16, arousable with verbal and physical stimulation, speech incomprehensible. Skin pale and clammy, peripheral pulses weak. Monitor shows bradycardia. Transcutaneous pacing initiated with posterior pacing electrode placed on left back, below scapula, and to the left of the spine and anterior electrode placed on left anterior chest over V_2 to V_5. Output set at 40 mA, rate of 60. Cardiac monitor shows 100% paced beats. AP 60, BP 94/60, RR 18. Pt. alert and oriented; no c/o chest pain, dyspnea, or dizziness. Peripheral pulses strong; skin warm and dry. ________ **PATIENT TEACHING/EDUCATION:** Explained to pt. that he may feel a thumping or twitching sensation during pacing and to report discomfort so that meds can be given. ________ ________ **Sally Hanes, RN**

PACEMAKER, INSERTION OF PERMANENT

A permanent pacemaker is a self-contained unit designed to operate for 3 to 20 years. In an operating room or cardiac catheterization laboratory, a surgeon implants the device in a pocket under the patient's skin in the pectoral region within the chest wall. A permanent pacemaker allows the patient's heart to beat on its own but prevents pacing from falling below a preset rate. Pacing electrodes can be placed in the atria, the ventricles, or both. Pacemakers may pace at a rate that varies in response to intrinsic conditions such as skeletal muscle activity and may also have antitachycardia and shock functions.

Candidates for permanent pacemakers include patients with myocardial infarction and persistent bradyarrhythmia and patients with complete heart block or slow ventricular rates stemming from congenital or degenerative heart disease or cardiac surgery. Patients who experience Stokes–Adams attacks, sick sinus syndrome, and those with Wolff–Parkinson–White syndrome may also benefit from a permanent pacemaker.

Essential Documentation

Record the time that the patient returned to the unit after insertion of the pacemaker. Document the type of pacemaker used, pacing rate, and health care provider's name. Record the pacemaker three-letter code. Verify that the chart contains information on the pacemaker's serial number, three-letter code, and its manufacturer's name. Note whether the pacemaker reduces or eliminates the arrhythmia and include other pertinent observations, such as the condition of the incision site and the percentage of paced or captured beats. Chart the patient's vital signs and level of consciousness every 15 minutes for the first hour, every hour for the next 4 hours, every 4 hours for the next 48 hours, and then once every shift, or according to facility policy or health care provider's order. Record these frequent assessments on a critical care or frequent vital signs flow sheet. Assess for and record signs and symptoms of complications, such as infection, lead displacement, perforated ventricle, cardiac tamponade, or lead fracture and disconnection. Record the name of the health care provider notified, the time of notification, interventions, and the patient's response. Document the patient and family teaching. This may be recorded on a patient-teaching flow sheet.

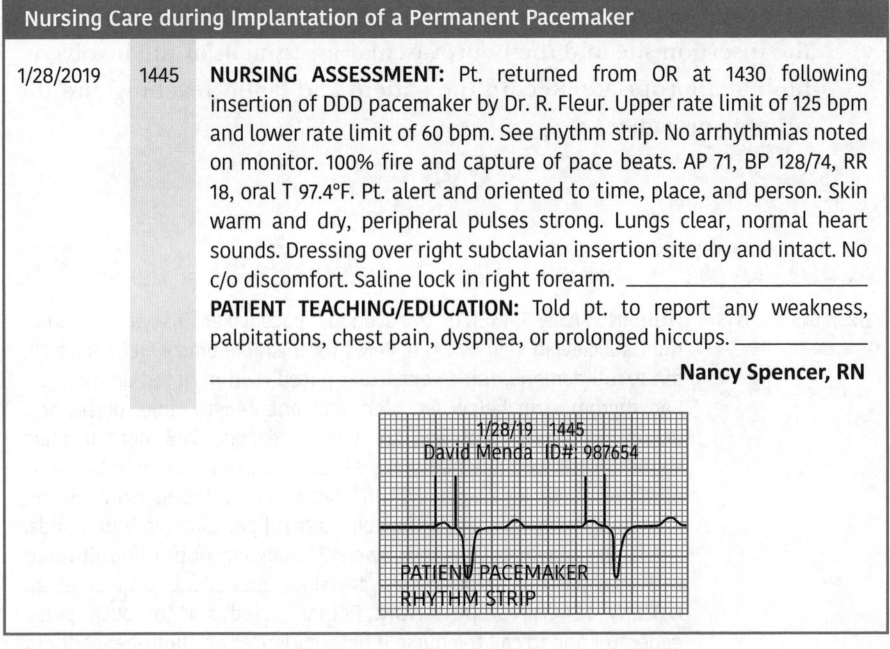

Nursing Care during Implantation of a Permanent Pacemaker

1/28/2019	1445	**NURSING ASSESSMENT:** Pt. returned from OR at 1430 following insertion of DDD pacemaker by Dr. R. Fleur. Upper rate limit of 125 bpm and lower rate limit of 60 bpm. See rhythm strip. No arrhythmias noted on monitor. 100% fire and capture of pace beats. AP 71, BP 128/74, RR 18, oral T 97.4°F. Pt. alert and oriented to time, place, and person. Skin warm and dry, peripheral pulses strong. Lungs clear, normal heart sounds. Dressing over right subclavian insertion site dry and intact. No c/o discomfort. Saline lock in right forearm. ________
		PATIENT TEACHING/EDUCATION: Told pt. to report any weakness, palpitations, chest pain, dyspnea, or prolonged hiccups. ________
		________ **Nancy Spencer, RN**

PACEMAKER, INSERTION OF TRANSVENOUS

A transvenous pacemaker is usually inserted in an emergency or during cardiac surgery by threading an electrode catheter through a vein, such as the brachial, femoral, subclavian, or jugular vein, and then into the patient's right atrium, right ventricle, or both. The electrodes are then attached to an external battery-powered pulse generator. Some pulmonary artery catheters have transvenous pacing electrodes.

Essential Documentation

The nurse should record the date and time that the pacemaker was inserted, the reason for pacing, and the location of the insertion site. Chart the pacemaker settings and the frequency of paced or captured beats. Document the patient's level of consciousness and cardiopulmonary assessment, including vital signs. Note the patient's response to the procedure, complications, and interventions. Include a rhythm strip in the note or the electronic health record will automatically record rhythm in chart. Document the assessment of the insertion site and the neurovascular assessment of the involved limb, if appropriate. Record the patient and family teaching and the support provided.

Nursing Care during Insertion of Transvenous Pacemaker		
2/25/2019	1115	**NURSING ASSESSMENT:** Transvenous pacemaker inserted through right subclavian vein by Dr. V. Peres for unstable bradycardia. Rate 70, mA 2, full demand. 100% ventricular paced rhythm noted on monitor. See rhythm strip below. Pt. alert and oriented to time, place, and person. Skin pale, cool, and dry. Lungs clear, no SOB, normal heart sounds, weak dorsalis pedis pulses, and no pedal edema bilaterally. AP 70, BP 98/58, RR 22, oral T 97.0°F. Radial pulses strong, hands warm, no numbness or tingling; pt. is able to feel light touch in both hands. Insertion site without redness, swelling, bleeding, or bruising. Covered with transparent semipermeable dressing. ___ **PATIENT TEACHING/EDUCATION:** Pt. instructed not to touch pulse generator and to call the nurse if he experiences any light-headedness or dizziness. Pt. resting in bed, chatting with wife. ___ ___ **Sam Mailor, RN**

PACEMAKER MALFUNCTION

Occasionally, a pacemaker fails to function properly. To determine whether the patient's pacemaker is malfunctioning, the nurse must know its mode of function and its settings. If a malfunction occurs, the nurse should notify the health care provider immediately, obtain a 12-lead ECG, call for a stat chest x-ray, begin continuous ECG monitoring, and prepare for temporary pacing.

Essential Documentation

The nurse should record the date and time of the malfunction. Record the patient's signs and symptoms, such as dizziness, syncope, irregular pulse, pale skin, dyspnea, chest pain, hypotension, heart rate below the pacemaker's set rate, palpitations, hiccups, and chest or abdominal muscle twitching. Place a cardiac rhythm strip in the chart, if possible, noting the percentage of captured beats or malfunctioning of the pacemaker, such as firing without capturing or the electronic health record will demonstrate patient heart rhythm. Note the name of the health care provider notified, the time of notification, and the orders given, such as obtaining a stat ECG, placing a magnet over a permanent pacemaker, and preparing for temporary pacing. If a temporary pacemaker malfunctions, chart the troubleshooting actions, such as repositioning the patient and checking connections and battery settings; the results of these efforts; and the patient's response. Be sure to include patient and family education and emotional support provided.

Nursing Care in Pacemaker Malfunction

7/30/2019	1135	**NURSING ASSESSMENT:** Pt. c/o feeling light-headed at 1100. P 54 and irregular, BP 92/58, RR 20, oral T 97.4°F. Skin pale, lungs clear, normal heart sounds, peripheral pulses palpable, no c/o chest pain or dyspnea. Pt. has VVI pacemaker set at rate of 68. Pt. attached to portable cardiac monitor; rhythm shows intermittent failure to capture. Rhythm strip attached below. ________
		NURSING INTERVENTION: Notified Dr. Steiger at 1105 and Dr. came to see pt. 12-lead ECG confirmed failure to capture. ________
		DIAGNOSTIC PROCEDURE: Stat CXR done at 1115. Results show lead fracture, which was reported to Dr. R. Steiger. Dr. Steiger to see pt. regarding pacemaker replacement. ________
		NURSING INTERVENTION: Pt. kept NPO. ________
		PATIENT TEACHING/EDUCATION: Situation explained to pt. and family. All questions answered. Reinforced to pt. that he was being monitored closely until he leaves for the OR. ________
		________ **Sarah Bigelow, RN**

PATIENT PACEMAKER RHYTHM STRIP

7/30/19 1135 Paul Trudeau ID#: 135789

PAIN MANAGEMENT

A person who feels pain typically seeks medical help not only because of a desire for relief, but also because the person believes the pain signals a serious problem. This perception produces anxiety, which in turn may increase the patient's perception of pain. The nurse's primary goal is to eliminate or minimize the patient's pain. The nurse can use a number of tools to assess pain. Always document the results of assessments. (See *Assessing and documenting pain,* pages 283 and 284.)

Interventions to manage pain include administering analgesics, providing emotional support and comfort measures, and using cognitive techniques to distract the patient. Patients with severe pain usually require an opioid analgesic. Invasive measures, such as epidural or patient-controlled analgesia, may also be required.

Essential Documentation

When charting pain levels and characteristics, the nurse should describe the location of the pain and note if it is internal, external, localized, or diffuse. Record whether the pain interferes with the patient's sleep or activities of daily living. In the chart, describe what the pain feels like in the patient's own words. Chart the patient's description of how long the pain lasts and how often it occurs. Record the patient's ranking of his pain using a pain rating scale.

Describe the patient's body language and behaviors associated with pain, such as wincing, grimacing, or restlessness. Note sympathetic responses commonly associated with mild to moderate pain, such as pallor, elevated blood pressure, dilated pupils, skeletal muscle tension, dyspnea, tachycardia, and diaphoresis. Record parasympathetic responses commonly associated with severe, deep pain, including pallor, decreased blood pressure, bradycardia, nausea and vomiting, dizziness, and loss of consciousness.

Chart situations that worsen the pain as well as interventions that relieve or decrease the pain, including heat, cold, massage, or drugs.

Document interventions taken to alleviate the patient's pain and the patient's responses to these interventions. Also, note patient teaching and emotional support provided.

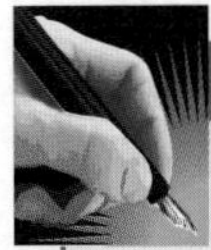

ACCUCHART

ASSESSING AND DOCUMENTING PAIN

Used appropriately, standard assessment tools such as the McGill-Melzack Pain Questionnaire and the Initial Pain Assessment Tool (developed by McCaffery and Beebe) provide a solid foundation for nursing diagnoses and care plans. If the health care facility does not use standardized pain questionnaires, the nurse can devise other pain measurement tools such as the pain flow sheet or the visual and graphic rating scales in the next section. Regardless of the pain assessment tool used, remember to document its use and include the graphic record in the patient's chart.

Pain Flow Sheet

Possibly the most convenient tool for pain assessment, a flow sheet provides a standard for reevaluating a patient's pain at regular intervals. It's also beneficial for patients and families, who may feel too overwhelmed by the pain experience to answer a long, detailed questionnaire.

If possible, incorporate the pain assessment into the flow sheet currently being used. Generally, the easier the flow sheet is to use, the more likely the nurse and the patient will use it.

PAIN FLOW SHEET

Date and time	Pain rating (0 to 10)	Patient behaviors	Vital signs	Pain rating after intervention	Comments
1/16/2019 0800	7	Wincing, holding head	186/88 98-22	2	Dilaudid 2 mg I.M. given
1/16/2019 1200	3	Relaxing, reading	160/80 84-18	0	Tylox tsp. P.O. given

Visual Analog Pain Scale

With a visual analog pain scale, the patient marks a linear scale containing words or numbers that correspond to the perceived degree of pain. The nurse should draw a scale to represent a continuum of pain intensity. Verbal anchors describe the pain's intensity; for example, "no pain" begins the scale and "pain as bad as it could be" ends it. Ask the patient to mark the point on the continuum that best describes the pain.

VISUAL ANALOG SCALE

No pain ——————————X—————————— Pain as bad as it could be

ASSESSING AND DOCUMENTING PAIN *(continued)*

Graphic Rating Scale

Other rating scales have words that represent pain intensity. The nurse should use one of these scales just as with the visual analog scale. Have the patient mark the spot on the continuum.

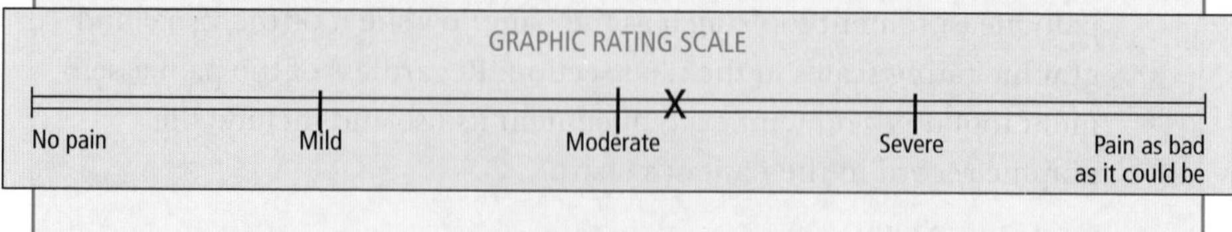

Nursing Care of Patient Pain		
3/19/2019	1600	**NURSING ASSESSMENT:** Pt. admitted to room 304 c/o severe pain in LLQ. Pt. states, "It feels like my insides are on fire." Pt. rates pain as 6 on a scale of 0 to 10. States pain keeps him from sleeping and eating. States he's been taking Percocet 2 tabs q4hr at home, but it's no longer providing relief. Pt. alert and oriented to time, place, and person. Curled in bed on left side, with arms wrapped around abdomen and moaning. Skin pale and diaphoretic, pupils dilated. ______ **NURSING INTERVENTION:** Dr. S. Martin notified. Dilaudid 2 mg ordered and given IV. P 92, BP 110/64, RR 22, oral T 99.0°F. ______ ______ **Kaylee Compton, RN**

PARACENTESIS

Paracentesis is a bedside procedure in which fluid from the peritoneal space is aspirated through a needle, trocar, or cannula inserted in the abdominal wall. Paracentesis is used to diagnose and treat massive ascites when other therapies have failed. Additionally, it is used as a prelude to other procedures, including radiography, peritoneal dialysis, and surgery. It is also used to detect intra-abdominal bleeding after traumatic injury and to obtain a peritoneal fluid specimen for laboratory analysis.

Essential Documentation

The nurse should document that the procedure and its risks have been explained to the patient and that a consent form has been signed. Chart patient teaching about the procedure. The facility may require documentation of patient education on a patient-teaching flow sheet. Record baseline vital signs, weight, and abdominal girth. Indicate that the abdominal area measured was marked with a felt-tipped marking pen.

The nurse should record the date and time of the procedure. Describe the puncture site and record the amount, color, viscosity, and odor of the aspirated fluid. Also, record the amount of fluid aspirated in the fluid intake and output record. Record the number of specimens sent to the laboratory. Note whether the wound was sutured and the type of dressing that was applied.

Record the patient's tolerance of the procedure, vital signs, and signs and symptoms of complications (such as shock and perforation of abdominal organs) that occur during the procedure. If peritoneal fluid leakage occurs, document that the notification of the health care provider, any orders given, nursing actions, and the patient's response.

The nurse should keep a record of the patient's vital signs and nursing activities related to drainage and dressing changes. Document drainage checks and the patient's response to the procedure every 15 minutes for the first hour, every 30 minutes for the next 2 hours, every hour for the next 4 hours, and then every 4 hours for the next 24 hours (or according to the facility's policy). This is best recorded on a flow sheet. Continue to document drainage characteristics, including color, amount, odor, and viscosity. Document daily patient weight and abdominal girth measurements after the procedure.

Nursing Care of Patient undergoing Paracentesis

Date	Time	Note
2/12/2019	0920	**PATIENT TEACHING/EDUCATION:** Procedure explained to pt. and consent obtained. ______ **DIAGNOSTIC PROCEDURE:** Dr. T. Novello performed paracentesis in RLQ. 1500 mL of cloudy pale-yellow fluid drained and sent to lab as ordered. Site sutured with one 3-0 silk suture. Sterile 4" × 4" gauze pad applied. ______ **NURSING ASSESSMENT:** No leakage noted at site. Abdominal girth 44" preprocedure and $42^3/_4$" postprocedure. VS and weight before and after procedure as per flow sheet. ______ **PATIENT TEACHING/EDUCATION:** Reinforced teaching related to the procedure and offered reassurances during the procedure. Pt. slightly anxious but resting comfortably in bed. ______ ______ **Carol Barsky, RN**

PARENTERAL NUTRITION ADMINISTRATION, LIPIDS

Lipid emulsions provide a source of calories and essential fatty acids. A deficiency in essential fatty acids can hinder wound healing, adversely affect the production of red blood cells and hormones, and impair prostaglandin synthesis. Typically given as separate solutions in conjunction with parenteral nutrition, lipid emulsions may also be given alone. They can be administered through a peripheral or central venous line.

Essential Documentation

Note the type of lipid solution, its volume, and the infusion rate. Document whether the lipids are being given peripherally or centrally, and note the location of the line. Record vital signs before starting the infusion, at regular intervals during the infusion (according to the facility's policy), and following the infusion. This is best recorded on a flow sheet. In the intake and output record, chart the amount of lipids infused. Document site care and describe the condition of the insertion site, cleaning the site, and the type of dressing applied. Also, record tubing and lipid solution changes. Monitor the patient for adverse reactions, and document observations, interventions, and the patient's response. Record patient teaching about lipids.

Nursing Care of Patient Receiving Parenteral Lipid Nutrition		
5/30/2019	1200	**NURSING ASSESSMENT:** P 92, BP 118/70, RR 23, oral T 98.4°F. ______ **NURSING INTERVENTION:** 500 mL of 10% lipids hung using new tubing with a 1.2 micron in-line filter at a rate of 60 mL/hr via infusion pump. Infusing via right subclavian CV line. See flow sheet for frequent VS assessments and I/O. Transparent dressing intact, site without redness, drainage, swelling, or discomfort. ______ **PATIENT TEACHING/EDUCATION:** Instructed pt. to report any pain or discomfort at insertion site. ______ ______ **David Felding, RN**

PARENTERAL NUTRITION ADMINISTRATION, TOTAL

Total parenteral nutrition (TPN) is the administration of a solution of dextrose, proteins, electrolytes, vitamins, trace elements, and (frequently) insulin in amounts that exceed the patient's energy expenditure, thereby achieving anabolism. Because this solution has about six times the solute concentration of blood, it requires dilution by delivery into a high-flow central vein to avoid injury to the peripheral vasculature. Typically, the solution is delivered to the superior vena cava through an indwelling subclavian vein catheter. Generally, TPN is prescribed for any patient who cannot absorb nutrients through the GI tract for more than 10 days.

Because TPN solution supports bacterial growth and the central venous (CV) line gives systemic access, contamination and sepsis are always a risk. Strict surgical asepsis is required during solution, dressing, tubing, and filter changes. Site care and dressing changes should be performed according to the facility's policy and whenever the dressing becomes wet, soiled, or nonocclusive. Tubing and filter changes should be performed every 24 hours or according to the facility's policy. Most facilities require that two nurses verify the contents of the TPN solution and the prescribed administration rate against the health care provider's order before hanging the solution.

Essential Documentation

Document the type and location of the CV line and the volume and rate of the solution infused. Record the amount of TPN infused on the intake and output record. Document site care, describing the condition of the insertion site, cleaning of the site, and the type of dressing applied. Many facilities document all of this information on an IV flow sheet. (See "IV flow sheet," page 227.) Monitor a patient receiving TPN for adverse reactions, such as hyperglycemia, hypoglycemia, air embolism, extravasation, phlebitis, pneumothorax, hydrothorax, septicemia, and thrombosis, and document observations, interventions, and the patient's response to them. Record patient teaching about TPN. When discontinuing a CV or peripheral IV line for TPN, record the date and time and the type of dressing applied. Also, describe the appearance of the infusion site.

Nursing Care of Patient Receiving Total Parenteral Nutrition		
8/31/2019	2020	**NURSING INTERVENTION:** 2 L bag of TPN hung at 2000. Infusing at 65 mL/hr via infusion pump through right subclavian CV line. ________ **NURSING ASSESSMENT:** Transparent dressing intact, and site is without redness, drainage, swelling, or tenderness. See I/O flow sheet for intake and output. ________ **PATIENT TEACHING/EDUCATION:** Reviewed reasons for TPN and answered pt.'s questions about its purpose. ________ ________ **Meg Callahan, RN**

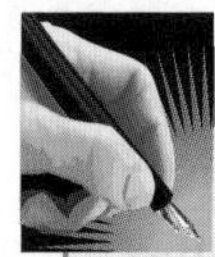

ACCUCHART

PCA FLOW SHEET

The form shown below is used to document the use of patient-controlled analgesia (PCA). PCA allows the patient to self-administer an opioid analgesic, as needed, within limits prescribed by the health care provider.

Patient name: Martin Smith Medical record #: 1234567 Date: 3/22/19

Medication: Morphine 50 mg in 50 ml (1 mg/ml)

	7a-7p Shift				7p-7a Shift	
Time (enter in box)	1200	1400			2000	
New cartridge inserted	OR					
PCA settings Lockout interval 10 (minutes)		10			10	
Dose volume 1 (ml/dose)___						
One-hour limit 10 mg___						
Basal dose 1 (mg/hr)___						
Respiratory rate	18	20			20	
Blood pressure	150/70	130/62			128/70	
Sedation rating 1. Wide awake 2. Drowsy 3. Dozing, intermittent 4. Mostly sleeping 5. Only awakens when stimulated	1	2			3	
Analgesia rts (1 – 10) Minimal pain – 1 Maximum pain – 10	7	8			6	
Additional doses given (optional doses)	3mL/OR					
Total ml delivered (total from ampule)	3	6			15	
ml remaining	27	24			15	

RN SIGNATURE (7a-7p SHIFT) Janet Green, RN Date 3/22/19

RN SIGNATURE (7p-7a SHIFT) Karen Singleton, RN Date 3/22/19

PATIENT-CONTROLLED ANALGESIA

Some patients receive opioids by way of a patient-controlled analgesia (PCA) infusion pump that allows patients to self-administer boluses of an opioid analgesic IV, subcutaneously, or epidurally within limits prescribed by the health care provider. To avoid overmedication, an adjustable lockout interval inhibits premature delivery of additional boluses. PCA increases the patient's sense of control, reduces anxiety, reduces drug use over the postoperative course, and gives enhanced pain control. Indicated for patients who need parenteral analgesia, PCA therapy is typically given to patients postoperatively, terminal cancer patients, and others with chronic diseases.

Essential Documentation

The nurse should document the name of the opioid used, lockout interval, maintenance dose, amount the patient receives when activating the device, and amount of opioid used during the shift. Record the patient's assessment of pain and pain relief and patient teaching performed. Document the patient's vital signs and level of consciousness according to facility policy. Record observations of the insertion site. See *PCA Flow Sheet,* page 288, for an example of documentation.

PATIENT REQUESTING ACCESS TO MEDICAL RECORDS

According to the Health Insurance Portability and Accountability Act (HIPAA) of 1996, the patient has the right to view and obtain copies of his or her medical records. Many states have since enacted laws allowing patients access to such records, and health care providers are required to honor such requests. HIPAA guarantees patients the right to obtain their medical records. The nurse should follow facility policy for provision of medical records to a patient.

PATIENT SELF-DOCUMENTATION OF CARE

Self-documentation can be effective for patients who must perform considerable self-care (those with diabetes, for example) or for those trying to discover what precipitates a problem such as chronic headaches.

By using self-documentation, a patient with diabetes may record information about his or her diet, insulin dose, self-tested blood glucose levels, and activity level. This information can help the patient avoid insulin reactions and delay, prevent, or even reverse complications of hyperglycemia or hypoglycemia. Self-documentation may provide valuable information for the health care provider or nurse, as well.

A patient with chronic headaches may be asked to record when a headache occurred, what warning signs were noticed, and what pain-relief measures were tried and their effect. Analyzing this information may help prevent headaches.

The patient can document entries on preprinted forms or in a journal. Such records can be used in both inpatient and outpatient care

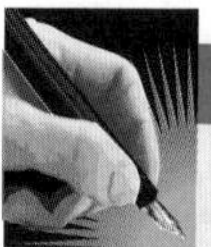

AccuChart

KEEPING A RECORD OF MONITORED ACTIVITIES

In many situations, the patient can provide information more accurately than a member of the health care team. A case in point is a patient who wears a Holter monitor to evaluate the effect of medication on his heart and his daily activities.

Keeping this in mind, some health care facilities prepare patient instructional materials to be used in conjunction with a diary-like chart (such as the one below), which the patient refers to and completes for the medical record.

Date	Time	Activity	Feelings
1/15/19	10:30 a.m.	Rode home from hospital in cab	Legs tired, felt short of
			breath
	11:30 a.m.	Watched TV in living room	Comfortable
	12:15 p.m.	Ate lunch, took propranolol	Indigestion
	1:30 p.m.	Walked next door to see neighbor	Felt short of breath
	2:45 p.m.	Walked home	Very tired, legs hurt
	3:00 to 4:00 p.m.	Urinated, took nap	Comfortable
	5:30 p.m.	Ate dinner slowly	Comfortable
	7:20 p.m.	Had bowel movement	Felt short of breath
	9:00 p.m.	Watched TV, drank one beer	Heart beating fast for about
			1 minute, no pain
	11:00 p.m.	Took propranolol, urinated,	Tired
		and went to bed	
1/16/19	8:15 a.m.	Woke up, urinated, washed	Very tired, rapid heartbeat
			for about 30 seconds
	10:30 a.m.	Returned to hospital	Felt better

settings. Depending on facility policy, these entries may or may not become a permanent part of the medical record. (See *Keeping a record of monitored activities,* page 290.)

Essential Documentation

The nurse should record the date and time of patient teaching about self-documentation. In the note, describe the instructions provided to the patient regarding measuring or timing or the symptoms to record and how frequently this should be done. Record the patient's response to this teaching. Describe the type of record keeping the patient is using. Document that the patient is able to verbalize understanding or give a return demonstration. Include any written materials given to the patient. Record that the patient knows who to call with questions or for emergency services.

Nursing Documentation of Patient Self -Management of Health Problem		
11/14/2019	1030	**PATIENT TEACHING/EDUCATION:** Pt. being discharged tomorrow morning. Taught pt. how to record his antihypertensive meds and daily BP readings. Wife brought in pt.'s electronic BP equipment from home. Readings correlate well with cuff readings. Pt. demonstrated proper technique for taking BP. Pt. correctly recorded date, time, BP reading, his position (seated or standing), any associated symptoms, and times meds taken in a notebook. Explained that home health nurse will review his notebook at each home visit. Reminded him to bring his notebook to his health care provider for follow-up visits. Pt. verbalized understanding of calling health care provider for SBP greater than 180 and DBP greater than 110 and to call EMS for s/s of stroke, such as difficulty speaking, numbness, difficulty moving, or weakness in arms or legs. ________ **Carolyn Buyers, RN**

PATIENT SELF–GLUCOSE TESTING

Patients with an established diagnosis of diabetes may prefer to use their own glucose meter to test his daily glucose levels. Per policy, the facility will require a health care provider's order stating that the patient may use his or her own glucose meter.

If the patient is permitted to use his or her own FDA approved glucose meter, the nurse must verify the patient's competency by having the patient demonstrate the procedure to ensure that the patient is performing it correctly and using the meter properly. Advise the patient to perform quality control testing on the meter each day. If the patient is using the meter for the first time during this admission, correlate the first glucose result from the meter with a fasting blood glucose level drawn by the facility's laboratory.

The nurse should confirm with the patient how to record his or her blood glucose levels and stress the importance of bringing results to all follow-up appointments. (See *Keeping a record of blood glucose levels* below) Review blood glucose levels that should be reported immediately. Frequency of testing is determined by whether the patient has type 1 or type 2 diabetes as well as the health care provider's instructions.

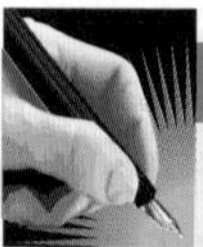

AccuChart

KEEPING A RECORD OF BLOOD GLUCOSE LEVELS

Recommendations for the best time of day to test the blood glucose level depend on the patient's medicine, meal times, and glucose control. On the chart below, the health care provider will check the times when the patient should test the glucose level. The health care provider may also suggest different goals, depending on the patient's situation.

Name: John Nichols **Dates:** 5/14/19-5/20/19

Time to test:	Fasting, before breakfast	1 to 2 hours after breakfast	Before lunch	1 to 2 hours after lunch	Before dinner	1 to 2 hours after dinner	Bedtime	3 a.m.
Target goal ranges:*	90-130 mg/dl	< 180 mg/dl	90-130 mg/dl	< 180 mg/dl	90-130 mg/dl	< 180 mg/dl		
Doctor's recommendation	90-110 mg/dl	160 mg/dl	90-110 mg/dl	160 mg/dl	90-110 mg/dl	160 mg/dl	100-130 mg/dl	70-100 mg/dl
Monday	93	159	95	147	97	158	118	84
Tuesday	88	158	98	143	101	161	112	81
Wednesday	89	161	103	156				
Thursday								
Friday								
Saturday								
Sunday								

*The target goals are based on recommendations from the American Diabetes Association. Talk with your doctor about what changes to make if your blood glucose levels are not within this range.

Essential Documentation

The nurse should verify the health care provider's order allowing the patient to use his or her glucose meter as well as the patient's ability to use his or her meter by demonstration. Compare the patient's first glucose meter reading with the fasting blood glucose level drawn by the facility's laboratory to correlate the patient's glucose meter accuracy. Then, record the date and time that the patient performs self-glucose monitoring. Be sure to document how often the patient tests the quality control of the meter. Also, document the results of the patient's glucose testing as ordered or per the facility's policy.

Nursing Documentation of Patient Self-Glucose Monitoring		
2/15/2019	1000	**PATIENT TEACHING/EDUCATION:** Pt. to use his own glucose meter to monitor glucose levels on discharge per order by Dr. James Wells using an Optium glucose meter. Pt. demonstrated his ability to properly use his meter. 0800 fasting blood glucose drawn by lab confirmed with pt.'s glucose meter results. Laboratory 0800 fasting blood glucose level was 93 mg/dl. Pt.'s glucose meter reading was 90 mg/dl. Pt. states he checks the quality of the meter every day in the morning and checks his blood glucose every day before meals, 2 hours after meals, and at bedtime and 0300 per dr.'s orders. Pt. verbalized how to record glucose levels and when to call the dr. or emergency services. ______ **Nancy Cooper, RN**

PATIENT TEACHING

Patient and caregiver teaching is essential for maintaining the patient's health, preventing or detecting early signs of complications, and promoting self-care and independence. Patient teaching is every patient's right in any setting. Teaching is most effective when it is specific to the patient's and family's physical, financial, emotional, intellectual, cultural, and social circumstances and when the patient and family are ready to learn, mentally alert, and free from discomfort and distraction.

The nurse should keep teaching sessions short and reinforce all instructions using verbal explanations, demonstrations, videos, and written materials. Evaluate the patient's understanding by asking the patient to restate material, answer questions, or give a return demonstration. Documentation of patient teaching is important and lets other

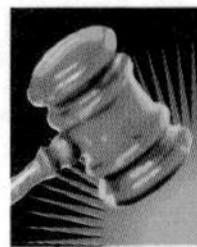

Legal Casebook

DOCUMENTING TEACHING

The nurse should always document the teaching provided to the patient and the family and their understanding of what was taught. The court in *Kyslinger v. United States (1975)* addressed the nurse's liability for patient teaching. In this case, a Veterans Affairs (VA) hospital sent a hemodialysis patient home with an artificial kidney. He eventually died (apparently while on the hemodialysis machine) and his wife sued, alleging that the hospital and its staff failed to teach either her or her late husband how to properly use and maintain a home hemodialysis unit.

After examining the evidence, the court ruled against the patient's wife, as follows: During those 10 months that plaintiff's decedent underwent biweekly hemodialysis treatment on the unit (at the VA hospital), both plaintiff and decedent were instructed as to the operation, maintenance, and supervision of said treatment. The Court can find no basis to conclude that the plaintiff or plaintiff's decedent were not properly informed on the use of the hemodialysis unit (*Kyslinger v. United States,* 1975).

health care team members know what the patient has been taught and what materials need to be reinforced. It also serves as a record if the patient files a lawsuit claiming injury due to lack of instruction. (See *Documenting teaching* above.)

Essential Documentation

The nurse should check facility policies and procedures regarding when, where, and how to document teaching. Despite their similar content, patient-teaching forms vary according to the health care facility. The forms may ask the nurse to document information by filling in blanks, checking boxes, or writing brief narrative notes. Typically, the nurse will need to document information about the patient's learning abilities, barriers to learning, learning needs, learning objectives, goals to be met, equipment or supplies used, specific content taught, teaching strategies, response to teaching, and skills to be acquired by the time of discharge. The nurse will also need to chart how the patient's

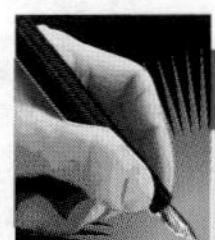

AccuChart

PATIENT-TEACHING RECORD

The nurse should use the model patient-teaching form below—for a patient with diabetes mellitus—as a guideline for documenting teaching sessions clearly and completely. The facility commonly has a form or place on the electronic health record for documentation of patient teaching and education, patient learning needs, patient learning objectives, teaching strategies, and evaluation of teaching and learning.

PATIENT TEACHING
Instructions for Patients with Diabetes

County Hospital, Waltham, MA

Bernard Miller
7 Main St.
Waltham, MA 04872

Admission date: 1/3/19 Anticipated discharge: 1/8/19 Diagnosis: TIA, type 2 DM

Educational assessment

Comprehension level

Ability to grasp concepts
- ☑ High
- ❑ Average
- ❑ Needs improvement

Comments: ______

Motivational level
- ☑ Asks questions
- ❑ Eager to learn
- ❑ Anxious
- ❑ Uncooperative
- ❑ Disinterested
- ❑ Denies need to learn

Comments: ______

Knowledge and skill levels

Understanding of health condition and how to manage it
- ❑ High (> 75% working knowledge)
- ❑ Adequate (50% to 75% working knowledge)
- ☑ Needs improvement (25% to 50% working knowledge)
- ❑ Low (< 25% working knowledge)

Comments: ______

Learning barriers
- ❑ Language (specify: foreign, impairment, laryngectomy, other): ______
- ❑ Vision (specify: blind, legally blind, other): ______
- ☑ Hearing (impaired, deaf)
  Need to speak loudly
- ❑ Memory
  - ❑ Change in long-term memory (specify): ______
  - ❑ Change in short-term memory (specify): ______
- ❑ Other (specify): ______
- ❑ No learning barriers noted

Instructor's initials: CW

Anticipated outcomes

Patient will be prepared to perform self-care at the following level:
- ☑ High (total self-care)
- ❑ Moderate (self-care with minor assistance)
- ❑ Minimal (self-care with more than 50% assistance)

PATIENT-TEACHING RECORD *(continued)*

Key

P =	Patient taught	N/A =	Not applicable	C =	Expressed denial, resistance
F =	Caregiver or family taught	A =	Asked questions	D =	Verbalized recall
R =	Reinforced	B =	Nonattentive, poor concentration	E =	Demonstrated ability

Date	1/4/19	1/5/19	1/5/19	1/5/19	1/6/19	1/7/19	1/7/19	1/8/19	
Time	1900	0800	1330	1830	1000	0800	1830	0800	
Assessed educational needs Assessment of patient's (or caregiver's) current knowledge of disease (include medical, family, and social histories)	A/CW								
Assessment of learner's reaction to diagnosis (verbal and nonverbal responses)	A/CW								
General diabetic education goals The patient (or caregiver) will:									
■ define diabetes mellitus.	P/A/CW	R/EG	D/ME					D/EG	
■ state hormone produced in the pancreas.	P/A/CW	R/EG	D/ME					D/EG	
■ identify three signs and symptoms of diabetes.	P/CW	R/EG	D/ME					D/EG	
■ discuss risk factors associated with diabetes.	P/CW	R/EG	D/ME					D/EG	
■ differentiate between type 1 and type 2 diabetes.	P/A/CW	R/EG	D/ME					D/EG	
Survival skill goals The patient (or caregiver) will:									
■ identify the name, purpose, dose, and time of administration of medication ordered.		P/EG	R/ME	D/LT				D/EG	
■ properly administer insulin.	N/A								
– draw up insulin properly.	N/A								
– discuss and demonstrate site selection and rotation.	N/A								
– demonstrate proper injection technique with needle angled appropriately.	N/A								
– explain correct way to store insulin.	N/A								
– demonstrate correct disposal of syringes.	N/A								
■ distinguish among types of insulin.	N/A								
– species (pork or recombinant DNA)	N/A								
– regular	N/A								
– NPH/Ultralente (longer acting)	N/A								

PATIENT-TEACHING RECORD *(continued)*

Key

P = Patient taught		N/A = Not applicable		C = Expressed denial, resistance			
F = Caregiver or family taught		A = Asked questions		D = Verbalized recall			
R = Reinforced		B = Nonattentive, poor concentration		E = Demonstrated ability			

Date	1/4/19	1/5/19	1/5/19	1/5/19	1/6/19	1/7/19	1/7/19	1/8/19
Time	1900	0800	1330	1830	1000	0800	1830	0800
■ properly administer mixed insulins.	N/A							
– demonstrate injecting air into vials.	N/A							
– draw up mixed insulin properly (regular before NPH).	N/A							
■ demonstrate knowledge of oral antidiabetic agents.								
– identify name of medication, dose, and time of administration.		P/EG	A/ME		D/EG	F/EG	R/LT	D/EG
– identify purpose of medication.		P/EG	A/ME		D/EG	F/EG	R/LT	D/EG
– state possible adverse effects.		P/EG	A/ME		D/EG	F/EG	R/LT	D/EG
■ list signs and symptoms, causes, implications, and treatments of hyperglycemia and hypoglycemia.		P/EG	A/ME			F/EG		D/EG
■ monitor blood glucose levels satisfactorily.								
– demonstrate proper use of blood glucose monitoring device.				P/LT	E/EG	E/EG	R/LT	E/EG
– perform fingerstick.				P/LT	E/EG	E/EG	R/LT	E/EG
– obtain accurate blood glucose reading.				P/LT	E/EG	E/EG	R/LT	E/EG
Healthful living goals The patient (or caregiver) will:								
■ consult with the nutritionist about meal planning.			P/ME	R/LT	A/EG			D/EG
■ follow the diet recommended by the American Diabetes Association.			P/ME	R/LT	A/EG			D/EG
■ state importance of adhering to diet.			P/ME	R/LT	A/EG			D/EG
■ give verbal feedback on 1-day meal plan.			P/ME	D/LT	A/EG			D/EG
■ state the effects of stress, illness, and exercise on blood glucose levels.			P/ME	D/LT	A/EG			D/EG
■ state when to test urine for ketones and how to address results.			P/ME	D/LT	A/EG			D/EG
■ identify self-care measures for periods when illness occurs.			P/ME	D/LT	A/EG			D/EG
■ list precautions to take while exercising.			P/ME	D/LT	A/EG			D/EG
■ explain what steps to take when patient doesn't want to eat or drink on proper schedule.			P/ME	D/LT	A/EG			D/EG
■ agree to wear medical identification (for example, a Medic Alert bracelet).			P/ME	A/LT				D/EG

PATIENT-TEACHING RECORD *(continued)*

Key

P	=	Patient taught	N/A =	Not applicable	C	=	Expressed denial, resistance
F	=	Caregiver or family taught	A =	Asked questions	D	=	Verbalized recall
R	=	Reinforced	B =	Nonattentive, poor concentration	E	=	Demonstrated ability

Date	1/4/19	1/5/19	1/5/19	1/5/19	1/6/19	1/7/19	1/7/19	1/8/19	
Time	1900	0800	1330	1830	1000	0800	1830	0800	
Safety goals The patient (or caregiver) will:									
■ state the possible complications of diabetes.	P/CW	R/EG		D/LT		F/EG		D/EG	
■ explain the importance of careful, regular skin care.	P/CW	R/EG		D/LT		F/EG		D/EG	
■ demonstrate healthful foot care.	P/CW	R/EG		D/LT		F/EG		D/EG	
■ discuss the importance of regular eye care and examinations.	P/CW	R/EG		D/LT					
■ state the importance of oral hygiene.	P/CW	R/EG		D/LT					
Individual goals									
Initial Signature CW Carol Witt, RN, BSN									
EG Ellie Grimes, RN, MSN									
ME Marianne Evans, RN									
LT Lynn Tata, RN, BSN									

learning was evaluated, such as by return demonstration or verbalization of understanding. Before discharge, document the patient's remaining learning needs, post-test, and note whether printed material or other patient-teaching aids were provided.

See *Patient-Teaching Record* (video, digital, or electronic), pages 295 to 298, for an example of how to document patient education.

PATIENT TEACHING, PATIENT'S REFUSAL OF

Although the Patient's Bill of Rights clearly outlines patients' right to receive information about their condition and treatment, and the Joint Commission requires that the patient and the family be provided with education, occasionally there will be a patient who does not want to be taught. If possible, the nurse should try to determine the reason for the patient's refusal. The nurse may be able to help the patient overcome some of the barriers to learning or provide instruction to other members of the family.

Essential Documentation

If a patient does not want to be taught, the nurse should be sure to document the incident. Include the patient's exact words in quotes. If the patient provides a reason for not wanting to be taught, include that information as well. Note whether teaching was provided to another family member or caregiver. Describe specifically what was taught, how it was taught, and the person's response to the teaching. Record the name of the health care provider who was notified of the patient's refusal to be taught.

Nursing Documentation of Patient Refusal of Teaching		
7/22/2019	1320	**FAMILY TEACHING/EDUCATION:** When giving pt. his meds at 1230, attempted to explain what each one was for. Pt. waved me away with his hands stating, "Tell my wife when she comes in. That's her department." Wife came in to visit at 1300 and was willing to learn about pt.'s meds. Gave her written information for each drug the pt. is taking. Reviewed indications for each drug, the dose, frequency, and adverse effects. Wife verbalized understanding of each med. and made out an appropriate schedule for giving her husband his meds at home. Notified Dr. G. Smith of pt.'s unwillingness to be taught. ________ **Thomas Daily, RN**

PATIENT THREAT OF SELF-HARM

A threat of self-harm may come as a refusal of care, a threat to injure oneself, or a threat to commit suicide. The best way to prevent self-harm is early recognition and treatment of depression and other mental illnesses, including substance abuse. (See "Suicidal intent," pages 384 to 386, for specific clues to monitor in a hospitalized patient who is at risk for self-harm or suicide.)

When a patient threatens or tries to harm himself, the nurse has a duty to protect him from harm. The nurse should use communication skills to try to calm the patient. Remove potentially harmful objects from the immediate area. If the patient is holding a dangerous object and is threatening to harm himself, send a coworker to call security, the nursing supervisor, and the patient's health care provider. Do not turn your back on the patient and stay with the patient until assistance arrives. If one-to-one observation is ordered, someone must stay with the patient at all times. Administer medications, as ordered. Restraints should be used as a last resort, according to the facility's policy.

Essential Documentation

The nurse should record the date and time of the entry. Record, in the patient's own words, his threat to harm himself. Objectively describe any behaviors that indicate a desire for self-harm. Note all steps taken immediately to protect the patient from harm, such as one-to-one observation and removal of any potential weapons from the immediate environment. Chart the names of the health care provider, nursing supervisor, and security officer, and who was notified and the time of notification. Document their responses, nursing interventions, and the patient's response. Record any explanations given to the patient and efforts to reduce anxiety.

Nursing Documentation of Patient Refusal of Teaching		
1/1/2019	1655	**NURSING ASSESSMENT:** Heard thumping noise in room at 1625 and found pt. beating his fist against wall. Asked pt. to stop beating right fist and tell me what was bothering him. Pt. replied, "I'm better, and my wife doesn't visit. If I was hurt, maybe she would visit." Asked pt. to sit on his bed and he complied. Sat on chair across from pt. and listened as he spoke of family problems. Pt. agreed to talk with social worker. Pt. able to move fingers of right hand, no bruising noted, no c/o pain. ________
		NURSING INTERVENTION: Called Meg Watkins, CNA, to sit with pt. and talk to him while doctor was called. Spoke with Dr. Sterling at 1635 who agreed to referral to social worker. Dr. Sterling will be by to see pt. at 1700. Andrew O'Toole, social worker, called at 1640 and will be by immediately to see pt. Will have CNA stay with pt. until social worker and doctor arrive. CNA instructed to speak calmly with pt. and to call nurse immediately if pt. resumes harmful behaviors.
		________ **Maria Perez, RN**

PATIENT THREAT TO HARM ANOTHER

When a patient threatens to harm someone else—whether verbally or by making threatening gestures—quick action is needed because a threat can turn to violence. The nurse should follow the facility's policy for dealing with a patient who threatens to harm someone else. Remove the person being threatened from the immediate area.

Use communication skills to calm the patient and reduce agitation. Call the health care provider, nursing supervisor, and security to inform them of the patient's threats. Some facilities use a specific code, such as "Mr. Strong," that can be announced throughout the facility to alert others that help is needed. Stay with the patient. If your own safety is threatened, have another coworker stay with you if necessary. Assess the patient for physical and psychosocial triggers to violence. Share the findings with the health care provider and nursing supervisor.

Essential Documentation

Chart the location of the incident. Describe the threat, quote exactly what the patient said, and record threatening behaviors or gestures. Record the immediate interventions and the patient's response. Chart the names of the people who were notified, such as the health care provider, nursing supervisor, and security; the time of notification; and their responses. Include the assessment results and the people with whom results were shared. Record any changes in the care plan. Do not name another patient in the patient's chart; this violates confidentiality. Use the word "roommate" or "visitor," or give a room and bed number to describe the person threatened.

The nurse should complete an incident report, repeating the exact information that is in the nurse's note. Include names, addresses, and telephone numbers of witnesses. This is the place to document the name of the threatened person.

Nursing Documentation of Patient Threat to Harm Another

5/29/2019	0315	**NURSING ASSESSMENT:** Pt. pacing back and forth in room at 0300, muttering phrases such as "I'll take care of it my way. I'll take care of him real good," while punching one hand into the other. Pt. alert, not oriented to time and date. Face red, diaphoretic, draws away from touch. Unable to obtain vital signs. ______ **NURSING INTERVENTION:** Pt.'s roommate moved to another room. At 0310 Dr. Chi, nursing supervisor Ron Hardy, RN, and security officer Tom Gulden were notified of pt.'s threats toward his roommate. ______ **Carla Aiken, RN**
5/29/2019	0345	**NURSING INTERVENTION:** Dr. Chi, Mr. Hardy, and Mr. Gulden arrived on unit at 0320. Assessment findings shared with them. ______ **PATIENT ASSESSMENT:** Pt. less agitated. Assisted back to bed. P 88 and regular, BP 136/94, RR 32. ______ **NURSING INTERVENTION:** Pt. given 1 mg Ativan IV as ordered by physician, Dr. Chi. ______ **Carla Aiken, RN**

PATIENT TRANSFER TO LONG-TERM CARE FACILITY

Most older adults are cared for at home, either by themselves or by their families. However, as many as 25% will need long-term care (LTC) assistance in their later years. Several types of LTC facilities are available. An assisted living facility provides meals, sheltered living, and some medical monitoring. This type of facility is appropriate for someone who does not need continuous medical attention.

An intermediate care facility provides custodial care for individuals unable to care for themselves due to mental or physical infirmities. Intermediate care facilities provide room, board, and regular nursing care. Physical, social, and recreational activities are provided, and some facilities have rehabilitation programs.

A skilled nursing facility provides medical supervision, rehabilitation services, and 24-hour nursing care by registered nurses, licensed practical nurses, and nurses' aides for patients who have the potential to regain function.

Essential Documentation

In the note, the nurse should record the date and time of the transfer, the health care provider's name, and that transfer orders were written. Note the long-term care facility's name and the name of the nurse who received the verbal report. Note that discharge instructions were written and that a copy was discussed with the patient and given to him. Have the patient sign a personal belongings form acknowledging that he has all his belongings. Remember to record that the form was completed and placed in the medical record. In the note, describe the condition of the patient at discharge, including vital signs, descriptions of wounds, and tubes or other equipment that is still in place. Record the time of discharge, who accompanied the patient, the mode of transportation, and the name of the person at the long-term care facility who will receive the patient. Indicate that the medical record was copied and sent with the patient or that electronic health records were sent.

Document that transfer forms have been completed. Also, indicate that one copy is being sent to the receiving facility. (See *Referral form*, pages 303 to 305.)

The transfer form may contain the following information:

- demographic patient information
- financial information

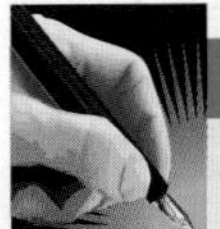

AccuChart

REFERRAL FORM

Documentation of the patient's condition before transfer and adequate communication between nursing staffs ensure continuity of nursing care and provide legal protection for the transferring facility and its staff. Referral forms such as the one below contain basic information about the patient and his care.

REFERRAL FORM

PATIENT INFORMATION

Last Name: Tomlin MR#: 1234
First Name: Vera MR#:
Address: 123 Main St.
City: Newtown State: VA Zip: 22222
County: Marital Status: W
Telephone: (123) 456-7890 S.S. #: 111-22-3333
Age: 90 Sex: F Height: 5'3" Weight: 126# DOB: 2/8/16
Adm. date: 2/26/19 Discharge date: 3/4/19

FINANCIAL INFORMATION

Primary: Medicare #:
Medicaid: County:
Policy #: Group #:
Secondary:
Precert #:
Level of Care: ❑ CORF ❑ ICF ❑ SNF ❑ Rehab Hospital ☑ Assisted ❑ Home Health ❑ ICF-MR

MEDICAL INFORMATION

Primary Dx: (date) Fx left arm 2/26/19
Secondary Dx: Type 2 DM
Surgery: (date) 2/27/19 open reduction
Allergies: none
Prior functional status: independent
Advance Directives: ☑ Living Will ☑ Power of Attorney ☑ DNR ❑ Legal Guardian ❑ PASSAR ❑ Level of Care

FAMILY or GUARDIAN

Last Name: Tomlin
First Name: Evelyn
Relationship: daughter
(H)#: (123) 456-7890 (W)#:

SERVICES REQUIRED

☑ PT ❑ OT ❑ ST ❑ IV. Therapy ❑ Hook Up
❑ Skilled Nursing ❑ Social Services ❑ Pain Management
❑ Home Healt ❑ Aid ❑ RT ❑ Wound Management
❑ Enteral Fdgs. ❑ TPN ❑ Nut. Tx. ❑ Palliative Care ❑ Hospice
❑ Dialysis: ❑ Peritoneal ❑ Hemo ❑ Ventilator Weaning/ Maintenance
Day/week:
Location:
Established Post Hospital LOS: ☑ < 30 days ❑ Other ❑ > 30 days

AGENCY ACCEPTING REFERRAL

Name: The Oaks Assisted Living Facility
Contact: Cathy O'Rourke, RN
Phone: (123) 987-6543 FAX:
Name:
Contact:
Phone: FAX:

PHYSICIAN

MD ordering: Dr. S. Chang Phone:
MD to follow: Dr. A. Meadows Phone:
Other: Phone:
Prognosis: good

To the best of my knowledge, all information provided about the individual is a true and accurate reflection of the patient's needs. I certify that inpatient care is required at: Level: ❑ Skilled ☑ Intermediate

Physician Signature: Dr. S. Chang
Date signed: 3/5/19

REFERRAL FORM *(continued)*

Patient Name: Vera Tomlin

LAB ORDERS

Labs: ______

Call or FAX results to: ______
Phone: ______ FAX: ______

Labs: ______

Call or Fax results to: ______
Phone: ______ FAX: ______

GENERAL PHYSICIAN ORDERS

PT to left arm
1800-cal ADA diet
DNR
Activity as tolerated

Home Medications	Last Dose Given	Dosage	Route	Frequency	Dosing Times	Start Date	End Date
Glucotrol	3/4/19 0730	5 mg	PO	daily	0730		
Lasix	3/4/19 0730	10 mg	PO	daily	0730		

❑ HIVAT (see Final HIVAT Script)

Comments/Delivery: ______

PHYSICAL THERAPY NOTES/PLAN

Assist for transfers supine to sit: ❑ Max ❑ Mod ❑ Min ❑ Contact Guard ❑ Superv ❑ Verbal Cue ❑ Tactile Cue ☑ Independ

Assist for transfers sit to stand: ❑ Max ❑ Mod ❑ Min ❑ Contact Guard ❑ Superv ❑ Verbal Cue ❑ Tactile Cue ☑ Independ

Ambulated ______ feet with: ❑ Walker ❑ Crutches ❑ Quad cane ❑ Straight cane ❑ W/o device ❑ Nonambulatory ❑ W/wheels ❑ W/platform attachments

Wit❑ assistance needed: ❑ Max ❑ Mod ❑ Min ❑ Contact Guard ❑ Superv ❑ Verbal Cue ❑ Tactile Cue ☑ Independ

Weight Bearing Status: ❑ NWB ❑ TDNWB ❑ TDWB ❑ PWB ❑ WBAT ❑ FWB ❑ On whic❑ leg: ❑ Right ❑ Left ❑ Both

Plan: strengthen left arm ❑ Therapy EX ❑ Bed Mobility Plan ❑ Transfer Training ❑ Gait Training

Goal: regain function left arm Demonstrates understanding of home safety precautions ☑ Yes ❑ No

PT Additional Comments:

Signature: Mary Jones Title: PT Phone: (123) 234-8290 Date: 3/4/19

REFERRAL FORM *(continued)*

Patient Name: Vera Tomlin

ASSESSMENT

Cardio-pulmonary	BP 148/84 Pulse 88 Temp 97.0°F Resp 22	☐ Oxygen Rate ____ Method ____ ☐ Secretions (describe): ____ ☐ Tracheostomy Size: ____	☐ Chest Tube(s) ☐ Vent Settings Type: ____	☐ CXR (date): ____ ☐ TB (date): ____
Nutrition and Hydration	Diet 1800 cal ADA Consistency regular ☐ Teeth ☐ No teeth ☑ Dentures type upper/lower ☐ Dentures wit☐ patient	☑ Feeds self ☐ Assist feed ☐ Total feed ☐ Hyperalimentation ☐ Feeding tube type ____ Date inserted ____	☐ Dehydration ☐ Edema ☐ Nausea ☐ Vomiting ☐ Dysphagia ☐ Poor appetite	Access device: ____ Insertion date: ____ Last flushed: ____

	VISION	HEARING	SPEECH	COMFORT	COMMENTS
Sensory-Comfort	☑ Adequate ☐ Poor ☐ Blind ☑ Glasses ☐ Contacts	☑ Adequate ☐ Poor ☐ Deaf ☐ Aid in ___ ear	☑ Good ☐ Difficult ☐ Unable Language: ____	Pain? ☐ Yes ☑ No Where? When?	

	MENTAL STATUS	BEHAVIOR	SUPPORTS
Pyscho-social	☑ Alert ☐ Lethargic ☐ Comatose ☐ Oriented ☐ Disoriented ☐ Confused ☐ Anxious	☐ Wanders ☑ Cooperative ☐ Combative ☐ Forgetful ☐ Sleep Problems ☐ Other (specify) ____	Supports: daughter - Evelyn Tomlin Safety:

	BLADDER	BOWEL	TOILETING	
Elimination	☑ Continent ☐ Incontinent ☐ Retention ☐ Frequency ☐ Dribbling	☑ Continent ☐ Incontinent ☐ Constipation ☐ Diarrhea ☐ Last BM: 3/4/19	☑ Independent ☐ Dependent ☐ Toilet ☐ Ostomy Type ____ Appliance ____	☐ Bedpan ☐ Catheter Type ____ Size ____ Date inserted: ____

Skin
Skin intact? ☑ Yes ☐ No
Describe any impairments: Incision left upper arm intact, healing well

		INDEPENDENT	ASSIST	TOTAL DEPENDENT	EQUIPMENT/# PERSONS USED
Hygiene	Oral Care	✓			
	Bathing		✓		needs help of 1 until arm heals
Mobility	Dressing		✓		
	Wheelchair				
	Transfer	✓			
	Ambulation	✓			

☐ Amputation ☐ Contractures ☐ Paralysis ☐ Paresis ☐ Other

	Test	Date	Result	Test	Date	Result	Test	Date	Result	
Labs										Isolation Precautions? Last culture date: Results:

- receiving facility information
- medical information, including diagnoses, surgeries, allergies, laboratory test values, and advance directives
- family contacts
- services needed, such as physical, occupational, or speech therapy; dialysis; or wound management
- health care provider's information and orders
- medication information, including last dose given
- assessment of body systems
- ability to perform activities of daily living

PATIENT TRANSFER TO SPECIALTY UNIT

Specialty units provide continuous and intensive monitoring of patients and constant and spontaneous care to persons who have limited tolerance for delay. Specialty units include perioperative units, labor and delivery units, burn units, and the many types of intensive care units.

Specialty units rely on close and continuous assessment by registered nurses as well as multiple uses of technologic monitoring. Medication administration is complex and frequent; measurements are performed hourly or more frequently.

Essential Documentation

The nurse should record the date and time of the transfer and the name of the unit receiving the patient. Document the receipt of transfer orders. Describe the patient's condition at the time of transfer, including vital signs, descriptions of incisions and wounds, and locations of tubes or medical devices still in place. Report significant events that occurred during the hospital stay. Be sure to note whether the patient has an advance directive and include special factors, such as allergies, special diet, sensory deficits, and language or cultural issues. List medications, treatments, and teaching needs. Note which goals were and were not met. Chart that a report was given to the receiving unit and include the name of the nurse who received the report. Note how the patient was transported to the specialty unit and who accompanied him. Include patient teaching given that related to the transfer such as explaining to the patient the reason for the transfer. Some facilities may use a transfer form to record this information.

PATIENT'S BELONGINGS, AT ADMISSION

The nurse should encourage patients to send home their money, jewelry, and other valuable belongings. If a patient refuses to do so, make a list of the belongings and store them according to the facility's policy.

The nurse should place personal belongings in approved bags and label them with the patient's identification number. Never use garbage containers, laundry bags, or other unauthorized receptacles for valuables because they could be discarded accidentally. Valuables such as money, credit cards, and jewelry should be stored by security. The facility provides a form for recording the patient's belongings on admission.

Essential Documentation

The nurse should make a list of the patient's valuables and include a description of each one. Most facilities provide an area on the nursing admission form to list the belongings. Ask the patient (or a responsible family member) to sign or witness the list that is compiled as documentation of mutual understanding about the items for which the facility is responsible. This provides protection for the nurse as well as the employer.

The nurse should use objective language to describe each item, noting its color, approximate size, style, type, and serial number or other distinguishing features. Do not assess the item's value or authenticity. For example, a diamond ring might be described as a "clear, round stone set in a yellow metal band."

In addition to jewelry and money, the nurse should include dentures, eyeglasses or contact lenses, hearing aids, prostheses, and clothing on the list. Belongings sent to security will be documented with a security form that is placed on the chart.

PERIPHERALLY INSERTED CENTRAL CATHETER SITE CARE

Proper peripherally inserted central catheter (PICC) site care and dressing changes are vital to preventing infection. The nurse should follow the facility's policy for the procedure and frequency of site care. Keep in mind, though, that a dressing should be changed any time it becomes wet or soiled or it loses integrity.

Twenty-four hours after the initial PICC insertion, the nurse should apply a new sterile, transparent, semipermeable dressing without using gauze because gauze may hold moisture and promote bacterial growth and skin maceration. Thereafter, change the dressing according to facility policy or as needed.

The nurse should assess the catheter insertion site through the transparent semipermeable dressing every shift, or per the facility's policy. Look at the catheter and cannula pathway and check for bleeding, redness, drainage, and swelling. Question the patient about pain at the site.

Essential Documentation

The nurse should record the date and time of PICC site care. Document explanation of the procedure to the patient and answer the patient's questions. Describe the condition of the site, noting any bleeding, redness, drainage, and swelling. Document pain or discomfort reported by the patient. Note the name of the health care provider who was notified of complications, the time of notification, orders given, nursing interventions, and the patient's response. Record how the site was cleaned and the type of dressing applied. Chart the patient's tolerance of the procedure and any patient teaching provided. Commonly this PICC site nursing care is recorded on a facility flow sheet or electronic health record.

Nursing Care of Peripherally Inserted Central Catheter Site		
10/31/2019	1100	**PATIENT TEACHING/EDUCATION:** Explained dressing change and site care for PICC to pt. Pt. verbalized understanding. ________ **NURSING INTERVENTION:** Pt. placed in seated position with left arm at 45-degree angle from body. Old dressing removed, no redness, bleeding, drainage, or swelling. No c/o pain at site. Using sterile technique, site cleaned with antimicrobial solution. Sterile, transparent, semipermeable dressing applied and tubing secured to edge of dressing with tape. ________ **PATIENT TEACHING/EDUCATION:** Reminded pt. to report pain or discomfort at insertion site or in left arm to nurse. ________ ________ **Lillian Mott, RN**

PERITONEAL DIALYSIS

Peritoneal dialysis is indicated for patients with chronic renal failure who have cardiovascular instability, vascular access problems that prevent hemodialysis, fluid overload, or electrolyte imbalances. In this procedure, dialysate—the solution instilled into the peritoneal cavity by a catheter—draws waste products, excess fluid, and electrolytes from the blood across the semipermeable peritoneal membrane. After a prescribed period, the dialysate is drained from the peritoneal cavity, removing impurities with it. The dialysis procedure is then repeated, using a new dialysate each time until waste removal is complete and fluid, electrolyte, and acid–base balances have been restored. Peritoneal dialysis may be performed manually or by using an automatic or semiautomatic cycle machine. Commonly this procedure will be documented on a facility provided standardized form.

Essential Documentation

The nurse should record the date and time of dialysis. There is a specific flow sheet used for documentation of peritoneal dialysis. During and after dialysis, monitor and document the patient's response to treatment. Record his vital signs every 10 to 15 minutes for the first 1 to 2 hours of exchanges and then every 2 to 4 hours or as often as necessary. If any abrupt changes in the patient's condition are detected, document them, notify the health care provider, and document the notification and any orders obtained.

The nurse should record the amount of dialysate infused and drained and medications added. Be sure to complete a peritoneal dialysis flow chart every 24 hours, or per facility policy. Keep a record of the effluent's characteristics and the assessed negative or positive fluid balance at the end of each infusion–dwell–drain cycle. Also, record each time the health care provider is notified of an abnormality. Chart the patient's weight (immediately after the drain phase) and abdominal girth daily. Note the time of day and variations in the weighing–measuring technique. In addition, document physical assessment findings and fluid status per shift.

The nurse should keep a record of equipment problems, such as kinked tubing or mechanical malfunction, and nursing interventions. Also, note the condition of the patient's skin at the dialysis catheter site, the patient's reports of unusual discomfort or pain, and nursing interventions. This information and all the parameters that require measurement will be commonly documented on a specific form provided by the facility or an electronic health record or flow sheet. The nurse would need to fill in blanks on a standard form for peritoneal dialysis.

PERITONEAL DIALYSIS, CONTINUOUS AMBULATORY

Continuous ambulatory peritoneal dialysis (CAPD) requires the insertion of a permanent peritoneal catheter to continuously circulate dialysate in the peritoneal cavity. Inserted when the patient is under local anesthetic, the catheter is sutured in place and its distal portion tunneled subcutaneously to the skin surface. There it serves as a port for the dialysate, which flows in and out of the peritoneal cavity by gravity. The bag of dialysate is attached to the tube entering the patient's abdominal area. The fluid flows into the peritoneal cavity over a period of 5 to 10 minutes. The dialysate remains in the peritoneal cavity, usually 4 to 6 hours. The patient can roll up the bag and place it under his shirt. After the prescribed dwell time is completed, the bag is unrolled and suspended below the pelvis, which allows the dialysate to drain from the peritoneal cavity back into the bag by gravity.

CAPD is used most commonly for patients with end-stage renal disease. It provides more patient independence, reduces travel for treatment, and helps stabilize fluid and electrolyte levels. Patients and family members can usually learn to perform CAPD after only 2 weeks of training.

Essential Documentation

The nurse should record the type and amount of fluid instilled and returned for each exchange, the time and duration of the exchange, and drugs added to the dialysate. Be sure to complete a peritoneal dialysis flow chart every 24 hours, or per facility policy. Note the color and clarity of the returned exchange fluid, and check it for mucus, pus, and blood. Also, note discrepancies in the balance of fluid intake and output as well as signs or symptoms of fluid imbalance, such as weight changes, decreased breath sounds, peripheral edema, ascites, and changes in skin turgor. Record the patient's weight, blood pressure, and pulse rate with his first and last fluid exchange of the day. This information and all the parameters that require measurement will be commonly documented on a specific form provided by the facility or an electronic health record or flow sheet. The nurse would need to fill in blanks on a standard form for peritoneal dialysis.

PERITONEAL LAVAGE (DIAGNOSTIC PERITONEAL ASPIRATION [DPA])

Used as a diagnostic procedure in a patient with blunt abdominal trauma, peritoneal lavage (diagnostic peritoneal aspiration) helps detect bleeding in the peritoneal cavity. This procedure is used infrequently since abdominal ultrasonography and abdominal CT scan are alternatively used.

Peritoneal aspiration may proceed through several steps. Initially, the health care provider inserts a catheter through the abdominal wall into the peritoneal cavity and aspirates the peritoneal fluid with a syringe. If the provider cannot see blood in the aspirated fluid, the provider then infuses a balanced saline solution and siphons the fluid from the cavity. The provider inspects the siphoned fluid for blood and also sends fluid samples to the laboratory for microscopic examination. This information and all the parameters that require measurement will be commonly documented on a specific form provided by the facility or an electronic health record or flow sheet. The nurse would need to fill in blanks on a standard form for peritoneal aspiration (peritoneal lavage).

Essential Documentation

The nurse should record the date and time of the procedure. Chart teaching done to prepare the patient for the procedure. Frequently monitor and document the patient's vital signs and signs and symptoms of shock (for example, tachycardia, hypotension, diaphoresis, or dyspnea).

Note whether an indwelling urinary catheter or nasogastric (NG) tube were inserted prior to the procedure. Record the size and type of urinary catheter or NG tube, and describe the amount, color, and other characteristics of the urine or NG drainage.

The nurse should keep a record of the incision site's condition, and document the type and size of catheter used, the type and amount of solution instilled and withdrawn from the peritoneal cavity, and the amount and color of fluid returned. Note whether the fluid flowed freely into and out of the abdomen. Record which specimens were obtained and sent to the laboratory. Note the patient's tolerance of the procedure. Also, note complications that occurred and the nursing actions taken to manage them. This procedure and all parameters are commonly documented on a standard form or electronic health record or flow sheet provided by the facility.

PERITONITIS

Peritonitis develops from a local or general inflammatory process in the peritoneal cavity caused by chemical irritation or infection. It may be an acute or chronic condition. Although the peritoneum is sterile, with peritonitis, bacteria and chemicals may enter the peritoneum as a result of such conditions as appendicitis; diverticulitis; peptic ulcer; ulcerative colitis; volvulus; strangulated obstruction; abdominal neoplasm; penetrating wound; peritoneal dialysis; rupture of the bowel, fallopian tube, or the bladder; or released pancreatic enzymes. Untreated, peritonitis can lead to complications such as septicemia, septic shock, abscess formation, and total body organ failure. Mortality is 10%, with death usually resulting from bowel obstruction.

If it is suspected that the patient has peritonitis, immediately contact the health care provider and anticipate administering IV fluids and antibiotics, inserting a nasogastric (NG) tube, and preparing the patient for surgery to repair organ perforation.

Essential Documentation

Document the assessment findings, such as sudden and severe abdominal pain, rebound tenderness, abdominal rigidity and spasm, abdominal distention, nausea or vomiting, fever, tachycardia, tachypnea, hypotension, pallor, cold skin, diaphoresis, decreased or absent bowel sounds, and signs of dehydration. Measure abdominal girth and mark placement of the measuring tape so that follow-up measurements are consistent. Note the name of the health care provider notified, the time of notification, and orders given, such as to obtain abdominal x-rays and blood work, insert an NG tube, and administer IV fluids, electrolytes, and antibiotics. Record nursing interventions, such as administering drugs and IV fluids, positioning for comfort and improved ventilation, providing analgesics and other comfort measures, keeping the patient from eating or drinking anything, preparing the patient for surgery, monitoring gastric decompression, and inserting a urinary catheter. Chart the patient's responses to these interventions. Use flow sheets to record the frequent assessments, vital signs, intake and output, IV therapy, and laboratory test values. Document patient teaching and emotional support rendered.

Nursing Care of Patient with Peritonitis

11/1/2019	1000	**NURSING ASSESSMENT:** Pt. c/o severe pain in left lower abdomen at 0930, rated as 6 on scale of 0 to 10. Pt. guarding abdomen with arms and moaning. Pt. placed on left side with legs flexed. No c/o nausea. Abdomen is rigid and distended, abdominal girth is 40 inches, bowel sounds hypo-active. No rebound tenderness noted. Skin cool, diaphoretic, and pale. Abdominal incision with purulent drainage, skin around wound red. P 118, BP 92/68, RR 24 and shallow, oral T 101.5°F. ______
		NURSING INTERVENTION: Dr. D. Fromm notified at 0940 and came to see pt.; orders given. Pt. made NPO, radiology called for stat abdominal X-ray, lab called for stat CBC w/diff, electrolytes, BUN, creatinine as ordered by physician, Dr. Fromm. Culture of wound drainage sent to lab as ordered by physician. IV line started in right antecubital space with 20G catheter on first attempt. 1000 mL NSS at 150 mL/hr infusing via infusion pump as ordered by physician. Receiving O_2 at 2 L by NC, with O_2 sat. by pulse oximetry 96% as ordered. NG tube inserted (placement confirmed by pH of aspirate) and attached to low intermittent suction by physician. Drained 100 mL dark green fluid, negative for blood. Morphine sulfate 2 mg given IV. at 0955 as per physician order, Dr. Fromm. See flow sheets for documentation of frequent vital signs, I/O, IV, and lab values.
		PATIENT TEACHING/EDUCATION: All procedures explained to pt.
		______ **Daniel Smith, RN**

PNEUMONIA

An acute infection of the pulmonary tissue, pneumonia often impairs gas exchange. The prognosis is generally good for people who have normal lungs and adequate host defenses before the onset of pneumonia; however, pneumonia is a leading cause of death in the United States, especially among older patients.

If the patient has pneumonia, the nurse should administer antibiotics, as ordered, and provide for good pulmonary hygiene.

Essential Documentation

Document the assessment findings, such as coughing, sputum production, pleuritic chest pain, shaking, chills, fever, malaise, anorexia, weakness, tachypnea, tachycardia, dyspnea, use of accessory muscles, abnormal breath sounds, pleural friction rub, dullness to percussion over consolidated areas, and tactile fremitus. Note the name of the health care provider notified, time of notification, and orders given, such as to obtain a chest x-ray and blood and sputum cultures, administer antibiotics, administer humidified oxygen therapy, and provide mechanical ventilation, if necessary. Respiratory therapists are commonly involved in monitoring the patient and administering breathing treatments. Note the attendance of the respiratory therapist, time, and intervention provided. Respiratory therapy commonly uses a flow sheet to chart their interventions.

The nurse should record nursing interventions, such as administering antibiotics and oxygen therapy, providing a high-calorie diet, promoting rest, and providing comfort measures and analgesics. Chart the patient's responses to interventions. Use flow sheets to record the frequent assessments, vital signs, intake and output, IV therapy, and laboratory test values. Record the patient teaching, including coughing and deep-breathing exercises, controlling the spread of infection, taking antibiotics properly, and encouraging vaccinations for influenza and pneumonia.

Nursing Care of Patient with Pneumonia		
12/24/2019	0900	**NURSING ASSESSMENT:** Pt. has cough productive for large amount of thick yellow sputum. Breath sounds diminished left base, crackles throughout all lung fields bilaterally. Dullness to percussion and tactile fremitus palpated over base of left lung. Pt. is SOB, using accessory breathing muscles. P 112, BP 152/88, RR 32 and shallow, rectal T 102.4°F. Pulse oximetry 91%. Pt. is shaking and c/o of chills, weakness, and malaise. Normal heart sounds. Skin hot, dry, peripheral pulses palpable, no edema. Pt. alert and oriented to time, place, and person. ————
		NURSING INTERVENTION: Notified Dr. A. Landers at 0845 of assessment findings. Per dr.'s orders, chest X-ray and blood cultures ordered. Sputum sent for culture and sensitivity. Placed pt. on 2 L humidified O_2 by NC as ordered by physician. Pulse oximetry 96%.
		PATIENT TEACHING/EDUCATION: Explained all procedures to pt. Taught pt. how to perform cough and deep-breathing exercises and encouraged him to perform them q2hr. Pt. able to give proper return demo. ————
		———— **Henry Porter, RN**

PNEUMOTHORAX

A pneumothorax is an accumulation of air in the pleural space, which leads to partial or complete lung collapse. A pneumothorax may be closed or open. A closed pneumothorax has no associated external wound. It is commonly caused by the rupture of small blebs in the lung's visceral pleural space. An open pneumothorax develops when air enters the pleural space through an opening in the external chest wall;

it is commonly associated with a stab or gunshot wound. With a tension pneumothorax, the intrathoracic pressure increases, causing the lung to collapse and the mediastinum to shift toward the side opposite the pneumothorax. These anatomic changes result in decreased venous return and compression of the great vessels, which decreases cardiac output. The respiratory and cardiovascular systems are affected, thus creating a life-threatening situation.

If the patient is suspected to have a pneumothorax, the nurse should contact the health care provider immediately and anticipate insertion of a chest tube. Commonly a standardized electronic health record or flow sheet would be used to document assessment and interventions regarding a pneumothorax.

Essential Documentation

Document the assessment findings of a pneumothorax, such as asymmetrical chest wall movement, absent or diminished breath sounds, shortness of breath, cyanosis, and sudden, sharp pleuritic pain exacerbated by movement. If the pneumothorax is moderate to severe, the nurse may assess and record such findings as profound respiratory distress, weak and rapid pulse, pallor, neck vein distention, shifting of the trachea and point of maximal impulse to the unaffected side, and anxiety. Note the name of the health care provider notified, time of notification, and orders given. Record nursing interventions, such as assisting with insertion of a chest tube or large-bore needle, managing the chest tube, close monitoring of vital signs and cardiopulmonary assessments, administering oxygen, and encouraging coughing and deep-breathing exercises. Chart the patient's responses to these interventions. Use flow sheets to record the frequent assessments, vital signs, intake and output, IV therapy, and laboratory values. Include the patient teaching and emotional support given. Commonly a standardized electronic health record or flow sheet provided by the facility would be used to document assessments and interventions regarding a pneumothorax.

Nursing Care of Patient with Pneumothorax

7/12/2019	0300	**NURSING ASSESSMENT:** Pt. entered ED at 0130 with c/o difficulty breathing and left-sided chest pain that worsened with movement; has history of COPD. Breath sounds absent on left side, clear breath sounds on right. Skin pale, cool. Normal heart sounds; however,

Nursing Care of Patient with Pneumothorax (*continued*)	
	PMI is shifted to right of midclavicular line. P 128 and weak, BP 112/62, RR 32, axillary T 99.0°F. Pulse oximetry 84% on room air. Dr. D. Hall in to see pt. at 0140 and orders given. __________ **NURSING INTERVENTION:** Portable CXR done as ordered by physician, and revealed 30% left pneumothorax. O_2 applied at 30% via facemask. Chest tube inserted by Dr. Hall and placed to 20 cm water suction with Pleurevac. Chest tube sutured to chest wall. Occlusive dressing applied. **NURSING ASSESSMENT:** Pt. states he's breathing easier, appears more comfortable P 110 and strong, BP 118/60, RR 24. See flow sheets for documentation of frequent VS, I/O, IV therapy, and lab values. __________ **Sue Jones, RN**

POISONING

Poisoning occurs after accidental or intentional contact with a harmful substance. Approximately 1 million poisonings occur in the United States every year. In children, accidental poisoning usually involves ingestion of salicylates, acetaminophen, or other medications, cleaning agents, detergent pods, batteries, insecticides, paints, or cosmetics. In adults, common workplace poisonings take place in companies that use chlorine, carbon dioxide, hydrogen sulfide, nitrogen dioxide, and ammonia and in companies that ignore safety standards. Other causes of poisoning in adults involve raw and contaminated foods; improper cooking, canning, and storage of food; ingestion of or skin contamination by plants; insect or animal bites; and drug overdose and carbon monoxide.

If it is suspected that the patient has been exposed to a poison, immediately notify the health care provider and provide emergency resuscitation and support, prevention of further poison absorption, continuing supportive or symptomatic care and, when possible, administration of the appropriate antidote. Specific interventions are based on the type of poison and the route of contact or ingestion, so every effort should be made to identify the poison involved. Consultation with the local poison control center will clarify the specific interventions based on the poison involved.

Essential Documentation

Record the type and amount of poison, route of poisoning, signs and symptoms exhibited, and interventions implemented before the patient's arrival at the facility. Chart a brief medical history, including allergies and current drugs. Document continued assessments of the patient, administration of an antidote or gastrointestinal decontaminant (such as activated charcoal, gastric lavage, cathartics, and whole-bowel irrigation), and supportive therapies. Include the patient's response to the nursing interventions. Use flow sheets or electronic health records to record the frequent assessments, vital signs, intake and output, IV therapy, and laboratory test values. Record any patient teaching, including strategies to prevent future poison exposure.

Nursing Care of Patient with Poisoning

7/14/2019	1700	**HISTORY OF PRESENT ILLNESS:** Pt. discovered by grandparents playing on the floor with a Tylenol bottle. Stated that they didn't know how many tablets the child may have consumed but did see a white powder around her mouth. Grandmother recalls that bottle was approximately 1/2 full (60 total count bottle). Grandparents report that the incident occurred approximately 30 minutes ago. Child is sleepy but responsive to questions. ______
		NURSING ASSESSMENT: Child states that "They tasted bad. I only tasted them." P 100, BP 90/60, RR 24, tympanic T 98.4°F. Wt. 30 lb. ______
		PAST MEDICAL HISTORY: Grandparents report no previous medical hx for child, no known allergies, and taking no drugs. ______
		NURSING INTERVENTION: Dr. L. Greene examined pt. at 1650 and ordered acetylcysteine (see MAR). Blood for LFTs and drug tox. drawn by lab as ordered by physician. See flow sheets for documentation of frequent VS, I/O, and lab values. Explained all procedures to grandparents and child. ______
		PATIENT FAMILY TEACHING/EDUCATION: Reinforced the need to keep all drugs out of reach of children and to use child-resistant bottles. Grandparents verbalized understanding. ______
		______ **Joyce Tomlin, RN**

POSTOPERATIVE CARE

When the patient recovers sufficiently from the effects of anesthesia, the patient can be transferred from the postanesthesia care unit (PACU) to the assigned unit for ongoing recovery and care. The nurse's documentation should reflect frequent assessments and interventions. A standardized flow sheet or electronic health record would be used here for continual assessments and interventions which would need to be required over a period of time. The patient is on telemetry and other digital devices and records of vital signs and other parameters are transmitted directly to health care providers.

Essential Documentation

The frequency of nursing assessments depends on the facility's policy, health care provider's orders, and the patient's condition. Compare nursing assessments to preoperative and PACU assessments. Documentation should include the following information:

- time the patient returned to the nursing unit
- assessment of airway and breathing, including breath sounds, positioning to maintain a patent airway, use of oxygen, and respiratory rate, rhythm, and depth
- vital signs
- neurologic assessment, including level of consciousness
- wound assessment, including the appearance of dressing, drainage, bleeding, and skin around site (Note the presence of drainage tubes and amount, type, color, and consistency of drainage; chart the type and amount of suction, if applicable.)
- cardiovascular assessment, including heart rate and rhythm, peripheral pulses, skin color and temperature
- renal assessment, including urine output, patency of catheter, and bladder distention
- gastrointestinal assessment, including bowel sounds, abdominal distention, and nausea or vomiting
- pain assessment, including the use of 0 to 10 rating scale, need for analgesics and patient's response, and use of other comfort measures
- safety measures, such as call bell within reach, bed in low position, proper positioning, and use of side rails
- fluid management, including intake and output, type and size of IV catheter, location of IV line, IV solution, flow rate, and condition of IV site
- use of antiembolism stockings, sequential compression device, early ambulation, and prophylactic anticoagulants
- patient education, such as turning and positioning, coughing and deep breathing, splinting the incision, pain control, and the importance of early ambulation, as well as emotional support given.

The nurse should document drugs given; the dosage, frequency, and route; and the patient's response. Record the name of the health care provider whom was notified of changes in the patient's condition, the time of notification, orders given, nursing actions, and the patient's responses. Use flow sheets or an electronic health record to record the frequent assessments, vital signs, intake and output, IV therapy, and laboratory values. Most commonly all these assessments, parameters, and interventions would be recorded digitally and electronically delivered to health care providers.

Nursing Care of Post-operative Patient		
12/8/2019	1100	**NURSING ASSESSMENT:** Pt. returned from PACU at 1030 S/P laparoscopic cholecystectomy. P 88 and regular, BP 112/82, RR 18 deep, regular, tympanic T 98.2°F. Pt. breathing comfortably, breath sounds clear on room air, skin pink and warm, capillary refill less than 3 sec. Sleeping but easily arousable and oriented to time, place, and person. Speech clear and coherent. PERRL. Normal heart sounds, strong radial and dorsalis pedis pulses bilaterally. Bladder nondistended, no indwelling urinary catheter, doesn't feel urge to void, positive bowel sounds in all 4 quadrants. Abdomen slightly distended, no c/o nausea. Has 4 abdominal puncture wounds covered with 4" × 4" gauze. Dressings without drainage. Pt. c/o of abdominal discomfort rated as 3 on a scale of 0 to 10, refusing analgesics at this time. ________
		NURSING INTERVENTION: Pt. placed in semi-Fowler's position, bed in low position, call bell within reach and pt. verbalized understanding of its use. IV of 1000 mL D5W/0.45NS infusing at 75 mL/hr in right forearm via infusion pump. See flow sheets for documentation of frequent VS, IV therapy, and I/O. ________
		PATIENT TEACHING/EDUCATION: Explained coughing and deep-breathing exercises to pt. and instructed how to splint abdomen with pillow when coughing. Pt. able to give return demo. Told her to call if she feels she needs pain medication. ________
		________ **Christina Gault, RN**

PREOPERATIVE CARE

Effective nursing documentation during the preoperative period focuses on two primary elements—the baseline preoperative assessment and patient teaching. Documenting these elements encourages accurate communication among caregivers. Most facilities use a preoperative checklist to verify that the required data have been collected,

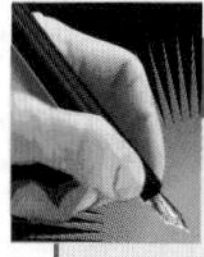

ACCUCHART

PREOPERATIVE CHECKLIST AND SURGICAL IDENTIFICATION FORM

To document preoperative procedures, data collection, and teaching, most facilities use a checklist such as the one below.

WOODVIEW
Hospital

Pre-Operative Checklist and Surgical Identification Form

Instructions: All items checked "No" requires follow up. Follow up is to be documented. In "Additional Information / Comment" section until resolved.

Patient name: Zachary, Timothy
Medical record number: 987654

Pre-Op Checklist	Yes	No	Resolved	Initials
ID Band On	✓			NRC
Allergies Noted / Bracelet	✓			NRC
History & Physical (Present & Reviewed)	✓			NRC
Surgical Informed Consent Signed	✓			NRC
Anesthesia Informed Consent	✓			NRC
Pre-Op Teaching	✓			NRC
Prep. as Ordered	N/A			
NPO After Midnight	✓	✓		NRC
Dentures, Capped Teeth, Cosmetics, Glasses, Contact Lenses, Wig Removed	N/A			
Voided/Catheter Inserted (Voided circled)	✓			NRC
Medical Clearance/Physician's Name	✓			NRC
TEDS, as Ordered	N/A			
SCD, as Ordered	N/A			
PCA Teaching, as Ordered	✓			NRC
Type & Cross/Screen Drawn (If Ordered Must Have Blood Informed Consent Signed)	N/A			
**Blood Informed Consent Signed				
*Lab Results on Chart	✓			NRC
*EKG on Chart	✓			NRC
*Chest X-ray on Chart	✓			NRC

*Abnormal Results Results Reported To H&H Dr. F. Schoblitz
Time & Date 4/28/19 0800
Reported By NRC

Temp. 98.6°F. Pulse 84 Resp. 18 B/P 132/82

Valuables
Destination: ☐ To Safe ☐ To Family, Name ______

✗ Norma R. Clay, RN — NRC
Signature of Nurse — Initials

✗ ______
Signature of Transferring RN — Date — Time

Additional Information /Comments
Pt has all own teeth

Surgical Patient Identification Form

Nursing Floor RN Patient Identification

☑ Patient I.D. Bracelet Personally Observed
☑ Patient Questioned Verbally Regarding I.D., Procedure & Site
☑ Patient's Chart Reviewed to Verify I.D., Procedure & Site

✗ Norma R. Clay, RN 4/28/19 0800
R.N.'s Signature — Date — Time

Pre-Op Anesthesia Patient Identification

☐ Patient's I.D. Bracelet Personally Observed
☐ Patient Questioned Verbally Regarding I.D., Procedure & Site
☐ Patient's Chart Reviewed to Verify I.D., Procedure & Site

✗ ______
Anesthesiologist/Anesthetist's Signature — Date — Time

Operating Room and Anesthesia Personnel Patient Identification

Operative Procedure & Site: ______

ANES	CIRC Nurse	
☐	☐	Patient I.D. Bracelet Personally Observed
☐	☐	Patient Questioned Verbally Regarding I.D., Procedure & Site
☐	☐	Patient's Chart Reviewed to Verify I.D., Procedure & Site
☐	☐	Surgical Site Confirmed

✗ ______
Anesthesiologist/Anesthetist's Signature — Time

✗ ______
CIRC Nurse's Signature — Time

Surgeon's Patient Identification Statement

☐ Patient I.D. Bracelet Personally Observed
☐ Patient Questioned Verbally Regarding I.D., Procedure & Site
☐ Surgical Site Marked

✗ ______
Surgeon's Signature — Time

preoperative teaching has occurred, and prescribed procedures and safety precautions have been implemented.

Essential Documentation

To use the preoperative checklist, the nurse should place a check mark in the appropriate column to indicate that a procedure has been performed (for example, checking that the patient is wearing an identification band or that the informed consent form has been signed). If an item does not apply to the patient, write "N/A," indicating that the item is not applicable. Initial the appropriate column to indicate that an item has been completed. Include full name, credentials, and initials on the form. Chart the patient's baseline vital signs on the form. Before the patient leaves for surgery, check the appropriate boxes to indicate that the patient has been properly and positively identified. (See "Surgical site identification," pages 391 to 393.)

The nurse should document the name of the person whom was notified of abnormalities that could affect the patient's response to the surgical procedure or deviations from facility standards.

See *Preoperative checklist and surgical identification form*, page 320, for an example of preoperative documentation. All facilities provide a standardized form for these assessments and intervention preoperatively and postoperatively.

PRESSURE ULCER (PRESSURE INJURY) ASSESSMENT

Pressure ulcers (pressure injuries) develop when pressure impairs circulation, depriving tissues of oxygen and life-sustaining nutrients. This process damages skin and underlying structures. The pressure may be of short duration with great force, or it may have been present for a longer period of time with lesser force.

Most pressure ulcers develop over bony prominences, where friction and shearing force combine with pressure to break down skin and underlying tissue. Common sites include the sacrum, coccyx, ischial tuberosities, and greater trochanters. In bedridden and relatively immobile patients, pressure ulcers develop over the vertebrae, scapulae, elbows, knees, and heels. (See Figure P.1.) Untreated pressure ulcers may lead to serious systemic infection.

To select the most effective treatment plan for pressure ulcers, the nurse first assesses the pressure ulcer and stages it based on the National Pressure Ulcer Advisory Panel and the Agency for Healthcare Research and Quality. (See *NPUAP pressure injury stages,* pages 323 and 324.)

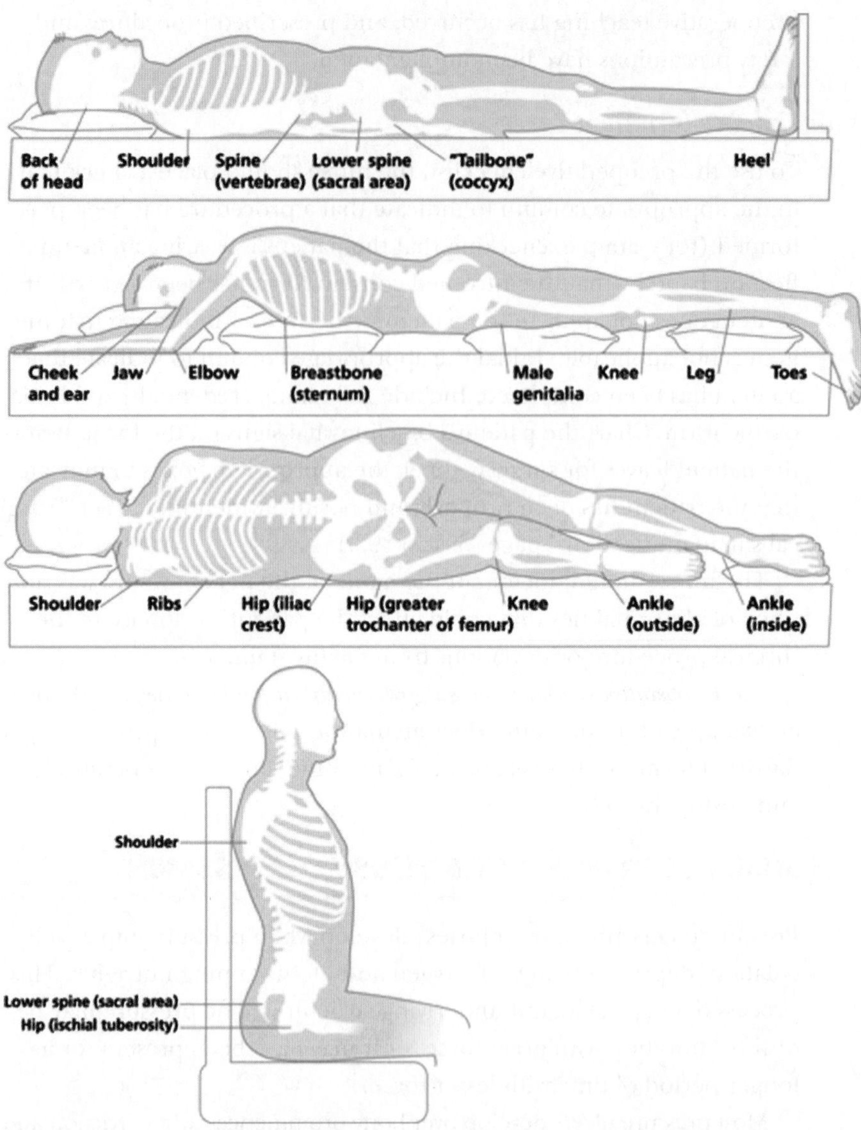

Figure P.1: Pressure points are areas where pressure ulcers are likely to form. (Reprinted with permission from Carter, P. [2015]. Lippincott textbook for nursing assistants. (84th ed.). Philadelphia, PA: Wolters Kluwer Health [LWW PE].)

NPUAP PRESSURE INJURY STAGES

The National Pressure Ulcer Advisory Panel redefined the definition of pressure injuries during the NPUAP 2016 Staging Consensus Conference that was held April 8 to 9, 2016, in Rosemont (Chicago), Illinois.

The updated staging definitions were presented at a meeting of over 400 professionals. Using a consensus format, Dr. Mikel Gray from the University of Virginia guided the Staging Task Force and meeting participants to consensus on the updated definitions through an interactive discussion and voting process. During the meeting, the participants also validated the new terminology using photographs.

The updated staging system includes the definitions in the following paragraphs.

Pressure Injury

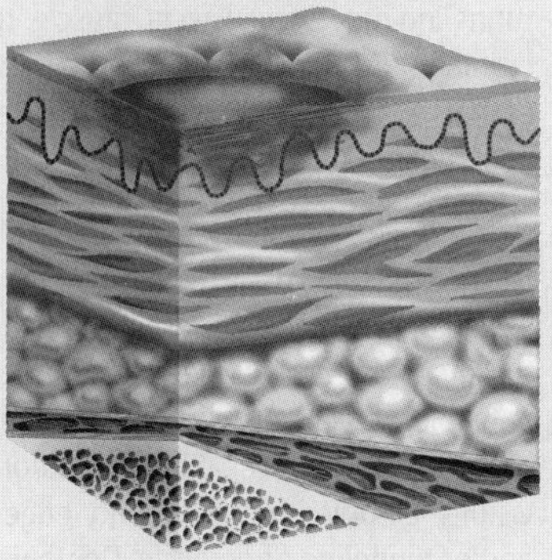

A pressure injury is localized damage to the skin and underlying soft tissue usually over a bony prominence or related to a medical or other device. The injury can present as intact skin or an open ulcer and may be painful. The injury occurs as a result of intense and/or prolonged pressure or pressure in combination with shear. The tolerance of soft tissue for pressure and shear may also be affected by microclimate, nutrition, perfusion, comorbidities, and condition of the soft tissue.

Stage 1 Pressure Injury: Nonblanchable Erythema of Intact Skin

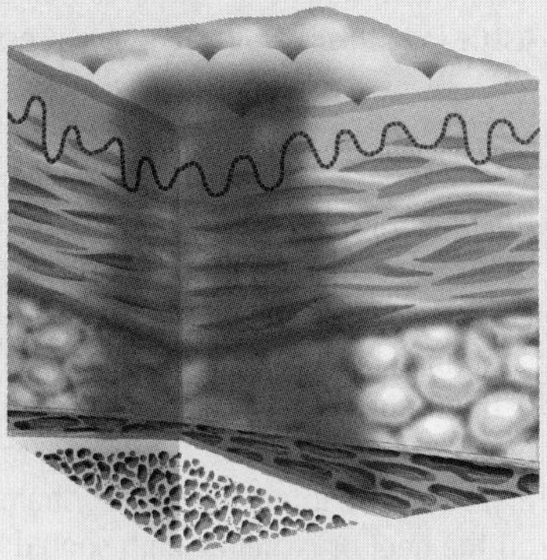

Stage 1 pressure injuries are characterized by intact skin with a localized area of nonblanchable erythema, which may appear differently in darkly pigmented skin. The presence of blanchable erythema or changes in sensation, temperature, or firmness may precede visual changes. Color changes do not include purple or maroon discoloration; these may indicate deep-tissue pressure injury.

Stage 2 Pressure Injury: Partial-Thickness Skin Loss With Exposed Dermis

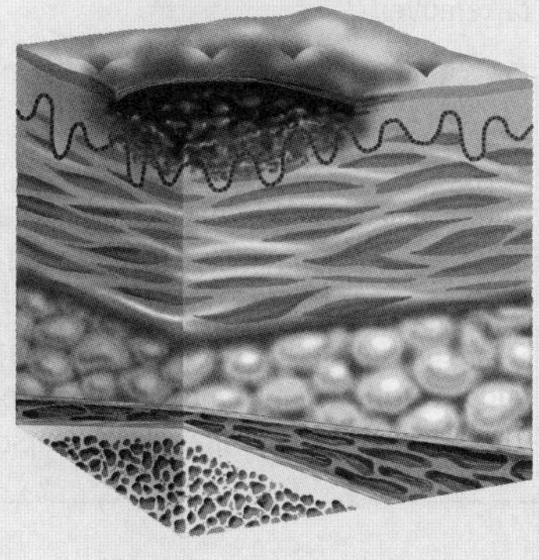

Stage 2 pressure injuries are characterized by partial-thickness loss of skin with exposed dermis. The wound bed is viable, pink or red, moist, and may also present as an intact or ruptured serum-filled blister. Adipose (fat) is not visible and deeper tissues are not visible. Granulation tissue, slough, and eschar are not present. These injuries commonly result from adverse microclimate and shear in the skin over the pelvis and shear in the heel. This stage should not be used to describe moisture-associated skin damage (MASD) including incontinence-associated dermatitis (IAD), intertriginous dermatitis (ITD), medical adhesive–related skin injury (MARSI), or traumatic wounds (skin tears, burns, abrasions).

(*continued*)

NPUAP PRESSURE INJURY STAGES *(continued)*

Stage 3 Pressure Injury: Full-Thickness Skin Loss

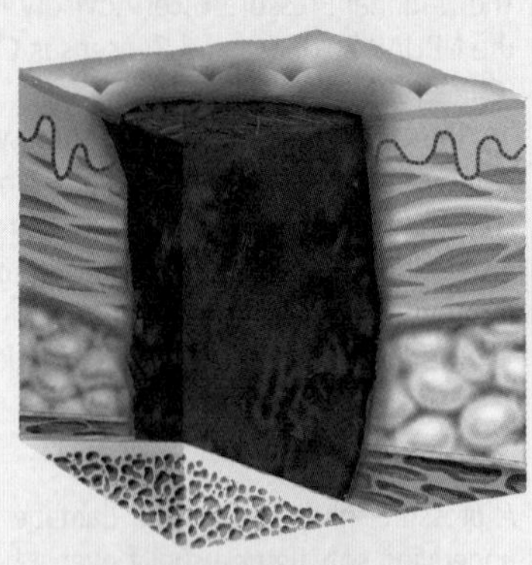

Stage 3 pressure injuries are characterized by full-thickness loss of skin, in which adipose (fat) is visible in the ulcer and granulation tissue and epibole (rolled wound edges) are often present. Slough and/or eschar may be visible. The depth of tissue damage varies by anatomic location; areas of significant adiposity can develop deep wounds. Undermining and tunneling may occur. Fascia, muscle, tendon, ligament, cartilage, and/or bone are not exposed. If slough or eschar obscures the extent of tissue loss, this is an unstageable pressure injury.

Stage 4 Pressure Injury: Full-Thickness Skin and Tissue Loss

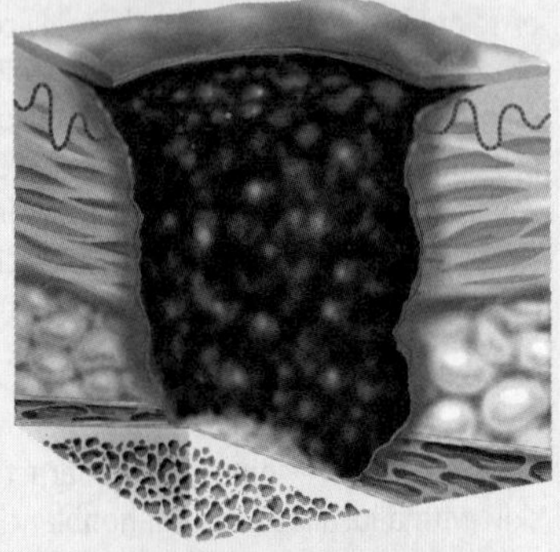

Stage 4 pressure injuries are characterized by full-thickness skin and tissue loss with exposed or directly palpable fascia, muscle, tendon, ligament, cartilage, or bone in the ulcer. Slough and/or eschar may be visible. Epibole (rolled wound edges), undermining, and/or tunneling often occur. Depth varies by anatomic location. If slough or eschar obscures the extent of tissue loss, this is an unstageable pressure injury.

Unstageable Pressure Injury: Obscured Full-Thickness Skin and Tissue Loss

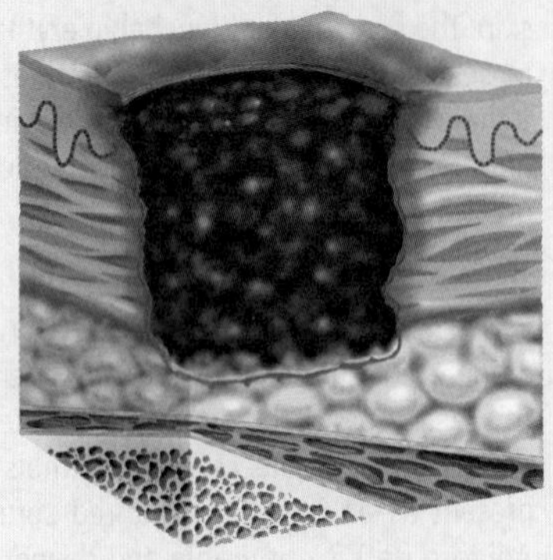

Unstageable pressure injuries are characterized by full-thickness skin and tissue loss in which the extent of tissue damage within the ulcer cannot be confirmed because it is obscured by slough or eschar. If slough or eschar is removed, a Stage 3 or Stage 4 pressure injury will be revealed. Stable eschar (i.e., dry, adherent, intact without erythema or fluctuance) on the heel or ischemic limb should not be softened or removed.

Deep-Tissue Pressure Injury: Persistent Nonblanchable Deep Red, Maroon, or Purple Discoloration

Deep-tissue pressure injuries are characterized by intact or nonintact skin with localized area of persistent nonblanchable deep red, maroon, purple discoloration or epidermal separation revealing a dark wound bed or blood-filled blister. Pain and temperature change often precede skin color changes. Discoloration may appear differently in darkly pigmented skin. This injury results from intense and/or prolonged pressure and shear forces at the bone–muscle interface. The wound may evolve rapidly to reveal the actual extent of tissue injury or it may

NPUAP PRESSURE INJURY STAGES *(continued)*

resolve without tissue loss. If necrotic tissue, subcutaneous tissue, granulation tissue, fascia, muscle, or other underlying structures are visible, this indicates a full-thickness pressure injury (unstageable, Stage 3, or Stage 4). Do not use deep-tissue pressure injury (DTPI) to describe vascular, traumatic, neuropathic, or dermatologic conditions.

Additional pressure injury definitions appear in the following paragraphs.

Medical Device–Related Pressure Injury

Medical device–related pressure injuries result from the use of devices designed and applied for diagnostic or therapeutic purposes. The resultant pressure injury generally conforms to the pattern or shape of the device. The injury should be staged using the staging system.

Mucosal Membrane Pressure Injury

Mucosal membrane pressure injuries are found on mucous membranes with a history of a medical device in use at the location of the injury. Due to the anatomy of the tissue, these ulcers cannot be staged.

In addition to assessing the pressure ulcer, the nurse should perform an assessment to determine the patient's risk of developing pressure ulcers. The Braden scale is one of the most reliable instruments. The Braden scale assesses sensory perception, moisture, activity, mobility, nutrition, and friction and shear. The lower the score, the greater the risk. (See *Braden scale: Predicting pressure ulcer risk,* pages 326 and 327.)

Documentation of pressure ulcer assessments assists the nurse in detecting changes in a patient's skin condition, determining the response to treatment, identifying at-risk patients, and reducing the incidence of pressure ulcers through early independent interventions and treatment.

Essential Documentation

Nursing documentation of pressure ulcer assessment should include the patient's history and risk factors leading to the formation of a pressure ulcer, using a tool such as the Braden scale. In the note, the nurse should describe the pressure ulcer, including its location, size and depth (in centimeters), stage, color, and appearance; presence of necrotic or granulation tissue, drainage, and odor; length of any undermining or tunneling; and condition of the surrounding tissue. A photograph of the wound may also be included. Describe any treatment and dressing applied. Assess the pressure ulcer with each dressing change or at least weekly for the patient at home.

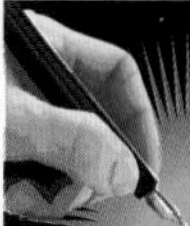

ACCUCHART

BRADEN SCALE: PREDICTING PRESSURE ULCER RISK

The Braden scale, shown below, is the most reliable of several instruments for assessing the older patient's risk of developing pressure ulcers. The lower the score, the greater the risk.

Patient's name Kevin Lawson Medical record # 654321

SENSORY PERCEPTION Ability to respond meaningfully to pressure-related discomfort	1. Completely limited: Is unresponsive (doesn't moan, flinch, or grasp in response) to painful stimuli because of diminished level of consciousness or sedation OR Has a limited ability to feel pain over most of body surface	2. Very limited: Responds only to painful stimuli; can't communicate discomfort except through moaning or restlessness OR Has a sensory impairment that limits ability to feel pain or discomfort over half of body
MOISTURE Degree to which skin is exposed to moisture	1. Constantly moist: Skin kept moist almost constantly by perspiration, urine, or other fluids; dampness detected every time patient is moved or turned	2. Very moist: Skin often but not always moist; linen must be changed at least once per shift
ACTIVITY Degree of physical activity	1. Bedridden: Confined to bed	2. Chairfast: Ability to walk severely limited or nonexistent; can't bear own weight and must be assisted into chair or wheelchair
MOBILITY Ability to change and control body position	1. Completely immobile: Doesn't make even slight changes in body or extremity position without assistance	2. Very limited: Makes occasional slight changes in body or extremity position but is unable to make frequent or significant changes independently
NUTRITION Is NPO or maintained on clear liquids or IV fluids for more than 5 days	1. Very poor: Never eats a complete meal; rarely eats more than one-third of any food offered; eats two servings or less of protein (meat or dairy products) per day; takes fluids poorly; doesn't take a liquid dietary supplement OR Is NPO or maintained on clear liquids or IV fluids for more than 5 days	2. Probably inadequate: Rarely eats a complete meal and generally eats only about half of any food offered; protein intake includes only three servings of meat or dairy products per day; occasionally will take a dietary supplement OR Receives less than optimum amount of liquid diet or tube feeding
FRICTION AND SHEAR Ability to assist with movement or to be moved in a way that prevents skin contact with bedding or other surface	1. Problem: Requires moderate to maximum assistance in moving; complete lifting without sliding against sheets is impossible; frequently slides down in bed or chair, requiring frequent repositioning with maximum assistance; spasticity, contractures, or agitation leads to almost constant friction	2. Potential problem: Moves feebly or requires minimum assistance during a move; skin probably slides to some extent against sheets, chair restraints, or other devices; maintains relatively good position in chair or bed most of the time but occasionally slides down

Evaluator's name Joan Norris, RN

		DATE OF ASSESSMENT	3/21/19			
3. Slightly limited: Responds to verbal commands but can't always communicate discomfort or need to be turned	4. No impairment: Responds to verbal commands; has no sensory deficit that would limit ability to feel or voice pain or discomfort		3			
3. Occasionally moist: Skin occasionally moist, requiring an extra linen change approximately once per day	4. Rarely moist: Skin usually dry; linen only requires changing at routine intervals		3			
3. Walks occasionally: Walks occasionally during day, but for very short distances, with or without assistance; spends majority of each shift in bed or chair	4. Walks frequently: Walks outside room at least twice per day and inside room at least once every 2 hours during waking hours		2			
3. Slightly limited: Makes frequent though slight changes in body or extremity position independently	4. No limitations: Makes major and frequent changes in body or extremity position without assistance		2			
3. Adequate: Eats more than half of most meals; eats four servings of protein (meat and dairy products) per day; occasionally refuses a meal but will usually take a supplement if offered OR Is on a tube feeding or total parenteral nutrition regimen that probably meets most nutritional needs	4. Excellent: Eats most of every meal and never refuses a meal; usually eats four or more servings of meat and dairy products per day; occasionally eats between meals; doesn't require supplementation		2			
3. No apparent problem: Moves in bed and in chair independently and has sufficient muscle strength to lift up completely during move; maintains good position in bed or chair at all times			2			
		Total	14			

Nursing Care of Patient with Pressure Ulcer (Pressure Injury)		
1/18/2019	1100	**PATIENT ASSESSMENT:** Pt. admitted to 6 South from Green Brier Nursing Home. Pt. has stage 2 pressure ulcer on coccyx, approx. 2 cm × 1 cm × 0.5 cm. No drainage noted. Base has deep pink granulation tissue. Skin surrounding ulcer pink, intact, well-defined edges. ______ **NURSING INTERVENTION:** Irrigated ulcer with NSS. Skin around ulcer dried and ulcer covered with transparent dressing. Braden score 14 (see Braden Pressure Ulcer Risk Assessment Scale). ______
		______ **Joan Norris, RN**

PRESSURE ULCER (PRESSURE INJURY) CARE

Successful pressure ulcer treatment involves relieving pressure, restoring circulation and, if possible, resolving or managing related disorders. Typically, the effectiveness and duration of treatment depend on the pressure ulcer's characteristics.

Ideally, prevention is the key to avoiding extensive therapy. Preventive measures include ensuring adequate nourishment and mobility to relieve pressure and promote circulation.

When a pressure ulcer develops despite preventive efforts, treatment includes methods to decrease pressure, such as frequent repositioning to shorten pressure duration and the use of special equipment to reduce pressure intensity. Treatment may also involve special pressure-reducing devices, such as beds, mattresses, mattress overlays, and chair cushions. Other therapeutic measures include risk-factor reduction and the use of topical treatments, wound cleansing, debridement, and dressings to support moist wound healing.

Nurses usually perform or coordinate treatments according to facility policy. Always follow the standard precautions guidelines of the Centers for Disease Control and Prevention.

Essential Documentation

The nurse should record the date and time of initial and subsequent dressing changes and treatments. Note the specific treatment and the patient's response. Detail preventive strategies performed. Document the pressure ulcer's location and size (length, width, and depth in centimeters); color and appearance of the wound bed; amount, color, odor, and consistency of drainage; and condition of surrounding skin. Reassess ulcers with each dressing change and at least weekly.

The nurse should update the care plan as required. Note changes in the condition or size of the pressure ulcer and elevation of skin temperature on the clinical record. Document when the health care provider was notified of pertinent changes. Record the patient's temperature daily on the graphic sheet to allow easy assessment of body temperature patterns. Chart patient education, such as the explanation of treatments, the need for turning and positioning every 2 hours, and proper nutrition. A facility-provided standard form or flow sheet is commonly used to make frequent assessments and interventions of pressure ulcers.

Nursing Care of Patient with Pressure Ulcer (Pressure Injury)		
4/20/2019	1230	**NURSING ASSESSMENT:** Pt. has stage 2 pressure ulcer on left heel. Approx. 2 cm × 5 cm × 1 cm. Base of ulcer has necrotic tissue, no drainage. Skin around ulcer intact. ______ **NURSING INTERVENTION:** Wet-to-dry dressing removed and ulcer irrigated with NSS. Gauze moistened with NSS, placed in wound bed, and covered with dry sterile 4" × 4" gauze. Pt. turned and repositioned. Heels elevated off bed with pillow placed lengthwise under legs. Dietitian in to see pt. High-protein, high-calorie shakes being encouraged with each meal. ______ **PATIENT TEACHING/EDUCATION:** Explained importance of proper nutrition for wound healing. ______ ______ **Harrriet Newman, RN**

PSYCHOSIS, ACUTE

Acute psychosis is a psychiatric disorder characterized by an inability to recognize reality. The person suffering from acute psychosis experiences hallucinations (such as auditory, visual, tactile, and olfactory) and delusions. The patient may also show paranoia, disordered thinking, and catatonia.

Acute psychosis may result from a psychiatric disorder, such as schizophrenia, schizoaffective disorder, bipolar disorder, and personality disorders. Other conditions that can lead to acute psychosis include drug intoxication, drug withdrawal, and a host of endocrine, metabolic, and neurologic abnormalities.

An acute psychosis may be delirium, which is an acute confusional state with agitation that can result from fever, sleep deprivation, critical illness, acute event that changes health status such as stroke or MI, metabolic imbalances, medication toxicity, malnutrition, immobilization or restraints, poor hearing or vision, polypharmacy, postoperative/postanesthesia reactions, decreased sensorium of intensive care settings, or unrecognized infection in the older adult. Delirium is usually reversible but can be mistaken for dementia or psychosis. Older adults are most susceptible to delirium, particularly during hospitalization. The time of recovery from delirium depends on the triggering stressor, effective resolution of stressor, and mental status of the patient prior to the acute confusional state.

If the patient exhibits manifestations of acute psychosis or delirium, the nurse should notify the health care provider immediately. Reassure the patient that he's in a safe and secure place. Acknowledge that the patient is experiencing what he says he's experiencing. Decrease the stimuli in the environment but do not decrease the patient's ability to see or hear. Treat patients' pain and provide their eyeglasses or hearing aids. A person sitting one on one with the patient is recommended. The attendant should have a calming and soothing tone of voice and demeanor. Never use restraints because this worsens delirium. Administer antipsychotic drugs, as ordered, and observe the patient's response.

Essential Documentation

Objectively document the patient's behavior. Describe what the patient says he is hearing or seeing (if auditory or visual hallucinations are present) and what the patient is being told to do if he is hearing voices. Record any delusions that the patient relates. Describe inappropriate behaviors or statements. Describe threats or thoughts of suicide or violence, nursing interventions, and the patient's response. Record a general assessment, vital signs, and history as best as possible. Record the name of the health care provider that was notified, the time of notification, orders given, nursing actions, and the patient's response to drugs administered, the environment, and caregivers.

Nursing Care of Patient with Acute Psychosis

9/3/2019	1500	**HISTORY OF PRESENT ILLNESS:** 23 y.o. male brought to ED by police at 1430. Officers state that pt. was found walking in the middle of Route 1 waving his arms and conversing with himself. ________ **NURSING ASSESSMENT:** Pt. states, "An angry voice told me to stop all traffic. I'm getting very upset about all this, and I've been very upset all week." Pt. states he has been hearing voices the last several days. Pt. interrupts conversation frequently, turns his head and cups his hand to his ear. When asked what he's hearing, he shakes his head and only says, "Terrible, terrible." ________ **NURSING INTERVENTION:** Told pt. that he was in the hospital and that he was safe. Dr. D. Clark in to see pt. at 1445 and orders written. Given oral liquid haloperidol and lorazepam as ordered by physician. Dr. Clark. See MAR. Pt. accepted meds. Pt. and belongings searched as per hospital policy and no weapons or sharp objects found. Pt. not allowing anyone to touch him to perform physical exam; at this time. ________ **Marion Tuttle, RN**

PULMONARY EDEMA

Pulmonary edema is a diffuse extravascular accumulation of fluid in the tissues and air spaces of the lungs due to increased pressure in the pulmonary capillaries. Normally, fluid that crosses the capillary membrane and enters the lung is removed by the pulmonary lymphatic system. If the left ventricle fails, blood backs up into the pulmonary vasculature, and capillary pressure increases. Fluid crosses the membrane in amounts greater than the lymphatics can drain. Fluid builds up in the interstitial tissues, then in the alveoli. Pulmonary edema can occur as a chronic condition, or it can develop quickly and rapidly become fatal.

Most cases of pulmonary edema are cardiogenic, and the causes include acute myocardial infarction, acute volume overload of the left ventricle, and mitral stenosis. Noncardiogenic pulmonary edema can also occur and is caused by increased capillary permeability, which also permits fluid leakage into the alveoli. Causes of noncardiogenic pulmonary edema include acute respiratory distress syndrome, increased intracranial pressure, shock, and disseminated intravascular coagulation.

If the patient shows signs of pulmonary edema, notify the health care provider immediately. Administer oxygen by nasal cannula or facemask or, if respiratory distress develops, prepare for intubation and mechanical ventilation. Administer drugs as ordered, such as diuretics, nitrates, morphine, inotropics, vasodilators, and angiotensin-converting enzyme inhibitors. Anticipate assisting with the insertion of hemodynamic monitoring lines. Reassure the patient and family and explain what is being done and the rationale. The patient with pulmonary edema is commonly on hemodynamic monitoring, which automatically sends digital measurements of patient parameters to health care providers and documents the measurements.

Essential Documentation

Document the assessment findings of pulmonary edema, such as dyspnea, orthopnea, use of accessory muscles, pink frothy sputum, diaphoresis, cyanosis, tachypnea, tachycardia, adventitious breath sounds (such as crackles, wheezing, or rhonchi), pleural rub, neck vein distention, and increased intensity of the pulmonic component of S_2 and S_3 heart sounds. Note the name of the health care provider notified, time of notification, and orders given, such as oxygen, chest x-ray, and drug administration. Record nursing interventions, such as positioning the patient with the head of the bed elevated, inserting IV lines, administering oxygen and drugs, assisting with the insertion of hemodynamic monitoring lines, and suctioning. Chart the patient's responses to these interventions. Use flow sheets to record the frequent assessments, vital signs, pulse oximetry readings, hemodynamic measurements, intake and output, IV therapy, and laboratory test and arterial blood gas values. Include patient teaching and emotional care given. The patient will be hemodynamically monitored and all vital signs and parameters will be digital and automatically sent to health care providers and documented on record.

PULMONARY EMBOLISM

A common pulmonary complication in hospitalized patients, pulmonary embolism is an obstruction of the pulmonary arterial bed by a dislodged thrombus or foreign substance. Massive pulmonary embolism obstructing more than 50% of the pulmonary arterial circulation can be rapidly fatal. In fact, approximately 10% of patients die within the first hour.

Pulmonary embolism generally results from dislodged thrombi originating in the leg veins. More than half of such thrombi arise in the deep veins of the legs and are usually multiple. Other less common sources of thrombi are the pelvic veins, renal veins, hepatic vein, right side of the heart, and upper extremities. Such thrombus formation results directly from vascular wall damage, venostasis, or hypercoagulability of the blood.

Predisposing risk factors to pulmonary embolism include immobility, prolonged sitting, chronic pulmonary disease, heart failure, thrombophlebitis, polycythemia vera, thrombocytosis, autoimmune hemolytic anemia, sickle cell disease, varicose veins, vascular injury, surgery, advanced age, pregnancy, lower extremity fractures or surgery, burns, obesity, malignancy, and use of hormonal contraceptives.

If it is suspected that the patient has a pulmonary embolism, notify the health care provider immediately. Prepare the patient for a computed tomography scan, pulmonary angiography, or a lung scan. Administer oxygen and anticipate IV administration of heparin. With massive pulmonary embolism, anticipate fibrinolytic therapy or an emergent thrombectomy. A patient would most likely be on telemetry and have oxygenation monitored digitally. An electronic health record or flow sheet would be used to document the pulmonary dysfunction of the patient and record it permanently.

Essential Documentation

Document the assessment findings of pulmonary embolism, such as dyspnea, tachypnea, tachycardia, crackles on lung auscultation, chest pain, productive cough, mild fever, change in mental status, and feelings of apprehension and impending doom. Note the name of the health care provider notified, the time of notification, and orders given, such as diagnostic testing, oxygen administration, and heparin and thrombolytic therapy. Record the interventions, such as positioning, inserting IV lines, giving drugs, administering oxygen, watching for bleeding, and monitoring coagulation studies. Chart the patient's responses to these interventions. Use flow sheets to record the frequent assessments, vital signs, pulse oximetry readings, intake and output, IV fluid therapy, and laboratory test and arterial blood gas (ABG) values. Include patient teaching and emotional support given. An electronic health record or flow sheet would be used to document the patient status with pulmonary embolism and record the patient's changing status and parameters permanently.

Nursing Care of Patient with Pulmonary Embolism		
4/19/2019	0745	**NURSING ASSESSMENT:** Pt. found SOB, pale, restless, and c/o chest pain described as "crushing." P 104, BP 150/90, RR 30 and shallow, SaO_2 88%, oral T 99.9°F. Crackles heard in lower lobes bilaterally. Occasional productive cough with pink-tinged sputum. Alert and oriented but very anxious, stating "Help me, I'm going to die." ____ **NURSING INTERVENTION:** Dr. B. Hope stat paged and came to see pt. immediately at 0725. O_2 started via nonrebreather mask and SaO_2 improved to 92% as ordered. IV line started as ordered in right forearm with 18G angiocath on first attempt. 500 mL NSS infusing at 30 mL/hr. Stat portable CXR done as ordered at 0735. ABGs, CBC, coagulation studies, and cardiac enzymes drawn as ordered and sent to lab stat. 12-lead ECG shows sinus tachycardia. $\dot{V}/\dot{Q}$ scan ordered stat as ordered. See flow sheets for documentation of frequent VS, pulse ox, assessments, I/O, IV therapy, and lab values. ____ **PATIENT TEACHING/EDUCATION:** Explaining all procedures to pt. as well as the need for lung scan. ____
		____ **George Stein, RN**

PULSE OXIMETRY

Pulse oximetry is a noninvasive procedure used to monitor a patient's arterial blood oxygen saturation (SaO_2) to detect hypoxemia. Lack of adequate oxygenation can cause permanent cellular damage and death.

A sensor containing two light-emitting diodes (LEDs)—one red and one infrared—and a photodetector placed opposite these LEDs across a vascular bed are attached to the skin with adhesive or clips. The sensor is placed across a pulsating arteriolar bed, such as a finger, toe, nose, or earlobe. Selected wavelengths of light are absorbed by hemoglobin and transmitted through tissue to the photodetector. The pulse oximeter computes SaO_2 based on the relative amounts of light that reach the photodetector. The normal value is between 95% and 100%. Pulse oximetry may be performed intermittently or continuously. Pulse oximetry is a digitalized monitoring device that would record measurements directly on an electronic health record or flow sheet.

Essential Documentation

The nurse should record the date and time of each pulse oximetry reading. Frequent SaO_2 readings may be documented on a flow sheet. Document the reason for use of pulse oximetry and whether readings are continuous or intermittent. If SaO_2 readings are continuous, record the alarm settings. Chart whether the reading is obtained while the patient is breathing room air or receiving supplemental oxygen. If the patient is receiving oxygen, record the concentration and mode of delivery. Describe events precipitating acute oxygen desaturation, nursing actions, and the patient's response. Record activities or interventions affecting SaO_2 values. Document patient teaching related to pulse oximetry. Pulse oximetry is a digitalized monitoring device that would send recorded results to the electronic health record or flow sheet.

Nursing Care of Patient on Pulse Oximetry		
3/13/2019	1100	**NURSING ASSESSMENT:** At 1040 pt. gasping and SOB. P 128, BP 140/96, RR 34, tympanic T 97.3°F. Lips and nail beds cyanotic. Able to speak only 2 or 3 words between breaths due to dyspnea. O_2 NC resting on bedside table. Wife states, "He took it off because it hurts his ears." SaO_2 86%. ______ **NURSING INTERVENTION:** NC reapplied at 6 L/min. ______ **NURSING ASSESSMENT:** Pt. less dyspneic, able to speak in sentences. P 100, BP 136/90, RR 26. SaO_2 93%. ______ **NURSING INTERVENTION:** Pt. and wife instructed to leave NC in place in nostrils. Tubing padded around earpieces for comfort. ______ **PATIENT AND FAMILY TEACHING/EDUCATION:** Pt. instructed to call the nurse if tubing becomes uncomfortable rather than removing it. Pt. and wife verbalized understanding of the need for the oximetry monitoring. ______ **Terry Delmonico, RN**

SELECTED READINGS

Aggarwal, A., & Chikara, A. (2018). Common principles of management of poisoning. *Indian Journal of Medical Specialties, 9*(3), 107–112.

Anderson, D. (2018). Enhancing acute hospital care for patients who have self-harmed. *Nursing Times, 114* (2), 41–41.

Aplin, N. (2017). Advanced nurse practitioner-led abdominal therapeutic paracentesis. *Emergency Nurse, 24*(10), 34–37.

Arshad, H., Young, M., Adurty, R., & Singh, A. C. (2016). Acute pneumothorax. *Critical Care Nursing Quarterly, 39*(2), 176–189.

Bernstein, A. D., Daubert, J. C., Fletcher, R. D., Hayes, D. L., Luderitz, B., Reynolds, D. W., ... Sutton, R. (2002). The revised NASPE/BPEG generic code for antibradycardia, adaptive-rate, and multisite pacing. *Pacing and Clinical Electrophysiology, 25*(2), 260–264.

Black, J. (2018). Take three steps forward to prevent pressure injury in medical-surgical patients: Nursing care is key to pressure injury prevention. *American Nurse Today,* May Supplement, 10–39.

Bowman, S. (2017). Understanding the HIPAA individual right of access to health information. *Health Management Technology, 38*(9), 16.

Buley, D. D. (1986). When the burden of proof falls on you: Searching a patient's belongings for evidence. *Nursing, 16(*2), 41.

Bulger-Noto, J. (2018). Leadless pacemakers: A new technology in cardiac pacing. *American Nurse Today, 13*(10), 18–26.

Burkart, J. M. (2018). *Peritoneal dialysis.* Retrieved from UpToDate website: https://www.uptodate.com/contents/peritoneal-dialysis-beyond-the-basics

Chemecky, C., Macklin, D., & Blackburn, P. (2015). Catheter-related bloodstream infections (CR-BSI) in geriatric patients in intensive care units. *Critical Care Nursing Quarterly, 38*(3), 280–292.

Chivinge, A., Wilkes, E., James, M., Ryder, S., Aithal, G., & Simpson, D. (2015). Implementing a nurse-led paracentesis service to improve patient care and experience in a day case unit. *Gastrointestinal Nursing, 2015 Liver Nursing Supplement, 13*(Sup10), S11–S15.

Cicolini, G., Simonetti, V., Comparcini, D., Labeau, S., Blot, S., Pelusi, G., & Di Giovanni, P. (2014). Nurses' knowledge of evidence-based guidelines on the prevention of peripheral venous catheter-related infections: A multicentre survey. *Journal of Clinical Nursing, 23*(17/18), 2578–2588.

Cooper, K. L. (2015). Biventricular pacemakers in patients with heart failure. *Critical Care Nurse, 35*(2), 20–28.

Cox, F. (2018). Advances in the pharmacological management of acute and chronic pain. *Nursing Standard, 33*(3), 37–42.

Cox, J., Roche, S., & Murphy, V. (2018). Pressure injury risk factors in critical care patients: A descriptive analysis. *Advances in Skin & Wound Care, 31*(7), 328–334.

Davis, L. L.(2014). Cardiovascular issues in older adults. *Critical Care Nursing Clinics of North America,* 26(1), 61–89.

EDUCATION: Pre-and post-operative care. (2017). *Australian Nursing & Midwifery Journal, 25*(2), 22–23.

Feliciano, D. V. (2017). Abdominal trauma revisited. *American Surgeon, 83(*11), 1193–1202

Fletcher, J. (2013). Parenteral nutrition: Indications, risks, and nursing care. *Nursing Standard, 27*(46), 50–57.

Francis, J., & Young, G. B. (2018). Patient education: Delirium (Beyond the Basics). Retrieved from UpToDate website: https://www.uptodate.com/contents/delirium-beyond-the-basics

Frederick, D. E. (2014). Pulmonary issues in the older adult. *Critical Care Nursing Clinics of North America, 26*(1), 91–97.

Golembiewski, J., Dasta, J., & Palmer, P. P. (2016). Evolution of patient-controlled analgesia: From intravenous to sublingual treatment. *Hospital Pharmacy, 51*(3), 214–229.

Haddock, G., Eisner, E., Davies, G., Coupe, N., & Barrowclough, C. (2013). Psychotic symptoms, self-harm and violence in individuals with schizophrenia and substance misuse problems. *Schizophrenia Research, 151*(1–3), 215–220.

Hicks, R. W., Hernandez, J., & Wanzer, L. J. (2012). Perioperative pharmacology: Patient-controlled analgesia. *AORN Journal, 95*(2), 255–265.

Jackson, A. (2010). An overview of permanent cardiac pacing. *Nursing Standard, 25*(12), 47–57.

Jacobsen, P., Hodkinson, K., Peters, E., & Chadwick, P. (2018). A systematic scoping review of psychological therapies for psychosis within acute psychiatric in-patient settings. *British Journal of Psychiatry, 213*(2), 490–497.

Jepsen, S. (2018). Managing alarms in acute care across the life span: Electrocardiography and pulse oximetry. *Critical Care Nurse, 38*(2), e16–e20.

Kalowes, P. (2018). Preventing pressure injuries in critically ill patients: Evidence-based care bundles improve patient safety and prevent pressure injuries. *American Nurse Today, May Supplement,* 14–40.

Leier, M. (2018). Advancements in pacemaker technology: The leadless device. *Critical Care Nurse, 37*(2), 58–65.

Li, W., Xu, R., & Fan, D. (2018). Clinical application of electrocardiogram-guided tip positioning in peripheral inserted central catheters placement. *Journal of Cancer Research & Therapeutics, 14*(4), 887–891.

Mendes, A. (2018). Becoming aware of patients at risk of self-harm or suicide. *British Journal of Community Nursing, 23*(5), 256–257.

Mesko, P. J., & Eliades, A. B. (2018). Using pictures to assess pain location in children. *Journal of PeriAnesthesia Nursing, 33*(3), 319–324.

Miner, M. B., Stephens, K., Swanson-Biearman, B., Leone, V., & Whiteman, K. (2018). Enhancing cancer pain assessment and management in hospice. *Journal of Hospice & Palliative Nursing, 20*(5), 452–458.

Moreland-Lewis, M. J. (2018). Nursing research: Pain control and nonpharmacologic interventions. *Nursing, 48*(9), 65–68.

National Pressure Ulcer Advisory Panel (NPUAP). (n.d.). Educational and clinical resources. Retrieved from http://www.npuap.org/

Oware-Gyekye, F. (2008). Pain management: The role of the nurse. *West African Journal of Nursing, 19*(1), 50–54.

Palmer, C. (2017). Providing self-management education to patients with type 2 diabetes mellitus: Addressing basic nutrition and hypoglycemia. *Nurse Practitioner, 42*(11), 36–42.

Palmer, S. J. (2014). Post-implantation pacemaker complications: The nurse's role in management. *British Journal of Cardiac Nursing, 9*(12), 592–598.

Q & A Legal Questions. (2000). Patient privacy: Unreasonable search? *Nursing, 30*(3), 66–67.

Rali, P., Gandhi, V., & Malik, K. (2016). Pulmonary embolism. *Critical Care Nursing Quarterly, 39*(2), 131–138.

Rowe, J., & Jaye, C. (2017). Caring for self-harming patients in general practice. *Journal of Primary Health Care, 9*(4), 279–285.

Runyon, B. A. (2018). Spontaneous bacterial peritonitis in adults: Treatment and prophylaxis. Retrieved from UpToDate website: http://www.uptodate.com

Runyon, B. A. (2018). Spontaneous bacterial peritonitis in adults: Diagnosis. Retrieved from UpToDate website: http://www.uptodate.com

Schreiber, M. L.(2016). Evidence-based practice. Peritoneal dialysis: Understanding, educating, and adhering to standards. *Medsurg Nursing, 25*(4), 270–274.

Wang, T., Pizziferri, L., Volk, L. A., Mikels, D. A., Grant, K. G., Wald, J. S., & Bates, D. W. (2004). Implementing patient access to electronic health records under HIPAA: Lessons learned. *Perspectives in Health Information Management, 1,* 11.

Wang, Y., Liao, C., & Kao, C. (2012). Nursing assessment and management of patients with cardiogenic pulmonary edema. *Journal of Nursing, 59*(1), 24–29.

Webb, J. A., & LeBlanc, T. W. (2018). Evidence-based management of cancer pain.

Seminars in Oncology Nursing, 34(3), 215–226.

Wyer, N. (2017). Parenteral nutrition: Indications and safe management. *British Journal of Community Nursing, Supplement 7,* (22), S22–S28.

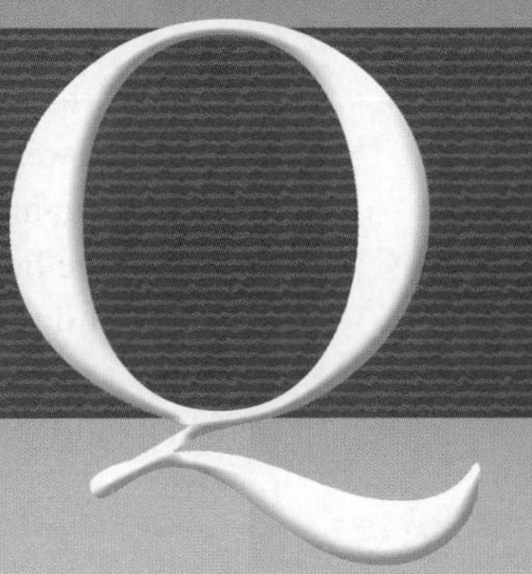

QUALITY OF CARE, FAMILY QUESTIONS ABOUT

At times, the family of a patient may have questions about the quality of care that a family member is receiving. These concerns should be taken seriously—ignoring them increases the risk of a lawsuit. Moreover, a nurse should not argue with the family or defend him- or herself, a coworker, the health care provider, or the facility. Active listening is the critical communication skill that must be applied at such times.

When family members question the quality of care, ask them to clarify what they believe to be the problem. The nurse needs to provide education about nursing routines, policies, procedures, and within the limits of confidentiality, the patient's care plan. If the concern is not a nursing issue, the family will find it helpful to be guided to the answers to their questions. A nurse can ask the health care provider, nursing supervisor, or another appropriate person to speak with the family, if appropriate. All unresolved concerns about the quality of care should be reported to the nursing supervisor or manager. This essential, professional communication is the national standard of ethical care as delineated in the American Nurses Association (2015) *Code of Ethics for Nurses with Interpretive Statements.* The nurse's capacity to listen carefully and respond appropriately without agreeing with family members' points of view may be all that it takes to resolve patient or family concerns.

Essential Documentation

The nurse needs to:

- Record the date and time of the initial conversation.
- Include the names of the family members present.

- Document the concerns using their own words, in quotes, if possible.
- Describe answers by the nurse and the family members' responses.
- Record the names of the people notified of the family's concerns, including the health care provider, nursing supervisor, and nursing manager, and the time of notification.
- Document the conversation and the responses, in quotes. It is critical to add a narrative, anecdotal note to the electronic health record.

Quality-of-Care Questions		
6/22/2019	1600	**NURSING ASSESSMENT:** Pt.'s daughter, Emily Jones, verbalized concerns regarding mother's hygiene. She stated, "I don't think my mother is receiving her showers. Her hair and fingernails are dirty." ________ **PATIENT TEACHING:** After reviewing the shower schedule, explained to Mrs. Jones that her mother has been refusing showers since admission and has been receiving sponge baths instead. Reassurance given that additional efforts will be made to provide pt. with a shower or additional bathing as needed. ________ **Liz Mazerka, RN**

SELECTED READINGS

American Nurses Association. (2015). *Code of ethics for nurses with interpretive statements.* Silver Spring, MD: Author. Retrieved from https://www.nursingworld.org/coe-view-only

Ratwani, R. M., Moscovitch, B., & Rising, J. P. (2018). Improving pediatric electronic health record usability and safety through certification. *JAMA Pediatrics, 172*(11), 1007–1008. doi:10:1001/jamapediatrics.2018/2784

R

RAPE-TRAUMA SYNDROME

The term *rape* refers to nonconsensual sexual intercourse. Rape inflicts varying degrees of physical and psychological trauma. Rape-trauma syndrome typically occurs during the period following the rape or attempted rape. It refers to the victim's short- and long-term reactions and the methods used to cope with the trauma. Traditionally, the victim of rape is a woman, and the abuser is a man. However, rape does occur between persons of the same sex. Additionally, women may also be rapists. Children are often victims of rape; most of the time, these cases involve manual, oral, or genital contact with the child's genitalia. Commonly the rapist is a member of the child's family.

The prognosis is promising if the rape victim receives physical and emotional support and counseling to help deal with feelings. Patients who articulate feelings can cope with fears, interact with others, and return to normal routines faster than those who do not. Objective and precise documentation of care for a patient who has been raped may be important if the notes are used as evidence in cases where the rapist is charged and brought to trial.

Essential Documentation

The nurse needs to:

- Record the patient's statements, using the patient's own words, in quotes.
- Also, document objective information provided by others.
- Include the time that the patient arrived at the facility, the date and time of the alleged rape, and the time of examinations performed.

- Ask the patient about recent illnesses (especially sexually transmitted disease) and allergies to medications.
- Ask a female patient about the possibility of pregnancy before the attack, the date of her last menstrual period, and details of her obstetric and gynecologic history.
- Describe the patient's emotional state and behaviors.
- Make sure the health care provider has obtained the patient's informed consent for treatment.
- Note whether she douched, bathed, or washed before coming to the facility.

If the case comes to trial, specimens will be used for evidence, so accuracy is essential. Most emergency departments have special kits for rape victims, with containers for specimens. During the examination, it is important for the nurse to:

- Make sure all specimens collected (including fingernail scrapings, pubic hair combings, semen, and gonorrhea culture) are labeled carefully with the patient's name, health care provider's name, and location from which the specimen was obtained.
- Place all the patient's clothing in paper, not plastic, bags. If clothing is placed in plastic bags, secretions and seminal stains will become moldy, destroying valuable evidence.
- Label each bag and its contents. List all specimens in the note, and record to whom these specimens were given.
- Follow agency protocol regarding the sealing of all evidence bags and containers.
- Document whether photographs were taken and by whom.

This examination is typically very distressing for the rape victim, so (a) provide reassurance, and (b) allow control of the interaction as appropriate. The victim may need to have periods of time out during the examination. If the patient wishes, a counselor may be asked to remain in the room throughout the examination. The nurse should:

- Document the names of witnesses to the examination.
- Counseling helps the patient identify coping mechanisms. The gender of the counselor may be of concern to the victim. Rapport may be easier to establish if the counselor is of the same sex.
- If the patient is wearing a tampon, remove it, wrap it, and label it as evidence.
- List all medications administered (e.g., antibiotics and birth control prophylaxis, such as morning-after pills) on the medication administration record.

- Explain possible adverse effects, what to expect of the medication, and signs and symptoms to report.
- Document all teaching administered, and provide the patient with written instructions before discharge.
- Record care given to such injuries as lacerations, cuts, or areas of swelling.
- Document whether the patient was offered and received testing for human immunodeficiency virus (HIV) or hepatitis B and C.
- Include whether prophylaxis for hepatitis was given.
- Chart that the nurse told the patient the importance of follow-up testing in 5 to 6 days for gonorrhea and syphilis.
- Record the names and telephone numbers of contact persons for local resources, including rape crisis centers, victims' rights advocates, and local law enforcement.
- Chart any other education and support given to the patient.

Rape Trauma Syndrome

8/10/2019	2250	**NURSING ASSESSMENT:** Pt. admitted to ED accompanied by police officers John Hanson (badge #1234) and Teresa Collins (badge #5678). Pt. states, "I was attacked in the supermarket parking lot. I think it was about 9 p.m. He pulled me into the bushes and raped me. When he ran away, I called 911 from my cell phone." Pt. trembling and crying but able to walk into ED on her own. Placed in private room. Police officers waited in waiting room. Pt. denies being pregnant, drug allergies, and recent illnesses including sexually transmitted disease (STD). LMP 7/28/19. States she didn't wash or douche before coming to the hospital. Chain of evidence maintained for all specimens collected (see flow sheet). ___ **NURSING INTERVENTION:** After obtaining written consent and explaining procedure, Dr. J. Smith examined pt. ___ **NURSING ASSESSMENT:** Pt. has reddened areas on face and anterior neck and blood on lips. Bruising noted on inner aspects of both thighs; some vaginal bleeding noted. ___ **NURSING INTERVENTION:** Pelvic exam performed by Dr. Smith. Specimens for STDs, blood, and vaginal smears collected and labeled. Evidence from fingernail scraping and pubic hair combing collected and labeled. Photographs of injuries taken. ___ **PATIENT TEACHING:** Stayed with pt. throughout exam, offering reassurance and comfort. Pt. cooperated with exam but was often teary. **NURSING INTERVENTION:** After explaining the need for prophylactic antibiotics to pt., she consented and ceftriaxone 250 mg I.M. was administered in left dorsogluteal muscle. Pt. declined morning-after pill. Pt. consented to blood screening for HIV and hepatitis. Blood samples drawn, labeled, and sent to lab. Pt. understands need for f/u tests for HIV, hepatitis, and venereal disease. States she will f/u with family dr. ___ **Susan Rose, RN**

Rape Trauma Syndrome (*continued*)

8/10/2019	2330	**PATIENT TEACHING:** June Jones spoke with pt. at length. Gave pt. information on rape crisis center and victims' rights advocate. Pt. phoned brother and sister-in-law who will come to hospital and take pt. to their home for the night. Police officers interviewed pt. with her permission regarding the details of the event. At pt.'s request, Ms. Jones and myself remained with pt. ——— **Susan Rose, RN**
8/10/2019	2350	Pt.'s brother, John Muncy, and his wife, Carol Muncy, arrived to take pt. to their house. Pt. will make appt. tomorrow to f/u with own dr. next week or sooner, if needed. ——— **PATIENT TEACHING:** Pt. has names and phone numbers for rape crisis counselor, victims' rights advocate, Ms. Jones, ED, and police dept. ——— **Susan Rose, RN**

REFUSAL OF TREATMENT

Any mentally competent adult can refuse treatment. In most cases, the health care personnel responsible for the patient's care can remain free from legal jeopardy as long as they fully inform the patient about the medical condition, the proposed testing or treatment, and the likely consequences of refusing treatment. The courts recognize a competent adult's right to refuse medical treatment, even when that refusal will clearly lead to death. (See *Respecting a patient's right to refuse care*, below.)

When treatment is refused, it is important to inform the patient of the risks involved in making such a decision. If possible, inform in writing. If refusal of treatment continues, the nurse should notify the health care provider, who will choose the most appropriate plan of action. If the patient has a language barrier, a translator should be provided per facility policy.

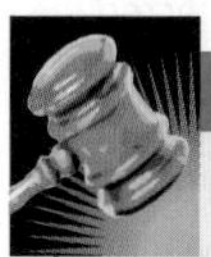

LEGAL CASEBOOK

RESPECTING A PATIENT'S RIGHT TO REFUSE CARE

A patient's request to refuse treatment should never be ignored. A patient can sue for battery—intentionally touching another person without authorization—for simply following a health care provider's orders.

To overrule the patient's decision, the health care provider or the facility must obtain a court order. Only then are health care providers legally authorized to administer the treatment.

Essential Documentation

The nurse needs to:

- Record the date and time of the patient's refusal of treatment.
- Be sure to document the patient's exact words in the chart as well as a neurologic assessment that describes the patient's mental status.
- Document that the prescribed treatment was not provided because the patient refused it. This action is necessary to protect the nurse legally.
- Ask the patient to sign a refusal-of-treatment release form. If the patient refuses to sign the release form, document this refusal in the progress notes along with the reason for refusal of treatment, if known. For additional protection, the facility's policy may require the nurse to ask the patient's spouse or closest relative to sign another refusal-of-treatment release form. If an interpreter is used, document the name of the translator, such as AT&T phone services.

Refusal of Treatment		
9/8/2019	2000	**NURSING ASSESSMENT:** Pt. refusing to have IV line inserted, stating that he's "sick and tired of being stuck." ______ **PATIENT TEACHING:** Explained to pt. the need for IV fluids and antibiotics and the likely result of refusing treatment. Dr. G. Eisenberg notified at 1930 and came to see pt. Dr. Eisenberg spent 20 minutes with pt. explaining rationales for therapies and potential risks of refusing therapy. Pt. still refusing I.V. line. Pt. has agreed to take oral antibiotics. Pt. verbalized understanding that oral antibiotics aren't as effective in treating his condition. ______ **Jack Bard, RN**

ACUTE KIDNEY INJURY

Acute kidney injury (AKI) is a clinical syndrome characterized by a rapid decline in renal function with progressive azotemia and increasing levels of serum creatinine in the blood. Obstruction, reduced circulation, and renal parenchymal disease can all cause the sudden interruption of renal function. Most commonly, AKI follows ischemic changes to renal cells due to severe, prolonged hypotension or hypovolemia, or renal cell changes due to contact with nephrotoxic agents. AKI is frequently reversible with medical treatment; however, it may progress to end-stage renal disease, uremic syndrome, and death.

If the nurse suspects that the patient has AKI, the health care provider must be contacted immediately. Diuretic therapy; fluid restrictions; electrolyte monitoring; treatment of hyperkalemia; and a diet low in protein, sodium, and potassium should be anticipated.

Essential Documentation

The nurse needs to:

- Document the assessment findings of AKI, such as oliguria, azotemia, anorexia, nausea, vomiting, bleeding, drowsiness, irritability, confusion, dry skin and mucous membranes, pruritus, Kussmaul's respirations, pulmonary edema, and hypotension early in AKI. Later in the disease, document such assessment findings as hypertension, arrhythmias, fluid overload, heart failure, systemic edema, anemia, and altered clotting.
- Note the name of the health care provider notified, the time of notification, and orders given, such as diagnostic testing; diet high in calories and low in protein, sodium, and potassium; fluid restrictions; and treatment of hyperkalemia with such therapies as dialysis, hypertonic glucose and insulin infusions, or sodium polystyrene sulfonate.
- Record the interventions, such as cardiac monitoring, initiating an intravenous (IV) line, inserting an indwelling urinary catheter, monitoring daily weights, assessing for pericarditis, monitoring electrolytes and fluid balance, maintaining proper nutrition, reporting abnormal laboratory test values to the health care provider, and monitoring for bleeding.
- Chart the patient's responses to these interventions. Use flow sheets to record the frequent assessments, vital signs, hourly intake and output, daily weight measurements, IV fluid therapy, drug administration, and laboratory test values.
- Chart all patient teaching and emotional care provided. Depending on the facility's policy, education may be recorded on a patient-teaching flow sheet.

Acute Kidney Injury		
12/18/2019	1300	**NURSING ASSESSMENT:** Answered call light at 1230 and found pt. SOB. Crackles and wheezes heard bilaterally, S_3 heart sound present, but no murmurs. Peripheral pulses palpable, skin warm and dry. Restless, moving about in bed. Drowsy, but alert and oriented to time, place, and person. No c/o nausea, vomiting, numbness, or tingling. P 118 and regular, BP 92/58, RR 22 and deep, tympanic T 99.0°F, weight 187 lb, up 3 lb since last weight on 12/17/19. ________________

Acute Kidney Injury (*continued*)		
		NURSING INTERVENTION: Dr. B. Kirsch notified of assessment findings at 1240 and came to see pt. Orders given. Lab called to draw stat CBC w/diff., BUN, creatinine, electrolytes, and coagulation studies. Urine sample sent to lab for UA. **Bob Harkin, RN**
12/18/2019	1430	**NURSING INTERVENTION:** #18 French Foley catheter inserted w/o difficulty to gravity drainage, initially drained 40 mL straw-colored urine. Renal ultrasound scheduled for 1500. 1500 mL fluid restriction started. See flow sheets for documentation of frequent VS, assessments, I/O, IV therapy, weights, and lab values. Furosemide 40 mg P.O. daily ordered and given at 1330. **PATIENT TEACHING:** Explained fluid restriction, dietary change, and indications and action of furosemide to pt. and wife. **Bob Harkin, RN**

REPORTS TO HEALTH CARE PROVIDER

The nurse needs the following reports to communicate to the health care provider: changes in the patient's condition, laboratory and other test results, and patient concerns. If the patient's care comes into question, the health care provider could claim not being notified. Such a claim, clearly, needs to be countered with proper documentation of the communication.

Nurses often write, "Notified health care provider of lab results." This statement is too vague. In the event of a malpractice suit, it allows the plaintiff's lawyer (and the health care provider) to imply that the nurse did not communicate reports to the health care provider. (See "Critical test values, reporting", page 84.)

Essential Documentation

The nurse needs to:

- Include in the note the date and time of notifying the health care provider, the means used to communicate (e.g., telephone or fax), the health care provider's name, and what was reported. If a message was left for the health care provider or a result was given to someone else such as a receptionist, record that person's name as well.
- Record the health care provider's response and any orders given. If no orders were given, that fact should also be documented.

Reports to Health care Provider		
9/13/2019	2215	**NURSING INTERVENTION:** Called Dr. W. Spencer at 2200 to report increased serous drainage from pt.'s left chest tube. Dr. Spencer's order was to observe the drainage for 1 more hr and then call him back. ______________________ **Danielle Bergeron, RN**

RESPIRATORY ARREST

Respiratory arrest is defined as the absence of respirations. If a patient is found without respirations, rapid intervention is critical because brain death occurs within 6 minutes after respirations cease. The nurse should immediately call for help and send a coworker to call the code team and the health care provider. After assessing the patient's airway and breathing, check for a pulse. If detected, rescue breathing is begun (using an Ambu bag) and continued until respirations return spontaneously or ventilatory support via endotracheal intubation and mechanical ventilation can be instituted.

Essential Documentation

Documenting the actions taken during a resuscitative effort may use a "code sheet." (For more on code sheets, see "Cardiopulmonary arrest and resuscitation," pages 61 to 63.) The documentation in the chart should:

- Include the date and time that the patient was found unresponsive and without respirations, the name of the person who found the patient, and whether the event was witnessed.
- Record the name of the person who initiated cardiopulmonary resuscitation (CPR) and the time CPR was initiated as well as the names of the other members of the code team.
- Document all interventions (e.g., drugs administered, cardiac monitoring, endotracheal intubation, and arterial blood gas analysis), the time they occurred, and the patient's response.
- Describe the outcome of the code. For example, patient resumption of spontaneous respirations, mechanical ventilation of the patient, or death.
- Note whether the family was present or the time that the family was notified of the event.
- Record the events leading to the respiratory arrest, the assessment findings that prompt the nurse to call a code, and any other interventions

performed before the code team arrived (e.g., the time that CPR was initiated). Include the patient's response to the interventions.

- Indicate in the note that a code sheet was used to document the events of the code.

Respiratory Arrest		
10/3/2019	1440	**NURSING INTERVENTION:** Pt. unresponsive and without spontaneous respirations. Code called at 1428. Ventilation attempt via Ambu bag unsuccessful. Head repositioned to open airway but still unable to deliver breath. No foreign bodies noted in mouth. After delivery of 3rd abdominal thrust, piece of meat was expelled. Pt. still without respirations; carotid pulse palpable. Rescue breathing initiated. Code team arrived at 1433 and continued resuscitative efforts. See code record. ________ **Fran Vitello, RN**
10/3/2019	1450	**NURSING ASSESSMENT:** Pt. resumed respirations and opened eyes. P 68, BP 102/52, RR 32 unlabored and deep. Placed on O_2 2 L/min via NC. Monitor showing sinus tachycardia. Pt. being transferred to ICU for observation. Report called to Peggy Wallace, RN, at 1445. Family notified of pt.'s condition and transfer to ICU. ________ **Fran Vitello, RN**

RESPIRATORY DISTRESS

Respiratory distress occurs when abnormalities of oxygenation or carbon dioxide are severe enough to endanger the function of vital organs. Causes of respiratory distress may be pulmonary or nonpulmonary in origin and may be a failure of oxygenation, ventilation, or both. Common causes of respiratory distress include acute respiratory distress syndrome, pneumonia, cardiogenic pulmonary edema, pulmonary embolism, asthma, chronic obstructive pulmonary disease, sedative and opioid overdose, hypersensitivity pneumonitis, head injury, chest trauma, massive obesity, amyotrophic lateral sclerosis, phrenic nerve or cervical cord injury, Guillain–Barré syndrome, and multiple sclerosis.

Respiratory distress can develop suddenly or gradually and is a life-threatening emergency. If the patient develops respiratory distress, the health care provider should be notified immediately. The nurse should anticipate interventions to treat the underlying condition and improve oxygenation, such as administering oxygen; mobilizing secretions; initiating endotracheal intubation and mechanical ventilation; and administering drug therapy to relieve bronchospasm, reduce airway inflammation, reverse opioid overdose, and alleviate severe anxiety and restlessness.

Essential Documentation

The nurse needs to:

- Record assessment findings of respiratory distress, such as dyspnea, use of accessory breathing muscles, abnormal breath sounds, cyanosis, restlessness, confusion, anxiety, delirium, tachypnea, tachycardia, hypertension, and arrhythmias.
- Provide information from the patient's reports of activities associated with or preceding the episodes of respiratory distress.
- Note the name of the health care provider notified, the time of notification, and the orders given, such as oxygen and drug administration.
- Record the interventions, such as the insertion of IV lines, administering oxygen and drugs, monitoring pulse oximetry and arterial blood gas (ABG) studies, assisting with the insertion of hemodynamic monitoring lines, assisting with endotracheal intubation, maintaining mechanical ventilation, and suctioning.
- Chart the patient's responses to these interventions.
- Use flow sheets to record the frequent assessments, vital signs, hemodynamic measurements, intake and output, IV therapy, and laboratory and ABG values.
- Document the instructions and explanations given to the patient, such as for coughing and deep-breathing exercises.
- Describe emotional support given to the patient.

Respiratory Distress		
11/3/2019	1500	**NURSING INTERVENTION:** At 1430 while receiving mechlorethamine via implanted port, pt. c/o chills and reported, "I have tightness in my chest. It feels like my throat is closing up." Drug infusion stopped and NSS infusing at 20 mL/hr. Pt. dyspneic, diaphoretic, and restless. P 122 and regular, BP 169/90, RR 34. O_2 sat. by pulse oximetry 88%. Expiratory wheezes noted bilaterally on posterior and anterior chest auscultation. Accessory muscle use observed. ______
		NURSING INTERVENTION: Dr. B. Jones stat paged at 1437 and told of assessment findings. Orders given. Non-rebreather mask applied. Pt. placed in high Fowler's position to facilitate breathing. Stat ABGs drawn by Dr. Jones. I.V. methylprednisolone given. See MAR. ______
		NURSING ASSESSMENT: At 1450 P 104, BP 140/84, RR 20. Pulse oximetry 95%. Pt. states her breathing is easier, no further chills. Breath sounds clear, no longer using accessory muscles. See flow sheets for documentation of frequent VS, I/O, and lab values. Reassured pt. that she will be closely monitored. ______
		______ **Rita Clarke, RN**

RESTRAINTS

Restraints are defined as any method of physically restricting a person's freedom of movement, physical activity, or normal access to the body; a drug that manages a patient's behavior or restricts a patient's movement and is not the standard treatment for that condition is also considered a restraint. Restraints can cause numerous problems, including limited mobility, skin breakdown, impaired circulation, incontinence, psychological distress, and strangulation.

There are two types of reasons for restraint use: behavioral (mental) health reasons (related to a patient's uncontrolled, dangerous behavior) and medical-surgical reasons (related to actions caused by a medical condition).

In 2009, The Joint Commission issued revised standards that were intended to reduce the use of restraints. The Joint Commission Policy on Restraint and Seclusion can be found at https://www.crisisprevention.com/CPI/media/Media/Resources/alignments/Joint-Commission-Restraint-Seclusion-Alignment-2011.pdf. According to the revised standards, restraint use is to be limited to emergencies in which the patient is at risk for harming him- or herself or others. Restraint types include physical, chemical, and seclusion. Restraint use is not to be used as a form of discipline. However, because restraints may be needed in emergencies, a facility may authorize qualified registered nurses to initiate their use. The standards emphasize staff education. It's important to know and follow the facility's policy on the use of restraints.

Time limitations have also been set on the use of restraints. For behavioral restraints, a face-to-face assessment from the ordering health care provider must be done every 4 hours. For medical-surgical restraints, a licensed independent practitioner must give an order for restraints within 12 hours of placing a patient in restraints; however, if the need for restraints is due to a significant change in the patient's condition, the licensed independent practitioner must examine the patient immediately. This order must be renewed every 24 hours or every calendar day.

The revised standards of The Joint Commission require continuous monitoring to ensure patient safety, including monitoring the patient's vital signs, nutrition and hydration needs, circulation, and hygiene and toileting needs. Documentation of restraint use must be done every 15 minutes if the patient is on a medical-surgical unit. Patients with restraints in an intensive care unit require documentation of restraint monitoring every 2 hours. The patient's family members must also be notified of the use of restraints if the patient consented to have them informed of his medical care. Moreover, the patient must be informed of the conditions necessary for release from restraints.

Essential Documentation

The nurse needs to:

- Document each episode of the use of restraints, including the date and time they were initiated. the facility may have a special form or flow sheet for this purpose.
- Record the circumstances resulting in the use of restraints and alternative interventions attempted first.
- Describe the rationale for the specific type of restraints used. Alternatives to restraint use should be documented.
- Chart the name of the licensed independent practitioner who ordered the restraints.
- Include the conditions or behaviors necessary for discontinuing the restraints and that these conditions were communicated to the patient.
- Record 15-minute assessments of the patient if the patient is on a medical-surgical unit, including signs of injury, nutrition, hydration, circulation, range of motion, vital signs, hygiene, elimination, comfort, physical and psychological status, and readiness for removing the restraints.
- Record the interventions to help the patient meet the conditions for removing the restraints. Note that the patient was continuously monitored.
- Document any injuries or complications that occurred, the time they occurred, the name of the health care provider notified, and the results of the interventions or actions.

Restraints		
8/28/2019	1400	**NURSING INTERVENTION:** Pt. extremely confused and pulled IV out at 1245. Attempted to calm patient through nonthreatening verbal communication. No IV access available. Dr. B. Miller notified at 1250 and came to see pt. at 1330. Ativan 2 mg IM given per Dr. Miller's order. After evaluation, Dr. Miller ordered soft wrist restraints applied to prevent harm to patient. Pt. informed that restraints would be removed when he could remain calm and refrain from trying to remove IV. See restraint monitoring sheet for frequent assessments and intervention notations. ______ **Carol Sacks, RN**

SELECTED READINGS

American Nurses Association. (2015). *Code of ethics for nurses with interpretive statements.* Silver Spring, MD: Author. Retrieved from https://www.nursingworld.org/coe-view-only

Andersen, L. W., Holmberg, M. J., Berg, K. M., Donnino, M. W., & Granfeldt, A. (2019). In-hospital cardiac arrest: A review. *JAMA,* 321(12), 1200–1210.

Chen, Y., & Tsai, H. (2008). The nursing experience of caring for a sexual assault victim. *Journal of Nursing, 55*(1), 99–104.

Hosohata, K., Inada, A., Oyama, S., Furushima, D., Yamada, H., & Iwanaga, K. (2019). Surveillance of drugs that most frequently induce acute kidney injury: A pharmacovigilance approach. *Journal of Clinical Pharmacy & Therapeutics, 44*(1), 49–53.

Marco, C. A., Brenner, J. M., Kraus, C. K., McGrath, N. A., Derse, A. R., & ACEP Ethics Committee. (2017). Refusal of emergency medical treatment: Case studies and ethical foundations. *Annals of Emergency Medicine, 70*(5), 696–703.

Misumida, N., Abdel-Latif, A., Smyth, S. S., Messerli, A., Ziada, K. M., Ogunbayo, G. O., & Shrout, T. A. (2019). Trends, management patterns, and predictors of leaving against medical advice among patients with documented noncompliance admitted for acute myocardial infarction. *Journal of General Internal Medicine, 34*(4), 486–488.

Parker, C. (2015). An innovative nursing approach to caring for an obstetric patient with rape trauma syndrome. *Journal of Obstetric, Gynecologic & Neonatal Nursing, 44*(3), 397–404.

Stinson, K. J. (2016). Nurses' attitudes, clinical experience, and practice issues with use of physical restraints in critical care units. *American Journal of Critical Care, 25*(1), 21–26.

University of Toledo, Office of University Communications. (2016). *Patient privacy laws and the media.* Retrieved from http://www.utoledo.edu/media/patient_privacy.html http://www.utoledo.edu/media/patient_privacy.html

Yu, M. K., Kamal, F., & Chertow, G. M. (2019). Updates in Management and Timing of Dialysis in Acute Kidney Injury. *Journal of Hospital Medicine, 14*(4), 232–238.

S

SBAR

Documentation Format

The situation, background, assessment, recommendation (SBAR) documentation format was introduced by rapid response teams at Kaiser Permanente in Colorado in 2002 to investigate patient safety. The SBAR technique can be used to facilitate prompt and appropriate communication between health care professionals. It allows for important information to be transferred accurately in a concise, organized, and predictable manner. The main purpose of the SBAR technique is to improve the effectiveness of communication through standardization of the communication process.

Nurses often take more of a narrative and descriptive approach to explaining a situation, whereas physicians and nurse practitioners need to hear only the main aspects of a situation. The SBAR technique closes the gap between these two approaches, allowing communicators to understand each other better. It includes a summary of the patient's current medical status, recent changes in condition, potential changes to watch for, resuscitation status, recent laboratory values, allergies, problem list, and recommendations.

SBAR is a useful communication strategy when there is a change in patient condition or between nurses during patient transfers to a new department or during shift change. The SBAR communication method is an evidence-based strategy for improving interprofessional communication. Studies show that it improves the quality of patient care and enhances patient safety.

The SBAR framework for communication between members of the health care team about a patient's condition is as follows:

- **S = Situation** (a concise statement of the current problem)
- **B = Background** (pertinent and brief information related to the current patient situation)
- **A = Assessment** (analysis of the patient problem; possible etiology and reasoning)
- **R = Recommendation** (action that is being requested/recommended)

Situation

This is a brief summary of the patient's current condition, which includes patient complaint and/or problem, symptoms, and physical assessment findings. It is important to begin with patient name, age, gender, and current diagnosis or reason for seeking health care.

Background

This is a brief summary of the patient's current condition during hospitalization or clinical encounter and past medical/surgical history that is related to the current patient situation.

Assessment

This includes analysis and inference regarding the current patient complaint, symptoms, and physical assessment findings. A nursing diagnosis can be stated here.

Recommendations/Request

This is a recommendation for action that can resolve the current patient problem. Alternatively, it can be a request for an order, medication, or treatment that can resolve the situation.

Example of SBAR Communication

The following is an example of the SBAR method of communication between a physician and nurse caring for the patient. The scenario involves a home health care nurse who is contacting the patient's physician regarding a new patient problem that has arisen.

Situation

I am the home health care nurse currently visiting Mrs. Maria Rodgers, who is a 76-year-old patient discharged from St. Peter's Medical Center 2 days ago after treatment for systolic heart failure. She is currently experiencing shortness of breath when walking short distances.

Background

Mrs. Rodgers has a past history of heart failure with pulmonary edema for which she was hospitalized in 2016 and 2017. Mrs. Rodgers was discharged 2 days ago with a diagnosis of heart failure and is currently taking Lasix 20 mg po daily, Digoxin 0.125 mg po daily, and Ramipril 5 mg po daily.

Assessment

Mrs. Rodgers is dyspneic on exertion, with evident circumoral cyanosis. Vital signs are 98.4 T-P 78- RR 18- BP 130/80. She has no jugular venous distension but has audible crackles bilaterally in both lung bases. She has +2/4 ankle edema bilaterally. The patient is likely suffering worsening heart failure.

Recommendations/Request

I have sat the patient upright in a chair with her legs elevated and applied thromboembolic stockings. I am requesting your advice as to how to proceed with the nursing care of Mrs. Rodgers. Would it be appropriate to increase the dosage of any of her current medications?

SECLUSION

During seclusion, a patient is separated from others in a safe, secure, and contained environment with close nursing supervision to protect him- or herself, other patients, and staff members from imminent harm. Seclusion is perceived as a contentious practice, and with the move toward treating people with mental health issues in the least restrictive environment, it has received much criticism. Consequently, there has been considerable debate about its therapeutic value and a call for it to be phased out. Alternative methods are preferred to seclusion, such as de-escalation, which attempts to safely communicate with the patient to reduce agitation and violent behavior. Staff education on de-escalation communication techniques is essential to reduce the use of seclusion and restraint practices. A restrictive environment commonly escalates patient distress. A "comfort versus control" paradigm can be instituted that can decrease the use of seclusion and restraint. Seclusion is used when nonphysical interventions are ineffective and there are concerns for the safety of others. Seclusion should not be implemented as a form of punishment. Patients in seclusion must be under observation to prevent self-harm. The nurse should follow the facility's policy when placing a patient in seclusion and be familiar with The Joint Commission's standards on the use of seclusion for behavioral health care reasons in nonbehavioral health care settings.

Seclusion is based on three principles: containment, isolation, and decreased sensory input. In containment, the patient is restricted to an area in which he or she can be protected from harm. Moreover, others are protected from impulsive acts by the patient. Isolation permits the patient to withdraw from situations that are too intense for the patient to handle at that point. Decreased sensory input reduces external stimulation and sensory overload, allowing the patient to regroup and reorganize coping skills.

Essential Documentation

Record the date and time of each episode as well as the rationale for and circumstances leading up to the use of seclusion. Describe the nonphysical interventions that were tried first. In the nurse's notes, chart the time of notification of family members and their names. Document that the notification of the health care provider and the verbal or written order obtained. Enter the verbal order in the health care provider's orders, according to the facility's policy. Record each time the order for seclusion is renewed. Record the health care provider's visit and the provider's evaluation of the patient. Criteria for ending seclusion should be charted. Document what the patient was told about seclusion, including the behavior criteria for stopping seclusion. Chart frequent assessments of the patient, such as nutrition, hydration, circulation, range of motion, mobility, hygiene, elimination, comfort, and psychological status. Record nursing interventions to help the patient meet these needs. Describe nursing interventions to help the patient reduce the need for seclusion and the patient's responses to these interventions. Document that the patient is receiving continuous monitoring while in seclusion and by whom.

Seclusion		
10/26/2019	2000	**NURSING ASSESSMENT:** Approached by pt. at 1930, crying and saying loudly, "I can't stand it, they will get me." Repeated this statement several times. Unable to say who "they" were. Pt. asked to sit in a seclusion room saying, "it's quiet and safe there. That's what I do at the psych. hospital."
		NURSING INTERVENTION: Called Dr. R. Wright at 1935 and told him of pt. request. Verbal order given for seclusion as requested by pt. Dr. Wright will be in to evaluate pt. at 2030. Pt. placed in empty pt. room on unit in close proximity to nurses' station.
		PATIENT TEACHING: Told her that since seclusion was voluntary, she was free to leave seclusion when she felt ready. Rita Summers, CNA, assigned to continuously observe pt.
		NURSING ASSESSMENT: P 82, BP 132/82, RR 18, oral T 98.7°F.
		NURSING INTERVENTION/PATIENT AND FAMILY TEACHING: Family notified of pt.'s request for seclusion, that pt. is free to leave seclusion on her own, will be continuously observed by CNA and assessed frequently by RN, and that doctor will be by to see her at 2030. Family stated they were comfortable with this decision.
		Donna Blau, RN

SEIZURE MANAGEMENT

Seizures are paroxysmal events associated with abnormal electrical discharges of neurons in the brain. Partial seizures are usually unilateral, involving a localized or focal area of the brain. Generalized seizures involve the entire brain.

When the patient has a generalized seizure, observe the seizure characteristics to help determine the area of the brain involved; administer anticonvulsants as ordered; protect the patient from injury; and prevent serious complications, such as aspiration and airway obstruction. When caring for a patient at risk for seizures, take precautions to prevent injury and complications in the event of a seizure.

Essential Documentation

If a patient is at risk for seizures, document all precautions taken, such as padding the side rails, headboard, and footboard of the bed; keeping the bed in low position; raising the side rails while the patient is in bed; and having suction equipment nearby. Record that seizure precautions have been explained to the patient.

If the patient has a seizure, record the date and time it began as well as its duration and any precipitating factors. Provide a safe environment.

Remove any objects in the environment that can cause patient injury. Do not place anything in the patient's mouth. The patient can be turned on his or her side to avoid aspiration in case of vomiting. Describe involuntary behavior occurring at the onset, such as lip smacking, chewing movements, or hand and eye movements. Record any incontinence, vomiting, or salivation during the seizure. Describe where the movement began and the parts of the body involved. Note any progression or pattern to the activity. Document whether the patient's eyes deviated to one side and whether the pupils changed in size, shape, equality, or reaction to light. Note if the patient's teeth were clenched or open. Seizure activity that extends beyond 5 minutes is termed *status epilepticus.* This type of seizure signals an emergency that will need medical and pharmacologic intervention because it may be fatal.

The nurse should document the patient's response to the seizure, drugs given, complications, and interventions. Record the name of the health care provider notified, the time of notification, and any orders given. Finally, record the assessment of the patient's postictal mental and physical status every 15 minutes for 1 hour, every 30 minutes for 1 hour, and then hourly as long as there are no further complications or according to facility policy.

Document patient teaching provided for the patient or family members, including instructions given about preventing and managing seizures (See *Preventing seizures* below.).

PREVENTING SEIZURES

Teach the patient the following measures to help control and decrease the occurrence of seizures:

- Take the exact dose of medication at the times prescribed. Missing doses, doubling doses, or taking extra doses can cause a seizure.
- Eat balanced, regular meals. Low blood glucose levels (hypoglycemia) and inadequate vitamin intake can lead to seizures.
- Be alert for odors that may trigger an attack. Advise the patient and family members to inform the health care provider of any strong odors they notice at the time of a seizure.
- Limit alcohol intake. The patient should check with the health care provider to find out whether he or she can drink alcoholic beverages at all.
- Get enough sleep. Excessive fatigue can precipitate a seizure.
- Treat a fever early during an illness. If the patient can't reduce a fever, the patient should notify the health care provider.
- Learn to control stress. If appropriate, suggest learning relaxation techniques such as deep-breathing exercises.
- Avoid trigger factors, such as flashing lights, hyperventilation, loud noises, heavy musical beats, video games, and television.

Seizure Management

11/19/2019	1730	**NURSING ASSESSMENT:** At 1712, pt. had whole body stiffening, followed by alternating muscle spasm and relaxation, teeth clenched. Seizure lasted two minutes. Breathing was labored during seizure, no cyanosis noted. Pt. sleeping at time of onset. Pt. incontinent during seizure, but no vomiting or salivation noted. Padded side rails, headboard, and footboard in place prior to seizure; bed in low position; suction in room but not needed. ____ **NURSING INTERVENTION:** Pt. placed on left side, airway patent, breath sounds clear bilaterally. Dr. F. Gordon notified of seizure at 1716 and came to see pt. at 1720. Diazepam 10 mg given IV as ordered. ________ **NURSING ASSESSMENT:** Pt. currently sleeping, confused when aroused, not oriented to time or place. P 94, BP 142/88, RR 18 and regular, tympanic T 97.7°F. See flow sheets for frequent VS and neurologic assessments, per policy. Wife in to visit at 1725. ____________ **PATIENT/FAMILY TEACHING:** Explained that pt. had a seizure and measures taken to treat it. Reviewed with wife how to prevent seizures and gave her copy of written material, "Preventing Seizures." Wife verbalized understanding. ____________________ **Gale Hartman, RN**

SHOCK

Shock is a systemic pathologic event characterized by diffuse cellular ischemia that can lead to cell, tissue, and organ death if not promptly recognized and treated. Shock is classified as hypovolemic, cardiogenic, or distributive. The distributive type is further divided into septic, neurogenic, and anaphylactic shock. (See *Classifying shock*, page 362.)

Because shock either causes or results from multisystem failure, it's typically treated in an intensive care unit. Nursing responsibilities related to shock center on prevention, early detection, emergent treatment, and support during recovery and rehabilitation.

Essential Documentation

Record the date and time of the entry. Document the assessment findings of shock, such as declining level of consciousness, hypotension, tachycardia in early shock and bradycardia in later shock, electrocardiogram (ECG) changes, weakened pulses, dyspnea, tachypnea, declining arterial oxygen saturation and partial pressure of arterial oxygen, rising partial pressure of arterial carbon dioxide, respiratory and metabolic acidosis, oliguria, rising blood urea nitrogen and creatinine, diminished or absent bowel sounds, and pale and cool skin. Note the time of notification of the health care provider, the provider's name, and

CLASSIFYING SHOCK

Type	Description
Hypovolemic	Results from a decrease in central vascular volume. Total body fluids may or may not be decreased. Causes include hemorrhage, dehydration, and fluid shifts (trauma, burns, anaphylaxis).
Cardiogenic	Results from a direct or indirect pump failure with decreasing cardiac output. Total body fluid isn't decreased. Causes include valvular stenosis or insufficiency, myocardial infarction, cardiomyopathy, arrhythmias, cardiac arrest, cardiac tamponade, pericarditis, pulmonary hypertension, and pulmonary emboli.
Distributive	Results from inadequate vascular tone that leads to massive vasodilation. Vascular volume remains normal and the heart pumps adequately, the but size of vascular space increases, causing maldistribution of blood within the circulatory system. It includes the following subtypes: ▪ Septic shock—A form of severe sepsis characterized by hypotension and altered tissue perfusion. Vascular tone is lost, and cardiac output may be decreased. ▪ Neurogenic shock—Characterized by massive vasodilation from loss or suppression of sympathetic tone. Causes include head trauma, spinal cord injuries, anesthesia, and stress. ▪ Anaphylactic shock—Characterized by massive vasodilation and increased capillary permeability secondary to a hypersensitivity reaction to an antigen.

orders given, such as drug, fluid, blood, and oxygen administration. Record nursing interventions, such as assisting with the insertion of hemodynamic monitoring lines, inserting intravenous (IV) lines, administering drugs, continuous ECG monitoring, providing supplemental oxygen, inserting an indwelling urinary catheter, airway management, and pulse oximetry monitoring. Chart the patient's responses to these interventions. Use flow sheets to record frequent assessments, vital signs, hemodynamic measurements, intake and output, IV therapy, and laboratory test and arterial blood gas values. Also, record patient and family teaching and emotional care given.

Shock		
1/7/2019	1930	**NURSING ASSESSMENT:** At 1905 noted bloody abdominal dressing and abdominal distention. No bowel sounds auscultated. Pt. slow to respond to verbal stimulation, not oriented to time and place, and not readily following commands. Pupil response sluggish. Cardiac monitor reveals HR of 128, no arrhythmias noted. Peripheral pulses weak. Skin pale and cool; capillary refill 4-5 sec, BP 88/52. Breath sounds clear. Normal heart sounds. Breathing regular and deep, RR 24. O_2 sat. 88% on room air. ________

Shock (*continued*)

NURSING INTERVENTION: Dr. J. Garcia notified of changes at 1910 and orders given. 100% nonrebreather mask applied, O_2 sat. increased to 92%. Foley catheter placed with initial 70 mL urine output. Stat ABG, hemoglobin, hematocrit, serum electrolytes and renal panel ordered. IV inserted in left antecubital space with 18G catheter on first attempt. 1,000 mL IV dextrose 5% in 0.45% NSS infusing at 100 mL/hr. ________
PATIENT TEACHING: Explained all procedures and drugs to pt. and wife. Wife verbalized understanding and fears. Reassured wife that pt. is being closely monitored. See flow sheets for documentation of frequent VS, I/O, IV fluids, neuro. checks, and lab values. ________
________ **Brian Wilcox, RN**

SICKLE CELL CRISIS

Sickle cell anemia is a genetic disorder that occurs primarily, but not exclusively, in African Americans. It results from a defective hemoglobin molecule (hemoglobin S) that causes red blood cells to roughen and become sickle-shaped. Such cells impair circulation, resulting in chronic ill health (characterized by fatigue, dyspnea on exertion, and swollen joints), periodic vaso-occlusive crises, long-term complications, and premature death.

Although sickle cell anemia is a chronic disorder, acute exacerbations or crises periodically occur. If it is suspected that the patient with sickle cell anemia is in a crisis, the nurse should notify the health care provider immediately and anticipate oxygen and IV fluid administration and pain control.

Essential Documentation

The nurse should record the date and time of the entry. Document the assessment findings of a sickle cell crisis, such as severe abdominal, thoracic, muscular, and joint pain; jaundice; fever; dyspnea; pallor; and lethargy. Note the time of notification of the health care provider, the provider's name, and orders given, such as oxygen administration, analgesics, antipyretics, fluid administration, and blood transfusions. Record nursing interventions, such as initiating IV therapy using a large-bore catheter for blood and fluid administration, encouraging bed rest, placing warm compresses over painful joints, and administering drugs and oxygen. Chart the patient's responses to these interventions. Use flow sheets to record frequent assessments as well as the patient's vital signs, intake and output, IV therapy, and laboratory test values. Document any patient teaching performed (crisis prevention, genetic screening) and emotional support given.

Sickel Cell Disease		
4/8/2019	0900	**NURSING ASSESSMENT:** 19 y.o. male with history of sickle cell disease admitted to ED at 0825 with weakness and severe abdominal and joint pain. He reports nausea, vomiting, and poor oral intake × 3 days. Skin and mucous membranes pale and dry. Joints warm, red, swollen, and painful to touch. Pt. is dyspneic with clear breath sounds. Heart sounds normal. Pt. is alert and oriented to time, place, and person. Abdomen is painful to touch; auscultated bowel sounds in all 4 quadrants. P 96 and regular, BP 120/74, RR 22 and labored, oral T 100.2°F. Pt. rates abdominal and joint pain at 7 on a 0 to 10 scale, w/10 being the worst pain imaginable. ______
		NURSING INTERVENTION: Dr. B. McBride in to evaluate pt. at 0833. Electrolytes, bilirubin, CBC, ABGs drawn and sent to lab. Placed on O_2 at 4 L/min by NC. IV line started in left forearm on first attempt with #18G catheter. 1,000 mL of D5/0.45 NSS at 125 mL/hr. Tylenol 650 mg P.O. given for fever. Morphine 2 mg given IV over 4 min for pain at 0843. Pt. positioned with joints supported by pillows. Warm compresses placed on elbow and knee joints. Voided 400 mL clear yellow urine. Urinalysis sent to lab. ______
		PATIENT TEACHING: Explained all procedures and drugs to pt. Reinforced need for good hydration and encouraged oral fluids at 0853.
		NURSING ASSESSMENT: Pt. rated pain as 3 out of 10, with 10 being the worst pain imaginable. See flow sheets for documentation of frequent VS, I/O, IV fluids, and lab values. To be admitted to 6 West for pain control and IV hydration. Report called to Pat Stoner, RN. ______
		______ **Helene Mumford, RN**

SKIN CARE

In addition to helping shape a patient's self-image, the skin performs many physiologic functions. It protects internal body structures from the environment and potential pathogens, regulates body temperature and homeostasis, and serves as an organ of sensation and excretion. As a result, meticulous skin care is essential to overall health.

Essential Documentation

Record the date and time of the entry. Assess the patient's skin and describe its condition, noting changes in color, temperature, texture, tone, turgor, thickness, moisture, and integrity. Describe nursing interventions related to skin care, and record the patient's response. Note the time of notification of the health care provider of any changes, the provider's name, the orders given, nursing actions, and the patient's response. Describe patient teaching given, such as proper hygiene and the importance of turning and positioning every 2 hours.

Skin Care		
3/22/2019	1000	**NURSING ASSESSMENT:** During a.m. care, noted pt.'s skin to be dry and flaking, especially the hands, feet, and lower legs. Pt. states skin feels itchy in these areas. Skin rough, intact, warm to touch. Skin tents when pinched. After bath, blotted skin dry and applied emollient. ______ **PATIENT TEACHING:** Explained the importance of drinking more fluids and using emollients. Encouraged pt. not to scratch skin and to report intense itching to nurse. ______ **NURSING INTERVENTION:** Care plan amended to include use of superfatted soap with baths and application of emollients t.i.d. Dr. S. Johnson notified at 0945 and order given for Benadryl 0.25 mg P.O. every 6hr prn for intense itching. ______ **NURSING ASSESSMENT:** Pt. states, "The itching is not that bad right now after the lotion was applied." ______
		______ **Jason Dickson, RN**

SKIN GRAFT CARE

A skin graft consists of healthy skin taken from either the patient (autograft) or a donor (allograft) that is then applied to a part of the patient's body. The graft resurfaces an area damaged by burns, traumatic injury, or surgery. Care procedures for an autograft or allograft are essentially the same. However, an autograft requires care for two sites: the graft site and the donor site.

Successful grafting depends on various factors, including clean wound granulation with adequate vascularization, complete contact of the graft with the wound bed, aseptic technique to prevent infection, adequate graft immobilization, and skilled care. Depending on the facility's policy, a health care provider or specially trained nurse may change graft dressings.

Essential Documentation

The nurse should record the date and time of each dressing change. Note the location, size, and appearance of the graft site. Document all drugs used, and note the patient's response to these drugs. Describe the condition of the graft, and note any signs of infection or rejection. Chart the name of the health care provider notified, the time of notification, and any concerns or complications discussed. Record the specific care given to the graft site, including how it was covered and dressed. Document any patient and family teaching that provided and evidence of their understanding. Note the patient's reaction to the graft.

Skin Care Graft		
8/18/2019	1300	**NURSING ASSESSMENT:** Dressings carefully removed from right anterior thigh skin graft site. Site is 4 cm × 4 cm, pink, moist, and without edema or drainage. ____ **NURSING INTERVENTION:** Area gently cleaned by irrigating with NSS. Xeroflo placed over site and covered with burn gauze and a roller bandage. **PATIENT TEACHING:** Pt. instructed not to touch dressing, to report if dressing becomes loose, and to avoid placing any weight on the site. Pt. verbalized understanding of the instructions. Pt. stated, "The site doesn't look as bad as I thought it would." ____ ____ **Brian Wilcox, RN**

SMOKING

It's a well-known fact that smoking has adverse effects on health. Yet people continue to smoke—even in the hospital. Smoking in the hospital poses special risks beyond the usual health risks: secondhand smoke can aggravate many illnesses, fire and explosion may occur when a person smokes in an area where oxygen is being used, and a smoldering cigarette dropped in a wastebasket or on bed linens can start a fire.

Explain the facility's smoking policy to the patient on admission, and provide the patient with a written set of facility rules, if available. A patient found smoking in a nonsmoking area should be reminded of the facility's smoking policy. Ask the patient to extinguish the smoking materials and to move to a designated smoking area, if possible. Alert the health care provider if the patient is smoking against medical advice.

The nurse should talk to the patient about smoking cessation. A new diagnosis of cardiovascular disease, acute myocardial infarction, or acute coronary syndrome or a cardiovascular procedure all serve as "teachable moments" that can motivate a smoker to attempt cessation.

Evidence-based smoking cessation treatments include medications and behavioral support. The combination of medication and counseling is the most effective approach because it allows the management of both nicotine dependence and the conditioned behavior of smoking. The U.S. Public Health Service's 5As model provides a framework for brief, office-based tobacco treatment. Its steps include *asking* about tobacco use, *advising* tobacco users to quit, *assessing* readiness to quit, *assisting* with quit attempts by providing medications or connecting individuals to counseling resources, and *arranging* follow-up to monitor success or roadblocks related to quitting. If the patient is interested in quitting, discuss strategies for smoking cessation, including smoking cessation programs and nicotine replacement therapy.

Essential Documentation

The nurse should document that the patient received facility policies regarding smoking on admission. Record the patient's statement about smoking, including the number of years the patient has smoked and the number of cigarettes smoked per day. Describe the patient's feelings about quitting and the patient's experience with smoking cessation programs. Record patient teaching, such as discussing the hazards of smoking, the use of nicotine replacement therapy, and available information on smoking cessation programs and support groups. Describe the patient's response to teaching and any smoking cessation plans. Include any written materials given to the patient.

If the patient is smoking against facility policy, chart the date and time of the incident and where the patient was found smoking. Record what was told to the patient and the patient's response. Document any education that took place regarding smoking cessation and the patient's response. Some facilities may require the nurse to complete an incident report.

Smoking		
9/1/2019	1400	**NURSING ASSESSMENT:** Upon entering room, found pt. smoking while sitting up in his chair. Pt. complied when asked to extinguish cigarette. Reinforced the facility's no smoking policy. Discussed health risks of smoking to pt. ___
		PATIENT TEACHING: Explained that if pt. wished to smoke, he would need his dr.'s order to be escorted outdoors to a designated area. ___
		NURSING ASSESSMENT: Pt. stated that he was aware of health risks and would like to try to quit. Pt. stated, "I've been smoking since my teens, I know it's bad and I want to quit but I can't." Pt. reports 2-pack/day, 30-year history of smoking. Pt. asked about the use of a nicotine patch. Dr. N. Pasad notified of pt.'s smoking habit and interest in the use of a nicotine patch. Order given for nicotine patch, see MAR. ___
		PATIENT TEACHING: Use of nicotine patch, frequency, dosage, adverse effects, dangers of smoking while wearing patch, and s/s to report to dr. explained to pt. Pt. information dispensed with patch given to pt. to read. Pt. agrees to follow-up with Dr. Pasad after discharge for monitoring of smoking cessation. Gave pt. names and contact numbers for community support groups and cessation programs. ___
		___ **Bruce Mailor, RN**

SOAP

Documentation Format

The predominant type of electronic health record (EHR) used in hospitals and other clinical facilities is an electronic version of the problem-oriented SOAP documentation tool. Documenting the essential components of the patient encounter, including the patient's history, physical exam, diagnosis, and plan of care, is necessary for providing safety, continuity, and quality care. Nursing documentation requires a systematic, ordered, and logical approach, which the SOAP format provides, whether using an EHR or paper-based record.

The acronym SOAP represents the four major categories of documentation that have become traditional for provider documentation: subjective (S), objective (O), assessment (A), and plan (P).

Subjective

As the first section of the SOAP, the S section begins with a chief complaint (CC). This represents the specific concerns/complaint(s) for which the patient is seeking care or the current specific problem. The CC may be a direct quote or a paraphrased statement from the patient regarding the reason for seeking care. Depending on the chief complaint, the S subjective portion of the documentation may require some information from the patient's reported history of the present illness, past medical or surgical history, family or psychosocial history, or review of systems. Significant patient statements should be documented in the record exactly as stated and marked as a direct quotation.

Objective

In contrast to the subjective (S) information, objective (O) data consist of information that can be directly verified or measured. This information includes vital signs, physical assessment findings, lab results, and imaging/procedure findings. These data should be related to the subjective patient information and collected for the next step, which is assessment.

Assessment

The third section of the SOAP note is assessment (A) and includes data analysis and synthesis. It is the clinician's impression of the patient problem based on the subjective and objective data. Here the clinician uses logic and critical thinking skills to arrive at an assessment of the patient that concisely states the patient problem. The assessment section also includes nursing or medical diagnoses.

Plan

The final section, plan (P), is the clinician's proposed strategy to address the problem listed in the assessment section. The clinician determines the plan based on the subjective information, objective data, and assessment of the patient.

Example of SOAP Documentation

Date	Time	Entry
10-30-2019	1300	**S:** Patient reports she has a "headache that feels like a migraine is coming on" ______
		O: Patient is post–laparoscopic cholecystectomy, which was 2 hours ago. VS: 98.6–P 78–RR 12–120/80. Patient reports she has a history of migraine headaches × 10 years. Pain is described as 7/10, throbbing, bilateral. Reports that she takes rizatriptan for migraine headaches. Physical exam: unremarkable except for 3 small 2-cm sutured incisions in upper R quadrant of abdomen. Heart: RRR at 78 bpm. Lungs: clear. No bleeding from incisions. Bowel sounds present in all 4 Q. Patient has no neurologic deficit. ______
		A: Postoperative laparoscopic cholecystectomy × 2 hours. Acute migraine headache. History of migraine headache × 10 years. ______
		P: Called physician to report patient headache and request prescription for migraine medication for patient. M Conner, RN. ______

SPINAL CORD INJURY

In addition to spinal cord damage, spinal injuries include fractures, contusions, and compressions of the vertebral column (usually a result of trauma to the head or neck). The real danger lies in possible spinal cord damage. Spinal fractures most commonly occur in the 5th, 6th, and 7th cervical; 12th thoracic; and 1st lumbar vertebrae.

Most serious spinal injuries result from motor vehicle accidents, falls, diving into shallow water, and gunshot wounds; less serious injuries result from lifting heavy objects and minor falls. Spinal dysfunction may also result from hyperparathyroidism and neoplastic lesions.

If the patient has a spinal cord injury, the nurse should limit the extent of the injury with immobilization, administer medications as ordered, and take actions to prevent complications.

Essential Documentation

Record the date and time of the entry. Document measures taken to immobilize the patient's spine as well as measures taken to maintain airway patency and respirations. Document a baseline neurologic assessment, and chart the results of the cardiopulmonary, gastrointestinal, and renal assessments. Note the time of notification of the health care provider, the provider's name, and orders given, such as spinal immobilization and administration of steroids, analgesics, or muscle relaxants. Record nursing interventions, such as administering drugs, maintaining spinal immobilization, preparing the patient for neurosurgery, positioning and logrolling the patient, assisting with rehabilitation, and providing skin and respiratory care. Chart the patient's responses to these interventions. Use flow sheets to record frequent assessments and the patient's vital signs, intake and output, IV therapy, and laboratory test values. Include patient teaching and emotional care support given.

Spinal Cord Injury		
11/20/2019	0930	**NURSING ASSESSMENT:** Pt. alert and oriented to time, place, and person. Speech clear and coherent. No facial drooping or ptosis, tongue midline, swallows without difficulty. Readily follows commands. PERRLA. Pt. reports "mild tenderness" in lower back and states, "It's better than yesterday." Can perform active ROM of upper extremities with 5/5 muscle strength bilaterally in arms and hands. No voluntary muscle movement inferior to the iliac crests and pt. reports no sensation to touch, pressure, or temperature. Lower body muscles flaccid, patellar and Achilles reflexes absent. P 82 and regular, BP 126/72, RR 12 and regular, oral T 98.2°F. Breath sounds clear, normal heart sounds. Indwelling catheter in place and draining clear, yellow urine. See I/O sheet. Active bowel sounds are present in all 4 quadrants. Had brown, formed mod. size BM this a.m. Skin warm, dry, and intact with no tenting when pinched. Body alignment maintained while pt. logrolled with assist of 2 into left side-lying position. Skin intact, no areas of redness noted. ________
		PATIENT TEACHING: Reinforced importance of using incentive spirometer q/hr while awake. Pt. gave proper demo of its use. Pt. instructed to report any pain or changes in sensations. Discussed plan to begin bladder training today and remove indwelling catheter early tomorrow. Pt. expressed understanding of teaching and plans. ________
		________ **Brain Wilcox, RN**

SPLINT APPLICATION

By immobilizing the site of an injury, a splint alleviates pain and allows the injury to heal in proper alignment. It also minimizes possible complications, such as excessive bleeding into the tissues, restricted blood flow caused by bone pressing against vessels, and possible paralysis from an unstable spinal cord injury. In cases of multiple serious injuries, a splint or spine board allows caretakers to move the patient without risking further damage to bones, muscles, nerves, blood vessels, and skin.

Essential Documentation

Record the date and time of splint application. Document the circumstances and cause of the injury. Record the patient's complaints, noting whether symptoms are localized. Chart the assessment of the splinted region, noting swelling, deformity, and tissue and skin discoloration. Also, record neurovascular status before and after splint application.

Assessment of neurovascular status includes the following:

- Pulses distal to splinted region should be equal to unsplinted extremity.
- Color of extremities distal to the splinted region should be pink.
- Capillary refill of distal extremity should be < 2 seconds.

ASSESSING NEUROVASCULAR STATUS

When assessing an injured extremity, always include the following steps and compare the findings bilaterally:

- Inspect the color of fingers or toes.
- Note the size of the digits to detect edema.
- Simultaneously touch the digits of the affected and unaffected extremities and compare temperature.
- Check capillary refill by pressing on the distal tip of one digit until it's white. Then release the pressure and note how soon the normal color returns. It should return quickly in the affected and unaffected extremities.
- Check sensation by touching the fingers or toes and asking the patient to describe what is felt. Note reports of any numbness or tingling.
- Tell the patient to close his or her eyes; then move one digit and ask the patient which position it is in to check proprioception.
- Tell the patient to wiggle the toes or move the fingers to test movement.
- Palpate the distal pulses to assess vascular patency.

Record the findings for the affected and unaffected extremities, using standard terminology to avoid ambiguity. Warmth, free movement; rapid capillary refill; and normal color, sensation, and proprioception indicate sound neurovascular status.

- Sensation of the extremity distal to the splinted region should be intact.
- Mobility of the extremity distal to the splinted region should be intact.

The nurse should note the patient's level of discomfort, using a 0-to-10 pain scale, with 0 representing no pain and 10 representing the worst pain imaginable. Describe the type of wound, if any, noting the amount of bleeding and the amount and type of any drainage. Document the type of splint being used, and describe where it has been placed. If the bone end should slip into surrounding tissue or if transportation causes any change in the degree of dislocation, be sure to note it. Record the time of notification of the health care provider, the provider's name, and any orders given. Record all patient education, noting whether written instructions were given. Note that the patient received instruction for follow-up care.

Splint Application		
7/11/2019	0900	**NURSING ASSESSMENT:** Pt. fell off bicycle and landed on left arm. Left wrist swollen, no deformity or discoloration noted. 6 cm × 1 cm abrasion noted along left medial forearm. Pt. reports "throbbing" of left wrist, rates pain as 6 on a scale of 0 to 10, w/10 being the worst pain imaginable. Pt. denies pain in left hand or fingers, left radial pulse strong, left hand warm, capillary refill less than 3 sec, able to wriggle fingers of left hand and feel light touch. No c/o numbness or tingling in left hand. ______
		NURSING INTERVENTION: Abrasion cleaned with NSS and covered with sterile gauze dressing. Rigid splint applied to left forearm, extending from palm of left hand to just below left elbow. ______
		PATIENT/FAMILY TEACHING: Mother and son given discharge instructions. Mother verbalized understanding and says she will take pt. to pediatrician for follow-up care. Report called to pediatrician, Dr. E. Feng. No orders or instructions given to this nurse. ______
		______ **Steven Bobeck, RN**

STATUS ASTHMATICUS

An acute, life-threatening obstructive lung disorder, status asthmaticus doesn't respond to conventional asthma therapy and requires more aggressive treatment. Uncontrolled, status asthmaticus can lead to respiratory arrest or heart failure. Status asthmaticus may be triggered by allergens, occupational and environmental irritants, infections such as pneumonia, cold weather, and exercise.

If the patient's asthma continues to worsen despite medical treatment, suspect status asthmaticus and call the health care provider immediately. Anticipate administration of inhaled beta$_2$-adrenergic or anticholinergic drugs, subcutaneous epinephrine, IV aminophylline, corticosteroids, and fluids; oxygen administration; or intubation and mechanical ventilation.

Essential Documentation

The nurse should record the date and time of the entry. Document the assessment findings of status asthmaticus, such as severe dyspnea, tachypnea, tachycardia, air hunger, chest tightness, labored breathing, use of accessory muscles of breathing, nasal flaring, restlessness, extreme anxiety, frequent position changes, skin color changes, feelings of suffocation, wheezes (wheezing may not be heard with severe airway obstruction), low arterial oxygen saturation, or stridor.

Note the time of notification of the health care provider, the provider's name, and orders given, such as drug and fluid administration or oxygen therapy. Also, chart the time of notification of the respiratory therapist, the therapist's name, the therapist's actions, and the patient's response. Record nursing interventions, such as administering inhaled, IV, and subcutaneous drugs; administering oxygen; providing IV fluids; placing the patient in an upright position; calming the patient; and assisting with endotracheal intubation and mechanical ventilation. Chart the patient's responses to these interventions. Use flow sheets to record the frequent assessments and the patient's vital signs, intake and output, IV therapy, and laboratory tests, and arterial blood gas values. Include patient teaching and emotional care given.

Status Ashtmaticus		
12/13/2019	0900	**NURSING ASSESSMENT:** Called to room at 0930 and found pt. severely dyspneic stating, "I'm . . . suffocating . . ." Unable to speak more than 1 word at a time. Anxious facial expression, using nasal flaring and accessory muscles to breathe, restless and moving around in bed, skin pale. P 112 and regular, BP 142/88, RR 32 and labored. Wheezes audible without stethoscope, heard in all lung fields on auscultation. O_2 sat. 87%. **NURSING INTERVENTION:** Pt. placed in high Fowler's position and 35% oxygen by facemask applied. Called Dr. M. Dillon at 0937 and reported assessment findings. Orders given by Dr. Dillon. Stat ABG drawn at 0945 by Mike Traynor, RRT. IV line started on first attempt with #22G angiocath in right hand. 1,000 mL NSS infusing at 100 mL/hr. Methylprednisolone 150 mg given I.V.P. Nebulized albuterol administered by Mr. Traynor, RRT. ________

Status Ashtmaticus (*continued*)		
		PATIENT TEACHING: Stayed with pt. throughout event, explaining all procedures and offering reassurances. See flow sheets for documentation of frequent VS, I/O, IV, and ABG values. ________ ________ **Tom Gardner, RN**
12/13/10	1010	**NURSING ASSESSMENT:** ABG results: pH 7.33, Pao_2 75 mm Hg, $Paco_2$ 50 mm Hg, O_2 sat. 89%. Wheezes still heard in all lung fields but not as loud. Wheezing no longer audible without stethoscope. Pt. still dyspneic but states breathing has eased. Can speak several words at a time. Skin still pale, use of accessory muscles not as prominent. RR 24 and less labored. P 104, BP 138/86. ________ **NURSING INTERVENTION:** Dr. Dillon notified at 1000 of ABG results and assessment findings. No new orders. Repeat nebulized albuterol treatment ordered and given by Mr. Traynor. ________ ________ **Tom Gardner, RN**

STATUS EPILEPTICUS

Status epilepticus is a state of continuous seizure activity that exceeds 5 minutes or the occurrence of two or more sequential seizures without full recovery of consciousness in between. It can result from abrupt withdrawal of anticonvulsant drugs, hypoxic encephalopathy, acute head trauma, metabolic encephalopathy, or septicemia secondary to encephalitis or meningitis.

Status epilepticus is a life-threatening event that requires immediate treatment to avoid or reduce the risk of brain damage. If the patient develops status epilepticus, notify the health care provider right away, maintain a patent airway, protect the patient from harm, and administer anticonvulsant drugs as ordered.

Essential Documentation

The nurse should record the date and time that the seizure activity started, its duration, and precipitating factors. Note whether the patient reported warning signs (e.g., an aura). Document the characteristics of the seizure and related patient behaviors, such as pupil characteristics, level of consciousness, breathing, skin color, bowel and bladder continence, and body movements. Record the time of notification of the health care provider, the provider's name, and orders given, such as IV administration of anticonvulsants. Document nursing actions, such as maintaining a patent airway, suctioning, patient positioning, loosening of clothing, monitoring vital signs, and neurologic assessment. Record the patient's response to treatment, and document ongoing assessments. Note that the nurse stayed with the patient throughout the seizure and record any emotional support given to family members. Finally, record the assessment of the patient's postictal and physical status. Chart frequent assessments, vital signs, and neurologic assessments on the appropriate flow sheets.

Status Epilepticus

1/4/2019	1730	**NURSING ASSESSMENT:** At 1655, housekeeper Mary Smith noticed pt. lost consciousness while eating dinner and called for help. Pt. had full body stiffness, followed by alternating episodes of muscle spasm and relaxation. Breathing was labored and sonorous. Pt. was incontinent of bowel and bladder. Skin ashen color. Seizure lasted approx. 2 min. ___
		NURSING INTERVENTION: Clothing loosened and pt. placed on left side. Pt. unconscious after seizure, not responding to verbal stimuli. Airway patent, pt. breathing on own. ___
		NURSING ASSESSMENT: P 92, BP 128/62, RR 18 and uneven. Approx. 1 min later seizure recurred and was continuous. ___
		NURSING INTERVENTION: Dr. G. Maddox notified of assessment findings at 1703; diazepam 5mg IV administered over 5 minutes. Started 35% O_2 via facemask. Seizure stopped at 1710. Stayed with pt. throughout seizures. ___
		NURSING ASSESSMENT: Pt. breathing on own, RR 20 and regular, O_2 sat. 95%. P 88 and regular, BP 132/74, tympanic T 98.2°F. Pt. sleeping and not responding to verbal stimuli. ___
		NURSING INTERVENTION: O_2 mask removed. Incontinence care provided. Will maintain on left side and monitor closely during recovery. See flow sheets for documentation of frequent VS, I/O, and neuro. signs. ___
		___ **Mary Stafford, RN**

STROKE

A stroke is a sudden impairment of cerebral circulation in one or more of the blood vessels supplying the brain. A stroke interrupts or diminishes oxygen supply and commonly causes serious damage or necrosis in brain tissues. Clinical features of a stroke vary with the artery affected and, consequently, the portion of the brain it supplies, the severity of damage, and the extent of collateral circulation. A stroke may be caused by thrombosis, embolus, or intracerebral hemorrhage and may be confirmed by computed tomography or magnetic resonance imaging. Treatment options vary, depending on the cause of the stroke. Early onset of treatment impacts prognosis.

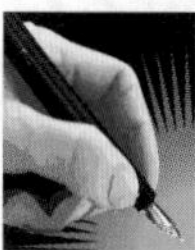

ACCUCHART

USING THE NATIONAL INSTITUTES OF HEALTH STROKE SCALE

The NIH Stroke Scale is widely used in conjunction with a neurologic examination to assess neurologic status and detect deficits in the patient suspected of having a stroke. For each item, choose the score that reflects what the patient can actually do at the time of assessment. Add the scores for each item and record the total. The higher the score, the more severe the neurologic deficits.

CATEGORY	DESCRIPTION	SCORE	BASELINE DATE/TIME	DATE/ TIME
1a. Level of consciousness (LOC)	Alert Drowsy Stuporous Coma	0 1 2 3	8/15/19 1100 1	
1b. LOC questions (Month, age)	Answers both correctly Answers one correctly Incorrect	0 1 2	0	
1c. LOC commands (Open/close eyes, make fist, let go)	Obeys both correctly Obeys one correctly Incorrect	0 1 2	1	
2. Best gaze (Eyes open — patient follows examiner's finger or face.)	Normal Partial gaze palsy Forced deviation	0 1 2	0	
3. Visual (Introduce visual stimulus/ threat to patient's visual field quadrants.)	No visual loss Partial hemianopia Complete hemianopia Bilateral hemianopia	0 1 2 3	1	
4. Facial palsy (Show teeth, raise eyebrows, and squeeze eyes shut.)	Normal Minor Partial Complete	0 1 2 3	2	
5a. Motor arm — left (Elevate extremity to 90 degrees and score drift/movement.)	No drift Drift Can't resist gravity No effort against gravity No movement Amputation, joint fusion (explain)	0 1 2 3 4 9	4	
5b. Motor arm — right (Elevate extremity to 90 degrees and score drift/movement.)	No drift Drift Can't resist gravity No effort against gravity No movement Amputation, joint fusion (explain)	0 1 2 3 4 9	0	

USING THE NATIONAL INSTITUTES OF HEALTH STROKE SCALE *(continued)*

CATEGORY	DESCRIPTION	SCORE	BASELINE DATE/TIME	DATE/ TIME
6a. Motor leg — left (Elevate extremity to 30 degrees and score drift/movement.)	No drift Drift Can't resist gravity No effort against gravity No movement Amputation, joint fusion (explain)	0 1 2 3 4 9	4	
6b. Motor leg — right (Elevate extremity to 30 degrees and score drift/movement.)	No drift Drift Can't resist gravity No effort against gravity No movement Amputation, joint fusion (explain)	0 1 2 3 4 9	0	
7. Limb ataxia (Finger-nose, heel-down shin testing)	Absent Present in one limb Present in two limbs	0 1 2	0	
8. Sensory (Pinprick to face, arm, trunk, and leg — compare side to side.)	Normal Partial loss Severe loss	0 1 2	R L 0 2	R L
9. Best language (Name items; describe a picture and read sentences.)	No aphasia Mild to moderate aphasia Severe aphasia Mute	0 1 2 3	1	
10. Dysarthria (Evaluate speech clarity by patient repeating listed words.)	Normal articulation Mild to moderate dysarthria Near to unintelligible or worse Intubated or other physical barrier	0 1 2 9	1	
11. Extinction and inattention (Use information from prior testing to identify neglect or double simultaneous stimuli testing.)	No neglect Partial neglect Complete neglect	0 1 2	0	
		Total	17	

Individual administering scale: Helen Hareson, RN

If the patient is suspected of having a stroke, the nurse should ensure a patent airway, breathing, and circulation. Perform a neurologic examination, and alert the health care provider of the findings.

Essential Documentation

Record the date and time of the nurse's note. Record the events leading up to the suspected stroke and the signs noted. If the patient can communicate, record symptoms using the patient's own words. Evaluate the patient's airway, breathing, and circulation. Document the findings, actions taken, and the patient's response. Record the neurologic and cardiovascular assessments, actions taken, and the patient's response. Document the name of the health care provider notified, the time of notification, and whether orders were given.

Assess the patient frequently, and record the specific time and the results of the assessments. Avoid using block charting. Use a frequent vital signs assessment sheet to document vital signs. (See "Vital signs, frequent," page 430.) A neurologic flow sheet such as the National Institutes of Health (NIH) Stroke Scale may be used to record the frequent neurologic assessments. (See *Using the National Institutes of Health Stroke Scale,* pages 376 and 377.)

Stroke		
11/10/2019	2030	**NURSING ASSESSMENT:** When giving pt. her medication at 2015, noted drooping of left eyelid and left side of mouth. Pt. was in bed breathing comfortably with RR 16, P 70, BP 142/72, axillary T 97.2°F. Breath sounds clear. Normal heart sounds. PERRL, awake and aware of her surroundings, answering yes and no by shake of head, speech slurred with some words inappropriate. Follows simple commands. Left hand grasp weaker than right hand grasp. Left foot slightly dropped and weaker than right. Glasgow Coma score of 13. See Glasgow Coma Scale flow sheet for frequent assessments. Skin cool, dry. Peripheral pulses palpable. Capillary refill less than 3 sec. ________ **NURSING INTERVENTION:** Called Dr. R. Lee at 2020. Stat CT scan ordered. Administered O_2 at 2 L/min by NC. IV infusion of NSS at 30 mL/hr started in right forearm with 18G catheter. Continuous pulse oximetry started with O_2 sat. of 96% on 2 L O_2. Dr. Lee in to see pt. at 2025. Pt. being prepared for transfer to ICU. Dr. Lee will notify family of transfer. ____ ________ **Luke Newell, RN**

SURGICAL AMPUTATION CARE

Patient care directly after limb amputation includes monitoring drainage from the wound, positioning the affected limb, assisting with exercises prescribed by a physical therapist, and wrapping and conditioning the wound. Postoperative care of the wound will vary slightly, depending on the amputation site (arm or leg) and the type of dressing applied to the wound.

After the wound heals, it requires only routine daily care, such as proper hygiene and continued muscle-strengthening exercises. The prosthesis—when in use—also requires daily care. As the patient recovers from the physical and psychological trauma of amputation, the patient will need to learn correct procedures for the routine daily care of the healed wound and prosthesis. There are a number of conditions that commonly accompany amputation. These conditions require nursing assessment, patient goals, nursing interventions, and evaluation. The nurse should document findings regarding the following conditions:

- Ineffective tissue perfusion
- Acute pain
- Impaired skin integrity
- Medication administration
- Wound care
- Neurovascular assessment
- Risk for infection
- Impaired physical mobility
- Risk for falls
- Deficient knowledge
- Anxiety ineffective coping
- Disturbed body image

Essential Documentation

Record the date, time, and specific procedures of all postoperative care. Chart the assessment of the wound in an EHR or flow sheet, such as appearance, type of drain, character and amount of drainage, appearance of suture line and surrounding tissue, and type of wound stabilizers (e.g., adhesive strips or sutures). Record the time of notification of the health care provider of any concerns or abnormal findings, such as irritation or signs of infection; the provider's name; and orders given. Document the specific care given to the wound, and consult the surgeon, physical therapist, and prosthetic specialist about the care of the remaining limb. Chart the patient's tolerance of exercises, pain level, and psychological reaction to the amputation. Record patient teaching about wound care. This may be charted on a patient-teaching flow sheet.

Stroke		
10/17/2019	0830	**NURSING ASSESSMENT:** Left BKA incision well-approximated, sutures intact. Slight redness and swelling along suture line. No drainage noted. Pt. reports stump pain of 2 on scale of 0 to 10. ________ **NURSING INTERVENTION:** Incision cleaned with NSS, blotted dry, dressed with dry sterile gauze, and covered with snug-fitting stump stocking. Foot of bed slightly elevated. Pt. instructed to keep knee extended to prevent flexion contractures, lie in right lateral position at least 4 hr/day, and report stump discomfort. Pt. looked at stump during care and asked many questions related to stump care and rehabilitation. ________ **Nick Heninger, RN**

SUBDURAL HEMATOMA

A potentially life-threatening condition, a subdural hematoma is the collection of blood in the space between the dura mater and the arachnoid membrane in the brain. Bleeding may be due to tears in the veins crossing the subdural space. Typically, a subdural hematoma is caused by severe blunt trauma to the head. Venous bleeding can accumulate rapidly or gradually over days to weeks.

If the patient is suspected of having a subdural hematoma, the nurse should alert the health care provider immediately. Perform frequent neurologic assessments, monitor for and take measures to prevent increased intracranial pressure (ICP), and maintain a patent airway and adequate ventilation. Anticipate surgery to evacuate the hematoma.

Essential Documentation

The nurse should record the date and time of the entry. Record the assessment findings of a subdural hematoma, such as a decline in the level of consciousness, seizures, headache, altered respiratory patterns, ipsilateral pupil fixed and dilated, hemiparesis, and hemiplegia. Monitor and record signs of increased ICP, such as increased systolic blood pressure, widened pulse pressure, and bradycardia. Note the time of notification of the health care provider, the provider's name, and orders given, such as transferring the patient to the intensive care unit, surgical intervention, osmotic diuretics, or endotracheal intubation and mechanical ventilation. Record nursing interventions, such as administering drugs, establishing IV access, administering oxygen, proper positioning, inserting an indwelling urinary catheter, maintaining a patent airway, following seizure precautions, maintaining mechanical ventilation, monitoring pulse oximetry values, and preparing the patient for diagnostic tests and surgery. Chart the patient's responses to these interventions.

If the patient has an ICP monitor, follow the documentation guidelines outlined in "Intracranial pressure monitoring", pages 219 and 220. Record frequent neurologic, cardiopulmonary, and renal assessments. A neurologic flow sheet such as the Glasgow Coma Scale may be used to record the frequent neurologic assessments. Use flow sheets to record frequent assessments, vital signs, hemodynamic monitoring, intake and output, IV therapy, and laboratory values. If the patient undergoes surgery, document postprocedural observations and care as well as the patient's tolerance of the procedure. Record patient and family teaching and emotional support given.

Subdural Hematoma		
12/30/2019	2000	**NURSING ASSESSMENT:** Pt.'s wife reports that pt. fell off a ladder 2 days ago and hit his head. States he didn't see a doctor at that time because he "felt fine." Wife states pt. is becoming confused and c/o headache. Pt. is drowsy and oriented to person but not time and place. Right pupil 5 mm with sluggish response to light, left pupil 3 mm with brisk response to light. Pt. opens eyes to verbal stimuli, answers questions inappropriately, and pushes away noxious stimuli. Glascow Coma score 12. Moving all extremities, hand grasps equal. P 58 and and regular, BP 130/62, RR 16 and regular, tympanic T 97.4°F. Breath sounds clear, no dyspnea noted, normal heart sounds. Skin warm and dry, peripheral pulses palpable. Pulse oximetry on room air 95%. ____ **NURSING INTERVENTION:** Dr. S. Kay notified of assessment findings at 1930, came to see pt. at 1935, and orders given for stat skull X-ray and CT scan. IV line started in right antecubital on first attempt with #18G angiocath. 1,000 mL of D5W infusing at 30 mL/hr. Pt. left for radiology at 1945 on stretcher, accompanied by this RN. Explained need for X-ray and CT scan to pt. and wife. Wife understands seriousness of pt.'s condition and the need for X-ray and CT scan to detect bleeding. See flow sheets for documentation of frequent VS, Glasgow Coma scores, I/O, IV fluids. ____ **Peter Mallory, RN**

SUBSTANCE ABUSE BY COLLEAGUE, SUSPICION OF

An estimated 10% to 15% of nurses are impaired or engaged in addiction recovery programs. This addiction may be a result of work-related stressors, injuries experienced in the workplace, access to medications, lack of education concerning substance abuse, lack of reporting in the workplace, or personal problems. The suspicion of substance abuse may not be limited to nursing colleagues but may include other members of the health care team, such as health care providers, assistive personnel, or multidisciplinary team members. (See *Reporting a colleague's substance abuse: The nurse's obligations* below.)

If signs of substance abuse are detected, the nurse should make sure that the suspicions are as accurate as possible. (See *Signs of drug or alcohol abuse in a colleague* below.) Be aware that allegations of substance

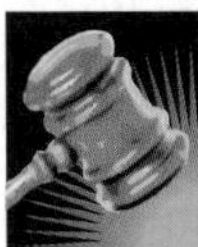

LEGAL CASEBOOK

REPORTING A COLLEAGUE'S SUBSTANCE ABUSE: THE NURSE'S OBLIGATIONS

Although the decision to report a coworker is never easy, the nurse has an ethical obligation to intervene if it is suspected that a colleague is abusing drugs or alcohol. Intervening enables the nurse to fulfill his or her moral obligation to the colleague: reporting abuse compels the colleague to take the first step toward regaining control over his or her life and undergoing rehabilitation. The nurse also fulfills his or her obligation to patients by protecting them from a nurse whose judgment and care do not meet professional standards.

SIGNS OF DRUG OR ALCOHOL ABUSE IN A COLLEAGUE

Signs of drug or alcohol abuse may include:

- rapid mood swings, usually from irritability or depression
- frequent absences, lateness, and use of private quarters such as bathrooms
- frequent volunteering to administer drugs
- excessive errors or problems with controlled substances, such as reports of broken vials or spilled drugs
- illogical or sloppy charting
- inability to meet deadlines or minimum job requirements
- increased errors in treatment
- poor personal hygiene
- inability to concentrate or remember details
- odor of alcohol on the breath
- discrepancies in opioid supplies
- slurred speech, unsteady gait, flushed face, or red eyes
- patient complaints of no relief from opioids supposedly administered when the nurse is on duty
- social withdrawal

abuse are serious and potentially damaging. Follow the facility's policy for reporting suspicions of substance abuse. Use the appropriate channels for the facility, and report the suspicions to the nursing supervisor. The nurse will be asked to document the suspicions on the appropriate form for the facility, possibly an incident or variance report.

Essential Documentation

The nurse should record the date, time, and location of the incident. Include a description of what was observed and what was said, using direct quotes. Write down the names of any witnesses. Record only objective facts, and make sure to leave out opinions and judgments. Document the name of the nursing supervisor notified of the incident, and record any instructions given.

INCIDENT REPORT

To: Theresa Stiller, RN
Nursing supervisor
From: Pamela Stevens, RN
Date: 6/3/19
Time: 2245
At about 2100 on 6/1/19, Janet Fox in room 501 told me "Your injections of morphine are much better than those the other nurse gives." I asked her what she meant. She told me, "Nurse Barrett's injections never do much for me, but yours always do." Two nights later, at 2215, I went to the restroom. When I opened the door, I saw Ms. Barrett injecting some solution into her thigh using a syringe. She told me to get out and I did. We didn't talk about the incident afterward. I immediately notified Theresa Stiller, RN, nursing supervisor, who advised me to write out this incident report so she could assess the situation. Ms. Stiller came to the unit at 2220 and met privately with Ms. Barrett. At 2230 Ms. Barrett and Ms. Stiller left the unit together, after which Ms. Stiller asked the other RNs and myself to assume Ms. Barrett's assignments.

SUBSTANCE WITHDRAWAL

Substance withdrawal occurs when a person who's addicted to a substance (alcohol or drugs) suddenly stops taking that substance. Withdrawal symptoms may include tremors, nausea, insomnia, and seizures. Substance withdrawal can result in death.

If the patient is at risk for substance withdrawal or shows signs of withdrawal, contact the health care provider immediately, and anticipate a program of detoxification, followed by long-term therapy to combat drug dependence.

Essential Documentation

The nurse should document the patient's substance abuse and addiction history, noting the substance, the amount and frequency of use, the date and time when last used, and any history of withdrawal. Note specific manifestations that the patient had during previous withdrawals. If available, use a flow sheet that lists the signs and symptoms associated with withdrawal from specific substances. Document current blood, urine, and breathalyzer results. Frequently monitor the patient for signs and symptoms of withdrawal, and document the findings. Record nursing interventions and the patient's response. Document the names of individuals notified regarding the patient, such as the health care provider, substance abuse counselor, and social worker, and the date, time, and reason of notification. Document orders or instructions given and nursing actions. Chart any patient education regarding withdrawal, such as manifestations that the patient should anticipate, nursing care that will be provided, and evidence of the patient's understanding.

Substance Withdrawal		
5/28/2019	1000	**NURSING ASSESSMENT:** Pt. admitted to Chemical Dependency Unit for withdrawal from ethanol. Has a 30-year history of alcohol dependence and states, "I can't keep this up anymore. I need to get off the booze." Reports drinking a fifth of vodka per day for the last 2 months and that her last drink was today shortly before admission. Her blood alcohol level is 0.15%. She reports having gone through the withdrawal process 4 times before but has never completed rehabilitation. Reports the following symptoms during previous withdrawals: anxiety, nausea, vomiting, irritability, and tremulousness. Currently demonstrates no manifestations of ethanol withdrawal. ________
		NURSING INTERVENTION: Dr. J. Jones notified of pt.'s admission and blood alcohol level results. Orders given. Lorazepam 2 mg P.O. given at 0930. Pt. instructed regarding S/S of ethanol withdrawal and associated nursing care. She expressed full understanding of the information. Will reinforce teaching when blood tests reveal no alcohol in blood. ________
		________ **Brian Winters, RN**

SUICIDAL INTENT

People with suicidal intent not only have thoughts about committing suicide, but they also have a concrete plan. People contemplating suicide commonly give evidence of their intent, either by displaying self-destructive behaviors or making comments about suicide. Take all self-destructive behaviors and comments about suicide seriously. Follow the facility's policy on caring for a patient with suicidal intent. If a patient is suspected of being at risk for self-destructive behavior or a suicide attempt, immediately notify the health care provider, and assess the patient for suicide clues. (See *Legal responsibilities when caring for a suicidal patient* below.)

Essential Documentation

The nurse should record the patient's statements or behaviors and any circumstances that led to the suspicion of suicidal intent. Use the patient's own words, in quotes. Document the patient's response to the inquiry about the patient's thoughts of harming or killing him- or herself and the presence and nature of a specific suicide plan. Document the patient's suicide history and the presence of suicide clues, such as:

- characteristics of depression (sad countenance, poor eye contact, declining self-care, isolation, lack of communication, poor appetite, and unkempt appearance)
- expressed or displayed feelings of hopelessness, unworthiness, futility, or lack of control over life
- suspicious questions, such as "How long does it take to bleed to death?"
- statements about the benefits of death, such as "My family won't have to worry about me anymore"
- giving away personal belongings and demonstration of an unusual amount of interest in death preparation, such as getting affairs in order and making funeral arrangements

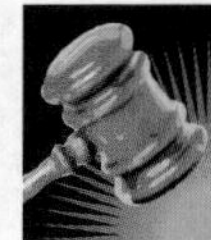

LEGAL CASEBOOK

LEGAL RESPONSIBILITIES WHEN CARING FOR A SUICIDAL PATIENT

Whether the nurse works on a psychiatric unit or a medical unit, the nurse will be held responsible for the decisions made about a suicidal patient's care. If the nurse is sued because the patient harms him- or herself while in the nurse's care, the court will judge the nurse on the basis of:

- whether the nurse knew (or should have known) that the patient was likely to harm him- or herself
- whether, knowing the patient was likely to harm him- or herself, the nurse exercised reasonable care in helping the patient to avoid injury or death

- hearing voices, especially those telling the patient to harm him- or herself
- history of significant personal loss
- withdrawal from those close to the patient
- loss of interest in persons, property, and pursuits previously important
- insomnia or hypersomnia
- substance abuse history

Record the results of the mental status examination of the patient, including the patient's appearance, orientation, cognition, speech, mood, affect, thought processes, and judgment. Record the time of notification of the health care provider of the patient's suicidal intent, the health care provider's name, and orders given. Include nursing interventions and the patient's response. (Also see *Suicide precautions,* pages 386 and 387.) Update the nursing care plan to reflect the patient's suicidal intent.

Suicidal Intent		
10/17/2019	1100	**NURSING ASSESSMENT:** Pt. reports that she lost her job yesterday. 3 months ago she had a miscarriage. She states, "I don't think I'm supposed to be here." Speaks with a low-toned voice, appears sad, avoids eye contact, and has an unkempt appearance. Reports getting no more than 3 hours of sleep per night for several weeks and states, "That's why I lost my job — I couldn't stay awake at work." Pt. reports having thoughts about suicide but declares, "I would never kill myself." She denies having a suicide plan. Has no history of previous suicide attempts. Pt. lives alone with no family nearby. Doesn't belong to a church and denies having any close friends. Denies having a history of drug or alcohol abuse or psychiatric illness. Pt. alert and oriented to person, place, and time. Speech clear and coherent. Answers questions appropriately. ________
		NURSING INTERVENTION: Dr. F. Patterson called at 1045 and told of this conversation with pt. She will see pt. for further evaluation at 1130. Will maintain constant observation of pt. until evaluated by health care provider.
		________________________ **Roger C. Trapley, RN**

SUICIDE PRECAUTIONS

Patients who have been identified as at risk for self-harm or suicide are placed on some form of suicide precautions based on the gravity of the suicidal intent. If the patient has suicidal ideations or makes a suicidal threat, gesture, or attempt, the nurse should contact the health care provider immediately and institute suicide precautions. Follow the facility's policy when caring for a potentially suicidal patient. Notify the nursing supervisor, other members of the health care team, and the risk manager, and update the patient's care plan.

Essential Documentation

The nurse should record the date and time that suicide precautions were initiated and the reasons for the precautions. Chart the time of notification of the health care provider, the provider's name, and orders given. Also, include the names of other people involved in making this decision. Document the measures taken to reduce the patient's risk of self-harm, for example, removing potentially dangerous items from the patient's environment, accompanying the patient to the bathroom, and placing the patient in a room by the nurses' station with sealed windows. Record the level of observation, such as close or constant observation, and who's performing the observation. Chart that the patient was instructed about the suicide precautions, and record the patient's response. Throughout the period of suicide precautions, maintain a suicide precautions flow sheet that includes mood, behavior, and location as well as nursing interventions and patient responses.

Suicide Precautions		
9/5/2019	1600	**NURSING ASSESSMENT:** Pt. stated, "Every year about this time, I think about offing myself." History of self-harm 1 year ago when he lacerated both wrists on the 3rd anniversary of his father's suicide. States that he has been thinking about cutting his wrists again. ——— **NURSING INTERVENTION:** Dr. F. Gordon notified and pt. placed on suicide precautions. Leah Halloran, RN, nursing supervisor, and Michael Stone, risk manager, also notified. Pt. placed in room closest to nurses' station, verified that the sealed window can't be opened. With pt. present, personal items inventoried and those potentially injurious were placed in the locked patient belongings cabinet. Instructed pt. that he must remain in sight of the assigned staff member at all times, including being accompanied to the bathroom and on walks on the unit. Betsy Richter, CNA is assigned to constantly observe pt. this shift. Pt. contracted for safety stating, "I won't do anything to hurt myself." See flow sheet for q15min assessments of mood, behavior, and location. ——— **Sandy Peres, RN**

SUICIDE PREVENTION CONTRACT

Nurses and other mental health practitioners often develop a contract for safety, also known as a *no-harm* or *no-suicide safety contract*, when a patient verbalizes suicidal thoughts or has plans to injure or kill him- or herself. Although a no-suicide contract isn't a legally binding document and doesn't guarantee against suicidal behavior, it's one tool that the nurse can use to help prevent suicide. A no-suicide contract is an agreement or pact between the patient and nurse outlining the actions that the patient will take if he or she becomes suicidal. By agreeing to the contract, the patient understands that the nurse will offer support and concern and remain available to help the patient address his or her feelings of hopelessness and depression. (Untreated depression is a major cause of suicide.)

Typically, a no-suicide safety contract is written with the patient and stated in simple, easily understood language. (See *Sample no-suicide safety-contract* below.)

SAMPLE NO-SUICIDE SAFETY CONTRACT

A no-suicide contract such as the one shown here can be used as part of the treatment plan for a patient who verbalizes suicidal thoughts or a plan to commit suicide.

NO-SUICIDE SAFETY CONTRACT

I, James Kelly, agree not to kill myself, attempt to kill myself, or injure myself.

I agree to come to my next appointment on September 7 at 9:00 am.

I agree to dismiss thoughts of harming and/or killing myself.

I agree to call 911 if I feel that I am in immediate danger of harming or killing myself.

I agree to call any and all of the people listed below at the following phone numbers if I am not in immediate danger of harming myself but am having suicidal thoughts.

John Kelly — Name; 123-456-7890 — Phone #
123 Broad Street — Address

Patty Williams — Name; 123-456-5555 — Phone #
123 Main Street — Address

I will call the 1-800-SUICIDE phone number, the 24-hour suicide prevention line, if I cannot reach any of the people listed above. I know this suicide prevention line can be called from anywhere in the United States at any time.

James Kelly
Signature of Client

Barbara Johnson
Signature of Nurse

John Kelly
Signature of family member/friend

Some points to emphasize when drafting a no-suicide safety contract include the following:

- The patient will agree not to die by suicide.
- The patient will contact an appropriate family member, supportive friend, or a local suicide hotline service to obtain help instead of committing suicide.

Including these points in the contract reinforces the idea that suicide is never an acceptable action and that the patient needs to seek immediate assistance whenever feeling suicidal. It is important to remember that a patient who is thinking about or planning suicide is in severe distress and emotional pain, feels hopeless, and is desperate to obtain relief from the suffering. Having essential information written down about what to do when feeling suicidal allows the patient to reach out to others for help when he or she is in an emotionally charged state and incapable of deciding what to do on his or her own.

Essential Documentation

Document that the patient and nurse have an unequivocal agreement that under no circumstances will the patient die by suicide and that it is never acceptable to die by suicidal means. Record the patient's negative life experiences that are contributing to the patient's depression, such as any serious losses, the breakup of a relationship, physical or sexual abuse, or feeling of being trapped. Also, document any signs and symptoms of mental illness that the patient may be experiencing.

If the patient's family or friends witnessed the agreement, have them sign it, and document their names and participation. Indicate that the patient has verbalized understanding of the contract, what it means, and what the patient will do if he or she feels suicidal. Document that the nurse instructed the patient where to keep the no-suicide contract for easy access, such as in a wallet or near the phone. Indicate that the no-suicide contract is one strategy used in the patient's care plan, making sure to document all relevant assessment data and the treatment plan. (See *Suicide precautions,* pages 386 and 387, for common procedures and documentation.) Make sure that both the nurse and the patient sign, date, and time the contract. If the patient does not want to sign the contract, document that the patient declined to sign the agreement and the specific actions taken to ensure the patient's safety. Include a copy of the no-suicide safety contract in the care plan and the patient's chart.

Suicide Prevention Contract		
1/2/2019	0830	**NURSING ASSESSMENT:** Pt'.s hx states that he recently lost his mother and father in a MVC. He states that he has been thinking about ending his life recently.
		NURSING INTERVENTION: No-suicide safety contract signed by pt. and me and witnessed by pt.'s brother, John Kelly. Pt. verbally expressed understanding of the contract. Pt. instructed to keep the contract where he can easily access it. Copy of contract placed in pt.'s chart.
		Barbara Johnson, RN

SURGICAL INCISION CARE

In addition to documenting vital signs and level of consciousness when the patient returns from surgery, the nurse must pay particular attention to maintaining records pertaining to the surgical incision and drains and the care provided. Also, read the records that travel with the patient from the postanesthesia care unit. Look for a health care provider's order indicating who will perform the first dressing change.

Essential Documentation

The nurse should chart the date, time, and type of wound care performed. Describe the wound's appearance (size, condition of margins, and necrotic tissue, if any), odor (if any), location of any drains, drainage characteristics (type, color, consistency, and amount), and the condition of the skin around the incision. Record the type of dressing and tape applied. Document additional wound care procedures provided, such as drain management, irrigation, packing, or application of a topical medication. Record the patient's tolerance of the procedure. Chart the time of notification of the health care provider of any abnormalities or concerns, the provider's name, and orders given. Note explanations or instructions given to the patient.

Record special or detailed wound care instructions and pain management measures on the nursing care plan. Document the color and amount of measurable drainage on an intake and output form. (See "Intake and output," pages 210 to 212.)

If the patient will need wound care after discharge, provide and document appropriate instructions. Record that the nurse explained aseptic technique, described how to examine the wound for signs of infection and other complications, demonstrated how to change the dressing, and provided written instructions for home care. Include the patient's understanding of the instructions. Have the patient demonstrate the change in wound dressing for the nurse prior to discharge.

Surgical Incision Care

5/10/2019	0830	**NURSING ASSESSMENT:** Dressing removed from 8-cm midline abdominal incision; no drainage noted on dressing. Incision well-approximated and intact with staples. Margin ecchymotic. Skin around incision without redness, warmth, or irritation. Small amt. of serosanguineous drainage cleaned from lower end of incision with NSS and blotted dry with sterile gauze. 3 dry sterile 4" × 4" gauze pads applied and held in place with paper tape. Jackson Pratt drain intact in LLQ draining serosanguineous fluid, emptied 40 mL. See I/O sheet for drainage records. Jackson Pratt insertion site without redness or drainage. ______
		NURSING INTERVENTION: Split 4" × 4" gauze applied around Jackson Pratt drain and taped with paper tape. Pt. stated he had only minor discomfort before and after discharge and that he didn't need any pain meds. Pt. instructed to call nurse if dressing becomes loose or soiled and for incision pain. Pt. demonstrated how to splint incision with pillow during C&DB exercises. ______
		______ **Grace Fedor, RN**

SURGICAL SITE IDENTIFICATION

To prevent wrong-site surgery and improve the overall safety of patients undergoing surgery, The Joint Commission launched the Universal Protocol for Preventing Wrong Site, Wrong Procedure, Wrong Person Surgery in 2004. This protocol encompasses three important steps:

- A *preoperative verification process* to ascertain that all important documents and tests are on hand before surgery and that these materials are evaluated and consistent with one another as well as with the patient's expectations and the surgical team's understanding of the patient, surgical procedure, surgical site, and any implants that may be used. All missing information and inconsistencies must be resolved before starting surgery.
- *Marking of the operative site*, by the surgeon performing the surgery and with the involvement of the awake and aware patient, if possible. The mark should preferably be the surgeon's initials with or without a line representing the proposed incision.
- Taking a *"time out"* immediately before surgery is started, in the location where the surgery is to be performed, so that the entire surgical team can confirm the correct patient, surgical procedure, surgical site, patient position, and any implants or special equipment requirements.

Essential Documentation

Most facilities use a detailed checklist to ensure that all steps of the verification process have been completed. Each member of the intraoperative team should document the checks that they performed to ensure proper surgical site identification. All documentation on the checklist should include the date, time, and initials of the team member providing the check. When using initials on a checklist, the nurse should be sure to sign his or her full name and initials in the signature space provided. Any discrepancies in the verification process should be noted on the checklist, with a description of actions taken to rectify the discrepancy. Include the names of any people notified and their actions. (See *Preoperative surgical identification checklist,* page 393.)

Preoperatively, the nurse should document identification of the patient using two identifiers. Confirm that the patient understands the procedure and that the patient can correctly describe the surgery being performed and identify the surgical site. Check that the consent form has been signed and that it includes the name of the surgery and the surgical site. The preoperative verification checklist also includes checking the medical record for the physical examination, medication record, laboratory studies, radiology and ECG reports, and anesthesia and surgical records and confirming that the medical record is consistent with the type of surgery planned and the identified surgical site.

In the intraoperative area, the checklist includes documenting that the patient was identified by staff as well as by the patient or family members. Documentation also includes confirmation of the surgical procedure by the staff as well as the patient or family members. The surgical site should be clearly marked, and the patient or family member should verify that the marked surgical site is correct. Ideally, site marking should be completed by the surgeon performing the surgery. The checklist should also indicate that the medical record is consistent with the planned surgery and surgical site. The availability of implants and special equipment, if relevant, should also be noted.

Documentation of "time out" occurs in the operating room, before the surgical procedure starts, and includes verbal consensus by the entire surgical team of identification of the patient, surgical site, and surgical procedure and the availability of implants and special equipment, if needed. Document any discrepancies in verification during "time out" and interventions taken to correct the discrepancy.

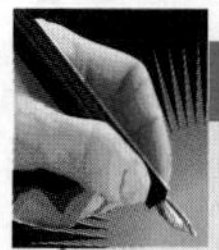

ACCUCHART

PREOPERATIVE SURGICAL IDENTIFICATION CHECKLIST

A preoperative surgical identification checklist such as the one shown here is commonly used to ensure the safety of patients undergoing surgery.

PREOPERATIVE SURGICAL IDENTIFICATION CHECKLIST

Patient's name Thomas Smith Date 1/6/19 Time 1032
Medical record number 123456 Initials MC

	HEALTH TEAM MEMBER INITIALS	DATE	TIME
Preoperative verification			
Patient identified using two identifiers	MC	1/6/19	1032
Informed consent with surgical procedure and site (side/level) signed and in chart	MC	1/6/19	1045
History and physical complete and in chart	MC	1/6/19	1045
Laboratory studies reviewed and in chart	MC	1/6/19	1045
Radiology and ECG reports reviewed and in chart	MC	1/6/19	1045
Medications listed in chart	MC	1/6/19	1045
Patient/family member/guardian verbalizes surgical procedure and points to surgical site	MC	1/6/19	1055
Surgical site marked	HD	1/6/19	1100
Patient, surgery, and marked site verified by patient/family/guardian	MC	1/6/19	1100
Surgical procedure and site, medical record, and tests are consistent	MC	1/6/19	1100
Proper equipment and implants available	MC	1/6/19	1100
Describe any discrepancies and actions taken:	N/A		
"Time out" verification			
Patient verification with two identifiers	BT	1/6/19	1135
Surgical site verified	BT	1/6/19	1135
Surgical procedure verified	BT	1/6/19	1135
Implants and equipment available	N/A		
Verbal verification of team obtained	BT	1/6/19	1135
Describe any discrepancies and actions taken:	N/A		

Signature Mary Cooke, RN Initials MC Signature Beverly Thomas, RN Initials BT
Signature Howard Dunn, MD Initials HD Signature _____ Initials _____

SUTURE REMOVAL

The goal of suture removal is to remove skin sutures from a healed wound without damaging newly formed tissue. The timing of suture removal depends on the shape, size, and location of the sutured incision; the absence of inflammation, drainage, and infection; and the patient's general condition. Usually, for a sufficiently healed wound, sutures are removed 7 to 10 days after they were inserted. Techniques for removal depend on the method of suturing; however, all techniques require sterile procedure to prevent contamination. Although sutures are usually removed by a health care provider, a nurse may remove them in some facilities on the health care provider's order.

Essential Documentation

The nurse should record the date and time of suture removal and note that the nurse explained the procedure to the patient. Include the type and number of sutures, appearance of the suture line, and whether a dressing or butterfly strips were applied. Document signs of wound complications, the name of the health care provider notified, the time of notification, and orders given. Record the patient's tolerance of the procedure.

Surgical Site Identification		
10/14/2019	1030	**NURSING ASSESSMENT:** Order written by Dr. E. Feng for nurse to remove sutures from left index finger. Suture line well-approximated and healed, site clean and dry, no redness or drainage noted. ______ **NURSING INTERVENTION:** Procedure for suture removal explained to pt. All 3 sutures removed without difficulty. Dry bandage applied to finger, according to dr.'s order. No c/o pain or discomfort following removal. Explained incision care to pt. and gave written instructions. Pt. verbalized understanding of instructions. ______ ______ **Amy Prima, RN**

SELECTED READINGS

Armstrong, D. G., & Meyr, A. J. (2018). *Basic principles of wound management.* Retrieved from UpToDate website: https://www.uptodate.com/contents/basic-principles-of-wound-management

Bonds, R. L. (2018). SBAR tool implementation to advance communication, teamwork, and the perception of patient safety culture. *Creative Nursing, 24*(2), 116–124.

Canady, V. A. (2018). Model-of-care effort reduces need for restraint, seclusion at BH facility. *Mental Health Weekly, 28*(34), 1–3.

Cares, A., Pace, E., Denious, J., & Crane, L. A. (2015). Substance use and mental illness among nurses: workplace warning signs and barriers to seeking assistance. *Substance Abuse, 36*(1), 59–66.

Drislane, F. W. (2018a). *Convulsive status epilepticus in adults: Classification, clinical features, and diagnosis.* Retrieved from UptoDate website: https://www.uptodate.com/contents/convulsive-status-epilepticus-in-adults-classification-clinical-features-and-diagnosis

Drislane, F. W. (2018b). *Convulsive status epilepticus in adults: Treatment and prognosis.* Retrieved from UpToDate website: https://www.uptodate.com/contents/convulsive-status-epilepticus-in-adults-treatment-and-prognosis

Epilepsy Foundation. (2014). *Status epilepticus.* Retrieved from https://www.epilepsy.com/learn/challenges-epilepsy/seizure-emergencies/status-epilepticus

Fanta, C. H. (2018). *Management of acute exacerbations of asthma in adults: Home and office management.* Retrieved from UpToDate website: https://www.uptodate.com/contents/acute-exacerbations-of-asthma-in-adults-home-and-office-management

Fehlings, M. G., Tetreault, L. A., Wilson, J. R., Kwon, B. K., Burns, A. S., Martin, A. R., . . . Harrop, J. S. (2017). A clinical practice guideline for the management of acute spinal cord injury: Introduction, rationale, and scope. *Global Spine Journal,* 7(Suppl. 3), 84S–94S.

Felicilda-Reynaldo, R. F. D. (2014). Recognizing signs of prescription drug abuse and addiction, part I. *Medsurg Nursing, 23*(6), 391–396.

Field, J. J., Vichinsky, E. P., & DeBraun, M. R. (2018). *Overview of the management and prognosis of sickle cell disease.* Retrieved from UpToDate website: https://www.uptodate.com/contents/overview-of-the-management-and-prognosis-of-sickle-cell-disease

Gulanick, M., & Myers, J. L. (2014). *Nursing care plans: Diagnoses, interventions, and outcomes* (8th ed.). Philadelphia, PA: Elsevier.

Gulanick, M., & Meyers, J. L. (2018). *Nursing care plans: Diagnosis, interventions, and outcomes* (9th ed.) Philadelphia, PA: Elsevier.

Kalkhoran, S., Benowitz, N. L., & Rigotti, N. A. (2018). Prevention and treatment of tobacco use: JACC health promotion series. *Journal of the American College of Cardiology, 72*(9), 1030–1045.

Kim, S. W., Kim, J. H., Kim, J. T., & Kim, Y. H. (2018). A simple and fast dressing for skin grafts: comparison with traditional techniques. *Journal of Wound Care, 23*(7), 417–420.

Kottner, J., & Surber, C. (2016). Skin care in nursing: A critical discussion of nursing practice and research. *International Journal of Nursing Studies, 61,* 20–28.

Lin, C. T., McKenzie, M., Pell, J., & Caplan, L. (2013). Health care provider satisfaction with a new electronic progress note format: SOAP vs APSO format. *JAMA Internal Medicine, 173*(2), 160–162.

Madison, J. M., & Irwin, R. S. (2017). *Identifying patients at risk for fatal asthma.* Retrieved from UpToDate website: https://www.uptodate.com/contents/identifying-patients-at-risk-for-fatal-asthma

Matarazzo, B. B., Homaifar, B. Y., & Wortzel, H. S. (2014). Therapeutic risk management of the suicidal patient: Safety planning. *Journal of Psychiatric Practice, 20*(3), 220–224.

Newman, J., Paun, O., & Fogg, L. (2018). Effects of a staff training intervention on seclusion rates on an adult inpatient psychiatric unit. *Journal of Psychosocial Nursing & Mental Health Services, 56*(6), 23–30.

Pearce, P. (2016). The essential SOAP note in an EHR age. *The Nurse Practitioner, 41*(2), 29–36.

Puskar, K., & Urda, B. (2011). Examining the efficacy of no-suicide contracts in inpatient psychiatric settings: Implications for psychiatric nursing. *Issues in Mental Health Nursing, 32*(12), 785–788.

Relias Media. (2009). *How you can avoid unsafe head injury discharges.* Retrieved from https://www.reliasmedia.com/articles/113189-how-you-can-avoid-unsafe-head-injury-discharges

Richards J. B., & Wilcox, S. R. (2014). Diagnosis and management of shock in the emergency department. *Emergency Medical Practice, 16*(3), 1–22.

Saitz, R. (2018). Medications for alcohol use disorder and predicting severe withdrawal. *Journal of the American Medical Association, 320*(8), 766–768.

Schrieber, M. L. (2016). Evidence-based practice. Neurovascular assessment: An essential nursing focus. *Medsurg Nursing, 25*(1), 55–57.

Schrieber, M. L. (2017). Lower limb amputation: Postoperative Nursing care and considerations. *Medsurg Nursing, 26*(4), 274–277.

Smith, G., Wagner, J. L., & Edwards, J. C. (2015). Epilepsy update, Part 2: Nursing care and evidence-based treatment. *American Journal of Nursing, 115*(6), 34–44.

Springer, G. (2015). How and when to use restraints. *American Nurse Today, 10*(1). Retrieved from https://www.americannursetoday.com/use-restraints/

Stewart, K. R. (2017). SBAR, communication, and patient safety: An integrated literature review. *Medsurg Nursing, 26*(5), 297–305.

Vacca, V. M. (2018). Chronic subdural hematoma: A common complexity. *Nursing, 48*(5), 24–32.

Wacogne, I., & Diwakar, V. (2010). Handover and note-keeping: The SBAR approach. *Clinical Risk, 16*(5), 173–175.

Wood, E., Albarqouni, L., Tkachuk, S., Green, C. J., Ahamad, K., Nolan, S., ... Klimas, J. (2018). Will this hospitalized patient develop severe alcohol withdrawal syndrome? The rational clinical examination systematic review. *Journal of the American Medical Association, 320*(8), 825–833.

Yoon, R. S., Alaia, M. J., Hutzler, L. H., & Bosco, J. A. (2015). Using "near misses" analysis to prevent wrong-site surgery. *Journal for Healthcare Quality: Promoting Excellence in Healthcare, 37*(2), 126–132.

T

TERMINATION OF LIFE SUPPORT

According to the right-to-die laws of most states, a patient has the right to refuse extraordinary life-supporting measures if there is no hope of recovery. If the patient cannot make this decision, the patient's next of kin is usually permitted to decide if life support should continue. A written statement of the patient's wishes is always preferable. Because of the Patient Self-Determination Act, each health care facility is required to ask the patient upon admission if the patient has an advance directive. (See "Advance directive," pages 8 to 10.) An *advance directive* is a statement of the patient's wishes that becomes valid if the patient is unable to make decisions independently. An advance directive may include a living will, which goes into effect when the patient cannot make independent decisions, as well as a durable power of attorney for health care, which names a designated person to make health care decisions when the patient cannot. The Patient Self-Determination Act also states that the patient must receive written information concerning the patient's right to make decisions about medical care.

If life support is to be terminated, the nurse must read the patient's advance directive to ensure that the present situation matches the patient's wishes and to verify that the risk manager has reviewed the document. The facility's policy on advance directives and termination of treatment have to be followed. Adequate time must be allowed for the family to interact with the medical staff to ensure that their questions and concerns are addressed. The nurse needs to check that the appropriate consent forms have been signed. Also, the nurse should ask the patient's family whether they would like to see the chaplain and whether they would like to be with the patient before, during, and after life-support termination.

Essential Documentation

The nurse needs to:

- Document whether an advance directive is present and whether it matches the patient's present situation and life-support wishes.
- Note that the facility's risk manager has reviewed the advance directive.
- Document that a consent form has been signed to terminate life support, according to facility policy.
- Document the names of persons who were notified of the decision to terminate life support and their responses.
- Describe physical care for the patient before and after life-support termination.
- Note whether the family was with the patient before, during, and after termination of life support.
- Record whether a chaplain was present.
- Document the time of termination, the name of the health care provider who turned off the equipment, and the names of people present.
- Record vital signs after extubation as well as the time the patient stopped breathing, the time pronounced dead, and who made the pronouncement.
- Document the family's response, the nurse's interventions for them, and postmortem care for the patient.

Termination of Life Support		
10/2/2019	1800	**NURSING ASSESSMENT:** Advance directive provided by pt.'s wife. Document reviewed by risk manager, Michael Stone, who verified that it matched the pt.'s present situation. Wife signed consent form to terminate life support. Wife spent approx. 10 min. alone with pt. before termination of life support. Declined to have anyone with her during this time. Life support terminated at 1730 by Dr. J. Brown, with myself, Chaplain Greene, and pt.'s wife present. VS after extubation: P 50, BP 50/20, no respiratory effort noted. Pronounced dead at 1737. Pt.'s wife tearful. ________
		NURSING INTERVENTION: Chaplain Greene and I stayed with her and listened to her talk about her 35 years with her husband. Pt. bathed and dressed in pajamas for family visitation. ________
		________ **Lucy Danios, RN**

THORACENTESIS

Thoracentesis involves the aspiration of fluid or air from the pleural space. It relieves pulmonary compression and respiratory distress by removing accumulated air or fluid that results from injury or such conditions as tuberculosis and cancer. It also provides a specimen of pleural fluid or tissue for analysis and allows the instillation of chemotherapeutic agents or other drugs into the pleural space.

Essential Documentation

The nurse needs to:

- Note that the procedure, its risks and advantages, alternative treatments, and the consequences of no treatment have been explained to the patient and that a consent form has been signed.
- Record the date and time of the thoracentesis and the name of the health care provider performing the procedure.
- Document the location of the puncture site, the volume and description (color, viscosity, and odor) of the fluid withdrawn, and specimens sent to the laboratory.
- Chart the patient's vital signs and respiratory assessment before, during, and after the procedure.
- Record any postprocedural tests, such as a chest x-ray.
- Note any complications (e.g., pneumothorax, hemothorax, or subcutaneous hematoma), the name of the health care provider notified and the time of notification, orders given, the nurse's interventions, and the patient's response.

After the procedure, the nurse should record the patient's vital signs every 15 minutes for 1 hour or according to facility policy. Then, as indicated by the patient's condition, the nurse should continue to record the patient's vital signs and respiratory status. These frequent assessments may be charted on a frequent vital signs flow sheet.

Thoracentesis		
9/10/2019	1100	**PATIENT TEACHING:** Procedure risks and benefits, alternatives, and consequences of no treatment explained to pt. and written consent obtained by Dr. D. McCall. —————————— **NURSING ASSESSMENT:** Breath sounds decreased in RLL and pt. SOB. Pulse oximetry 88% on 4 L O_2 by NC. P 102, BP 148/84, RR 32 and labored. Pt. positioned over secured bedside table. RLL thoracentesis

Thoracentesis (*continued*)

performed by health care provider without incident. Sterile 4" × 4" dressing applied to site. Site clean and dry, no redness or drainage present. 900 mL of blood-tinged serosanguineous fluid aspirated. Specimen sent to lab as ordered. During procedure P 108, BP 144/82, RR 30, pt. SOB, pulse oximetry 90%. Postprocedure P 98, BP 138/80, RR 16, breath sounds clear bilaterally, no dyspnea noted. Pt. denies SOB. Pulse oximetry 96% on 4 L O_2 by NC. No c/o pain or discomfort at puncture site. CXR done at 1045, results pending. See frequent VS sheet for q15min VS and respiratory assessments. ______________

______________ **Ellen Pritchett, RN**

THROMBOLYTIC THERAPY

Thrombolytic drugs are used to dissolve a preexisting clot or thrombus, commonly in an acute or emergency situation. Some of the thrombolytic drugs currently used include alteplase, reteplase, anistreplase, and streptokinase. Thrombolytic drugs are used to treat acute myocardial infarction, pulmonary embolism, acute ischemic stroke, deep vein thrombosis, arterial thrombosis, and arterial embolism and to clear occluded arteriovenous and intravenous (IV) cannulas. Patients receiving these drugs must be closely monitored for bleeding and allergic reactions.

Essential Documentation

The nurse needs to:

- Record the date and time of the nursing note.
- Chart the name, dosage, frequency, route, and intended purpose of the thrombolytic drug.
- Note whether the desired response is observed, such as cessation of chest pain, return of electrocardiogram changes to baseline, clearing of a catheter, or improved blood flow to a limb.
- Document the nurse's cardiopulmonary, renal, and neurologic assessments.
- Chart vital signs frequently, according to the facility's policy.
- Record partial thromboplastin time and other coagulation studies.
- Frequently assess and document signs and symptoms of complications, such as bleeding, allergic reaction, or hypotension.
- Note the time that the nurse notified the health care provider of complications and abnormal laboratory test values, the health care provider's name, orders given, nurse's interventions, and the patient's response.

- Document other nursing interventions related to thrombolytic therapy, such as measures to avoid trauma.
- Use flow sheets to record the nurse's frequent assessments, vital signs, hemodynamic measurements, intake and output, IV therapy, and laboratory test values.
- Include any patient teaching and emotional support provided.

Thrombolytic Therapy

5/18/2019	1010	**NURSING ASSESSMENT:** Pt. receiving streptokinase 100,000 International Units/hr by I.V. infusion for left femoral artery thrombosis. Left leg and foot cool, dorsalis pedis pulse now faintly palpable, poor capillary refill in left foot, able to wiggle left toes. P 82 and regular, BP 138/72, RR 18 unlabored, oral T 97.2°F. Breath sounds clear, no dyspnea. Normal heart sounds, skin warm and pink (except for left leg), no edema. Alert and oriented to time, place, and person. No c/o headache, hand grasps strong and equally bilaterally, PERRLA. Speech clear and coherent. Voiding on own, urine output remains greater than 75 mL/hour. Urine and stool negative for blood, no flank pain. No bruising, bleeding, or hematomas noted. No c/o itching, nausea, chills. No rash noted.
		NURSING INTERVENTION: Maintaining pt. on bed rest. Avoiding I.M. injections. See flow sheets for documentation of frequent assessments, VS, I/O, and lab values.
		PATIENT TEACHING: Reinforced the purpose of thrombolytic therapy in dissolving clot and the need to observe for bleeding. Pt. verbalized understanding that he's to report blood in urine or stool, headache, and flank pain.
		Cindy Trent, RN

TRACHEOSTOMY CARE

Tracheostomy care is performed to ensure airway patency of the tracheostomy tube by keeping it free from mucus buildup, maintain mucous membrane and skin integrity, prevent infection, and provide psychological support. The patient may have one of three types of tracheostomy tubes: uncuffed, cuffed, or fenestrated. An uncuffed tracheostomy tube, which may be plastic or metal, allows air to flow freely around the tube and through the larynx, reducing the risk of tracheal damage. A cuffed tube, made of plastic, is disposable. The cuff and the tube will not separate accidentally because they are bonded. A cuffed tube also does not require periodic deflating to lower pressures, and it reduces the risk of tracheal damage. A fenestrated tube, also made of plastic, permits speech through the upper airway when the external opening is capped and the cuff is deflated. It also allows easy removal of the inner cannula for cleaning. However, a fenestrated tracheostomy tube may become occluded. When using any of these tubes, the nurse needs to use aseptic technique to prevent infection until the stoma has healed. Caring for a recently performed tracheotomy requires using sterile gloves at all times. After the stoma has healed, clean gloves may be used.

Essential Documentation

The nurse needs to:

- Record the date and time of tracheostomy care.
- Document the type of care performed.
- Describe the amount, color, consistency, and odor of secretions.
- Chart the condition of the stoma and the surrounding skin.
- Note the patient's respiratory status.
- Record the duration of any cuff deflation, amount of any cuff inflation, and cuff pressure readings and specific body position.
- Note any complications, the time that the nurse notified the health care provider, the health care provider's name, and orders given.
- Record nursing interventions and the patient's response.
- Document the patient's tolerance of the procedure.
- Be sure to report any patient or family teaching and their level of comprehension.
- Depending on the facility's policy, patient teaching may be recorded on a patient-teaching record.

Tracheostomy Care		
10/19/2019	2200	**NURSING INTERVENTION:** Trach. care performed using sterile technique. Wiped skin around stoma and outer cannula with sterile gauze soaked in NSS. Dried area with sterile gauze and applied sterile trach. dressing. ________ **NURSING ASSESSMENT:** Skin around stoma intact, no redness. Inner cannula cleaned with hydrogen peroxide and wire brush. Small amount of creamy-white, thick, odorless secretions noted. Trach. ties clean and secure. Before procedure RR 18 and regular, unlabored. Breath sounds clear. After trach. care, RR 16 and regular, with clear breath sounds. Pt. verbalized no discomfort or respiratory distress. Pt.'s wife verbalized desire to assist with procedure when next scheduled to be performed. ________ **Laurie Wilkes, RN**

TRACHEOSTOMY OCCLUSION

On occasion, mucus may obstruct a tracheostomy tube, causing occlusion. When suctioning or withdrawing the inner cannula does not clear an occluded tube, the nurse needs to follow the facility's policy and stay with the patient while someone else calls the health care provider or the appropriate code. The nurse should continue to try to ventilate the patient by using whichever method works, for example, a handheld resuscitation bag. It is important *not* to remove the tracheostomy tube entirely because doing so may close the airway completely.

Essential Documentation

The nurse needs to:

- Record the date and time of the tracheostomy occlusion.
- Describe nursing efforts to clear the tube and the results.
- Note the time of notifying the health care provider (including name, interventions, and any orders given). If appropriate, record the time that a code was called.
- Use a code sheet to document the events of the code. (See "The code record," page 62.)
- Record the patient's respiratory status during the time of occlusion and after resolution of the occlusion.
- Note the patient's response to the event.

Tracheostomy Occlusion		
8/9/2019	2045	**NURSING ASSESSMENT:** Pt. noted to be cyanotic, with labored breathing at 2025. Diminished breath sounds in all lobes bilaterally. P 108, BP 102/64, RR 32 and shallow. Breathing not eased by suctioning or withdrawing inner cannula. ______
		NURSING INTERVENTION: Stayed with pt. and manually ventilated him with handheld resuscitation bag, meeting much resistance. Mary French, RN, called code at 2030. Code team arrived at 2032. Dr. J. Brown inserted new #18 Fr. trach. tube. ______
		NURSING ASSESSMENT: Pt. immediately began taking deep breaths, skin color pink, breath sounds heard in all lobes bilaterally. After 5 min. on room air, O_2 sat. 96%, P 84, BP 138/68, RR 16. ______
		PATIENT TEACHING: Explained all procedures to pt. and offered emotional support. See code flow sheet for code record. ______
		______ **Darcy Taylor, RN**

TRACHEOSTOMY SUCTIONING

Tracheostomy suctioning involves the removal of secretions from the trachea or bronchi by means of a catheter inserted through the tracheostomy tube. In addition to removing secretions, tracheostomy suctioning also stimulates the cough reflex. This procedure helps maintain a patent airway to promote the optimal exchange of oxygen and carbon dioxide and to prevent pneumonia that results from the pooling of secretions. Requiring strict sterile technique, tracheostomy suctioning should be performed as frequently as the patient's condition warrants.

Essential Documentation

The nurse needs to:

- Record the reason that the nurse performed tracheostomy suctioning as well as the date and time.
- Document the amount, color, consistency, and odor of the secretions.
- Note any complications as well as nursing actions taken and the patient's response to them.
- Record any pertinent data regarding the patient's response to the procedure.

Tracheostomy Suctioning		
7/19/2019	2145	**NURSING ASSESSMENT:** Pt. coughing but unable to raise secretions. Skin dusky P 98, BP 110/78, RR 30 noisy and labored. ______ **PATIENT TEACHING:** Explained suction procedure to pt. ______ **NURSING ASSESSMENT:** Using sterile technique, suctioned moderate amount of creamy, thick, odorless secretions from tracheostomy tube. After suctioning, skin pink, respirations quiet. P 88, BP 112/74, RR 16. Breath sounds clear. Pt. resting comfortably in bed; states he needs to cough and deep-breathe more frequently. ______ **Ken Wallings, RN**

TRACHEOSTOMY TUBE REPLACEMENT

Because a tracheostomy tube may be expelled accidentally, the nurse must make sure that a sterile tracheostomy tube and obturator of the same size and one size smaller than the one used (in case the trachea starts to close after the tube is expelled) are always kept at the patient's bedside. If the patient's tracheostomy tube is expelled, the nurse must stay with the patient and send a colleague to call the health care provider or a code, if necessary. Extreme caution needs to be exercised when attempting to reinsert an expelled tracheostomy tube because of the risk of tracheal trauma, perforation, compression, and asphyxiation. The institution usually has a procedure to follow because this is a medical emergency. It is imperative to follow the facility's policy when a tracheostomy tube is expelled. The nurse should reassure the patient until the health care provider arrives.

Essential Documentation

- Record the date and time that the tracheostomy tube was expelled and how it happened.
- Document the nurse's immediate interventions and the patient's response.
- Chart the time of notifying the health care provider (including name, time of arrival on the unit, actions and interventions, and any orders given).
- Note whether a code was called, and document the events of the code on a code flow sheet. (See "The code record," page 62.)
- Record the patient's respiratory status while the tube was out and after replacement.
- Document the patient's response to the procedure.

Tracheostomy Tube Replacement

6/18/2019	1835	**NURSING ASSESSMENT:** Answered pt.'s call light at 1810 and found pt. coughing vigorously and trach. tube lying on the blanket. _____ **NURSING INTERVENTION:** Attempted to reinsert same size (#25) trach. tube but stopped when resistance was met. _____ **NURSING ASSESSMENT:** Pt. gasping for breath, skin turning ashen color. Stayed with pt. and sent Martha Gray, RN, to call code at 1812. Pt. had labored breathing, skin pale. Code team arrived at 1814. #25 trach. tube inserted by Dr. J. Brown and fastened with trach. ties. Pt. breathing easily, clear breath sounds bilaterally. P 88, BP 158/84, RR 22, skin pink. Pt.'s health care provider, Dr. Buford, called at 1820 and notified of the event. _____ **NURSING INTERVENTION:** Dextromethorphan 10 mg P.O. q4hr p.r.n. for coughing ordered and given. New #25 trach. tube and obturator placed at bedside. Told pt. he may have cough medicine q4hr and to ask for it if coughing resumes. _____
		_____ **Tanya Holden, RN**

TRACHEOTOMY

A tracheotomy is the surgical creation of an external opening—called a *tracheostomy*—into the trachea and the insertion of an indwelling tube to maintain the airway's patency. If all attempts to establish an airway have failed, an emergency tracheotomy may be performed at the bedside to correct an airway obstruction resulting from laryngeal edema, foreign-body obstruction, or a tumor. An emergency tracheotomy may also be performed when endotracheal intubation is contraindicated. A nonemergency tracheotomy is typically performed during surgery.

The use of a cuffed tracheostomy tube provides and maintains a patent airway, prevents the unconscious or paralyzed patient from aspirating food or secretions, allows the removal of tracheobronchial secretions from a patient who is unable to cough, replaces an endotracheal tube when long-term mechanical ventilation is required, and permits the use of positive-pressure ventilation.

Essential Documentation

The nurse needs to:

- Record the reason for the tracheotomy, the date and time that it took place, and who performed it.
- Document that the health care provider explained the procedure to the patient, and document the preprocedure and time-out process if the patient's condition allows.
- Describe the patient's respiratory status before and after the procedure. Include any complications that occurred during the procedure, the amount of cuff pressure (if applicable), and the respiratory therapy initiated after the procedure. Also, note the patient's response to respiratory therapy.
- After insertion, assess the patient's vital signs and respiratory status every 15 minutes for 1 hour, every 30 minutes for 2 hours, and then every 2 hours until condition is stable, or according to the facility's policy. These frequent assessments may be charted on a flow sheet.
- Also, monitor the patient frequently for any signs of complications, and document any pertinent findings. (See *Assessing for complications of tracheotomy*, page 407.)

ASSESSING FOR COMPLICATIONS OF TRACHEOTOMY

Complication	Prevention	Detection
Aspiration	▪ Evaluate the patient's ability to swallow. ▪ Elevate the patient's head and inflate the cuff during feeding and for 30 minutes afterward.	▪ Assess for dyspnea, tachypnea, rhonchi, crackles, excessive secretions, and fever.
Bleeding at tracheotomy site	▪ Do not pull on the tracheostomy tube; do not allow the ventilator tubing to do so either. ▪ If dressing adheres to the wound, moisten with normal saline solution and gently remove it.	▪ Check the dressing regularly; slight bleeding is normal, especially if the patient has a bleeding disorder or if the tracheotomy was performed in the past 24 hours.
Infection at tracheotomy site	▪ Always use strict aseptic technique. ▪ Thoroughly clean all tubing. ▪ Change the nebulizer or humidifier jar and all tubing daily. ▪ Collect sputum and wound-drainage specimens for culture.	▪ Check for purulent, foul-smelling drainage from the stoma. ▪ Be alert for other signs and symptoms of infection, such as fever, malaise, increased white blood cell count, and local pain.
Pneumothorax	▪ Assess for subcutaneous emphysema, which may indicate pneumothorax. Notify the health care provider if this occurs.	▪ Auscultate for decreased or absent breath sounds. ▪ Check for tachypnea, pain, and subcutaneous emphysema.
Subcutaneous emphysema	▪ Make sure the cuffed tube is patent and properly inflated. ▪ Avoid displacement by securing the ties and using lightweight ventilator tubing and swivel valves.	▪ This complication is most common in mechanically ventilated patients. ▪ Palpate the neck for crepitus. Listen for air leakage around the cuff, and check the tracheostomy site for unusual swelling.
Tracheal malacia	▪ Avoid excessive cuff pressures. ▪ Avoid suctioning beyond the end of the tube.	▪ Assess for dry, hacking cough and blood-streaked sputum when the tube is being manipulated.

Tracheotomy

7/22/2019	1730	**PATIENT TEACHING/NURSING INTERVENTION:** Need for emergency tracheotomy due to laryngeal edema explained briefly to pt. while setting up for the procedure. ________ **NURSING ASSESSMENT:** Pt. nodded his assent. Breath sounds diminished bilaterally, using accessory muscles, anxious appearance, stridor audible on inspiration, skin pale and diaphoretic. P 132, BP 148/88, RR 34 and labored. Pulse oximetry 83%. ________ **NURSING INTERVENTION:** Assisted Dr. B. Jones with insertion of #18 Fr. tracheostomy tube using sterile technique. Sterile trach. dressing applied and tube secured with ties. ________ **NURSING ASSESSMENT:** Post-procedure, P 102, BP 138/82, RR 16 and unlabored, skin pink, clear breath sounds bilaterally. Placed on 40% O_2 by trach. collar. Pulse oximetry 95%. See frequent VS flow sheet for frequent post-procedure assessments. ________ ________ **David Kelly, RN**

TRACTION CARE, SKELETAL

Mechanical traction exerts a pulling force on a part of the body—usually the spine, pelvis, or long bones of the arms and legs. It can be used to reduce fractures, treat dislocations, correct or prevent deformities, improve or correct contractures, or decrease muscle spasms. Skeletal traction immobilizes a body part for prolonged periods by attaching weighted equipment directly to the patient's bones. This may be accomplished with pins, screws, wires, or tongs.

Essential Documentation

The nurse needs to:

- Record the amount of traction weight used, noting the application of additional weights and the patient's tolerance.
- Document equipment inspections and patient care, including routine checks of neurovascular integrity, skin condition, respiratory status, and elimination patterns.
- Note the condition of the pin site and any care given.
- Document patient education.

Skeletal Traction Care		
5/3/2019	0900	**NURSING ASSESSMENT:** Skeletal traction to left leg intact, with 5 lb of weight hanging freely without c/o discomfort. Pedal pulses strong bilaterally, no c/o numbness or tingling in legs or feet, skin of lower extremities warm and pink, able to move toes of both feet. Skin intact around pin sites; no redness, warmth, or drainage noted.
		NURSING INTERVENTION: Pin sites cleaned with peroxide, antibacterial ointment applied. Sterile gauze dressing applied. Traction connections tight, ropes and pulleys moving freely, no fraying noted, traction equipment in proper alignment. Breath sounds clear bilaterally. Moderate size, soft BM at 0830. Foley catheter patent, drained 200 mL in 2 hr. See I/O flow sheet. ________
		NURSING INTERVENTION: Assisted pt. with ROM exercises to unaffected extremities. ________
		NURSING ASSESSMENT: Skin intact, no redness or open areas noted. Pt. using trapeze to shift weight in bed every 1 to 2 hours. ________
		PATIENT TEACHING: Instructed pt. to report any pain or pressure from traction equipment. ________
		________ **Lily Evans, RN**

TRACTION CARE, SKIN

Mechanical traction exerts a pulling force on a part of the body, such as the spine, pelvis, or long bones of the arms and legs. Skin traction immobilizes a body part intermittently over an extended period through the direct application of a pulling force on the skin. The force may be applied using adhesive or nonadhesive traction tape or another skin traction device, such as a boot, belt, or halter. Adhesive attachment allows more continuous traction, whereas nonadhesive attachment allows easier removal for daily skin care.

Essential Documentation

The nurse needs to:

- Document the date, time, and amount of traction weight used.
- Note the application of additional weights and the patient's tolerance.
- Document equipment inspections and patient care, including routine checks of neurovascular integrity, skin condition, respiratory status, and elimination patterns.
- Document patient education provided.

Skin Traction Care		
4/28/2019	1400	**NURSING ASSESSMENT:** Skin traction to right leg intact, with 5 lb of weight hanging freely without c/o discomfort. Adhesive traction tape applied to lower right leg. Pedal pulses strong bilaterally, no c/o numbness or tingling in legs or feet, skin of lower extremities warm and pink, able to move toes of both feet. Traction connections tight, ropes and pulleys moving freely, no fraying noted, traction equipment in proper alignment. Breath sounds clear bilaterally. No BM today, last BM yesterday morning. Foley catheter patent, draining approx. 150 mL/hr. See I/O flow sheet. ____ **NURSING INTERVENTION:** Assisted pt. with ROM exercises to unaffected extremities. ____ **NURSING ASSESSMENT:** Skin intact, no redness or open areas noted. Pt. using trapeze to shift weight in bed every 1 to 2 hours. ____ **PATIENT TEACHING:** Instructed pt. to report any pain or pressure from traction equipment. ____ ____ **Rachel Hardwick, RN**

TRANSCUTANEOUS ELECTRICAL NERVE STIMULATION

Transcutaneous electrical nerve stimulation (TENS) involves a portable, battery-powered device that transmits a painless electrical current to peripheral nerves or directly to a painful area over large nerve fibers. By blocking painful stimuli traveling over smaller fibers, the patient's perception of pain is altered. TENS reduces the need for analgesic drugs when used after surgery or for chronic pain. A typical course of treatment is 3 to 5 days. (See *Current uses of transcutaneous electrical nerve stimulation*, below.)

Essential Documentation

In the medical record and nursing care plan, the nurse should record the electrode sites and control settings. It is necessary to document the (a) patient's tolerance to treatment and (b) during each shift, the nurse's evaluation of pain control.

Transcutaneous Electrical Nerve Stimulation		
1/2/2019	1730	**NURSING INTERVENTION:** TENS electrodes placed over right and left posterior superior iliac spines and right and left gluteal folds for lower back pain. Stimulation frequency set at 80 Hz. ____ **NURSING ASSESSMENT:** Pt. verbalizes discomfort as 3 on a scale of 0 to 10, w/10 being the worst pain imaginable. Pt. verbalizes satisfaction with level of pain control at this time. ____ ____ **Lydia Vrubel, RN**

CURRENT USES OF TRANSCUTANEOUS ELECTRICAL NERVE STIMULATION

TENS must be prescribed by a physician and is most successful if it is administered and taught to the patient by a therapist skilled in its use. TENS has been used for the temporary relief of acute pain, such as postoperative pain, and for ongoing relief of chronic pain, such as sciatica. Among the types of pain that respond to TENS are:

- arthritis
- bone fracture pain
- bursitis
- cancer-related pain
- lower back pain
- musculoskeletal pain
- myofascial pain
- neuralgias and neuropathies
- phantom limb pain
- postoperative incision pain
- sciatica
- whiplash

TRANSFUSION REACTION, DELAYED

A delayed transfusion reaction may occur 4 to 8 days after a blood transfusion and even up to 1 month later. This type of transfusion reaction occurs in people who have developed antibodies from previous blood transfusions, which cause red blood cell hemolysis during subsequent transfusions. Delayed transfusion reactions are typically mild and do not require treatment. If it is suspected that a patient is having a delayed transfusion reaction, the nurse needs to notify the health care provider and blood bank.

Essential Documentation

The nurse needs to:

- Record the date and time of the suspected delayed transfusion reaction.
- Note the signs of a delayed reaction, such as fever, elevated white blood cell count, and a falling hematocrit.
- Document the name of the health care provider notified, the orders given, nursing interventions, the patient's reaction, and the time that the health care provider came to see the patient.
- Record the time that the blood bank was notified, the name of the blood bank representative with whom the nurse spoke, and any orders given, such as obtaining blood or urine samples and sending them to the laboratory. Some facilities require the nurse to complete a transfusion reaction report. (See “Transfusion reaction report,” pages 45 and 46.)
- Record any patient education provided and the patient's reaction.

Delayed Transfusion Reaction		
5/8/2019	1215	**NURSING ASSESSMENT:** Oral T 102.4°F at 1200. Pt. states he has chills, but no itching, nausea, or vomiting. No flushing, facial edema, or urticaria noted. P 82 and regular, BP 128/72, RR 20 and unlabored. Lungs clear bilaterally. Labs from 0600 show Hct 35%, Hgb 12.4, WBC 15,000. **NURSING INTERVENTION:** Notified Dr. D. Small of elevated temp, assessment findings, and lab values at 1205. Dr. Small will see pt. at 1230. Notified Anna Cohen in blood bank of possible delayed transfusion reaction at 1210. Urine for UA and 2 red-top tubes of blood drawn and sent to lab. ________ **PATIENT TEACHING:** Explained to pt. that fever may be a possible delayed blood transfusion reaction and usually requires no treatment. ________ **Dave Burns, RN**

TRANSIENT ISCHEMIC ATTACK

Transient ischemic attacks (TIAs) are sudden, brief episodes of neurologic deficit caused by focal cerebral ischemia. They usually last 5 to 20 minutes and are followed by rapid clearing of neurologic deficits (typically within 24 hours). TIAs may warn of an impending stroke. About 50% to 80% of patients who experience a thrombotic stroke have previously suffered a TIA.

If a patient is suspected of having suffered a TIA, the nurse should immediately contact the health care provider and anticipate orders for antiplatelet or anticoagulant drugs. Surgery may be considered to treat carotid artery obstruction. To reduce risk factors, the nurse should recommend lifestyle changes, including weight loss, smoking cessation, proper nutrition, hypertension and diabetes management, and daily exercise.

Essential Documentation

The nurse needs to:

- Record the date and time that the signs and symptoms of a TIA occurred and the duration of the attack.
- Document the findings of the nursing assessment, such as dizziness; diplopia; dark or blurred vision; visual field deficits; ptosis; facial droop, difficulty speaking or swallowing; unilateral or bilateral weakness; staggered gait; transient blindness in one eye; altered level of consciousness; bruits on auscultation of the carotid arteries; hypertension; weakness, paralysis, or numbness in the fingers, arms, or legs.
- Track the level of consciousness, for example, with the use of the Glasgow Coma Scale. (See "Level of consciousness, changes in," pages 237 to 239.)
- Chart the time that the nurse notified the health care provider of the assessment findings (include the health care provider's name and any orders given, such as antiplatelet, thrombolytic,or anticoagulant drug administration).
- Record nursing interventions, such as preparing the patient for diagnostic tests, monitoring neurologic signs, tracking laboratory test values, giving drugs, and ensuring the patient's safety. Be sure to include the patient's response to these interventions.
- Document such patient teaching as lifestyle modification, signs and symptoms of stroke to report to the health care provider, and the importance of keeping follow-up laboratory appointments. Depending on the facility's policy, patient teaching may be recorded on a patient-teaching record.

Transient Ischemic Attack

1/6/2019	1015	**NURSING ASSESSMENT:** Pt. reports dizziness and numbness and tingling in right arm and fingers lasting 5 min. P 84, BP 162/84, RR 18, oral T 97.1°F. Peripheral pulses palpable. Skin pink, warm and dry. Normal heart sounds, clear breath sounds bilaterally. Bruits auscultated over both carotid arteries. Alert, oriented to time, place, and person. Speech clear and understandable, follows all directions. Strong hand grasps bilaterally, strong dorsi and plantar flexion against resistance, normal gait. PERRLA, no diplopia reported. See flow sheets for VS and neuro. assessments. ________ **NURSING INTERVENTION:** Dr. G. Luden notified of assessment findings and orders received for Carotid Doppler studies. ________ ________ **Carol Allen, RN**
1/6/2019	1025	**NURSING ASSESSMENT:** Pt. states dizziness and numbness and tingling in right arm and fingers has resolved. ________ **PATIENT TEACHING:** Explained S/S of TIA and stroke for pt. to report. Discussed reasons for Doppler study. ________ **NURSING INTERVENTION:** Dietitian called and will be in today to discuss low-cholesterol, low-fat diet with pt. and wife. See pt. teaching record. ________ ________ **Carol Allen, RN**

TUBE FEEDING (ENTERAL FEEDING)

Tube feeding involves the delivery of a liquid feeding formula directly to the stomach (gastrostomy), duodenum, or jejunum. A gastrostomy is typically indicated for a patient who cannot eat normally because of dysphagia or oral or esophageal obstruction or injury. Gastric feedings may also be given to an unconscious or intubated patient or to a patient recovering from gastrointestinal tract surgery who cannot ingest food orally.

Duodenal or jejunal feedings decrease the risk of aspiration because the formula bypasses the pylorus. Jejunal feedings reduce pancreatic stimulation; thus, the patient may require an elemental diet. Patients usually receive gastric feedings on an intermittent schedule. However, for duodenal or jejunal feedings, most patients tolerate a continuous slow drip.

Liquid nutrient solutions come in various formulas for administration through a nasogastric tube, small-bore feeding tube, gastrostomy or jejunostomy tube, percutaneous endoscopic gastrostomy or jejunostomy tube, or gastrostomy feeding button. Tube feedings are contraindicated in patients who have no bowel sounds or a suspected intestinal obstruction.

Essential Documentation

The nurse needs to:

- Record the date, volume of formula, and volume of water on the intake and output sheet. (See “Intake and output,” pages 210 to 212.)
- Document abdominal assessment findings (including tube exit site, if appropriate) in the nurse's note; the amount of residual gastric contents; verification of tube placement; amount, type, strength, and time of feeding; and tube patency.
- Discuss the patient's tolerance of the feeding, including complications, such as nausea, vomiting, cramping, diarrhea, or distention.
- Note the result of any laboratory tests, such as urine and serum glucose, serum electrolyte, and blood urea nitrogen levels, as well as serum osmolality.
- Document the time that the nurse notified the health care provider of complications, such as hyperglycemia, glycosuria, and diarrhea, as well as the health care provider's name. Be sure to include any orders given, the nurse's actions, and the patient's response.
- Record the patient's hydration status and any drugs given through the tube.
- Note any drugs or treatments to relieve constipation or diarrhea. Include the date and time of administration-set changes and the results of specimen collections.
- Describe any oral and nasal hygiene and dressing changes provided.

Tube (Enteral) Feeding

8/25/2019	0700	**NURSING ASSESSMENT:** Full-strength Pulmocare infusing via flexiflow pump through Dobhoff tube in right nostril at 50 mL/hr. Tube placement confirmed by aspirated gastric contents with pH of 5 and grassy-green color. 5 mL residual noted. HOB maintained at 45-degree angle. Pt. denies N/V, abdominal cramping. Active bowel sounds auscultated in all 4 quadrants, no abdominal distention noted. Mucous membranes moist, no skin tenting when pinched. Nares cleaned with cotton-tipped applicator dipped in NSS. Water-soluble lubricant applied to nares and lips. Skin around nares intact, no redness around tape noted. ______
		NURSING INTERVENTION: Helped pt. to brush teeth. Diphenoxylate elixir 2.5 mg given via tube feed for continuous diarrhea. Tube flushed with 30 mL H2O, as ordered. See I/O sheet for shift totals.
		NURSING ASSESSMENT: Urine dipstick neg. for glucose. Blood drawn this a.m. for serum glucose, electrolytes, and osmolality. Instructed pt to tell nurse of any discomfort or distention. ______
		______ **Sandra Mann, RN**

TUBERCULOSIS

Tuberculosis (TB) is an acute or chronic infection caused by *Mycobacterium tuberculosis.* TB is characterized by pulmonary infiltrates and the formation of granulomas with caseation, fibrosis, and cavitation. The disease spreads by inhalation of droplet nuclei when infected persons cough and sneeze. Sites of extrapulmonary TB include the pleura, meninges, joints, lymph nodes, adrenal gland, vertebrae, peritoneum, genitourinary tract, and bowel.

After exposure to *M. tuberculosis*, roughly 5% of infected people develop active TB within 1 year; in the remainder, microorganisms cause a latent infection. The host's immunologic defense system usually destroys the bacillus or walls it up in a tubercle. However, the live, encapsulated bacilli may lie dormant within the tubercle for years, reactivating later to cause an active infection.

If suspected of having TB, the patient needs to be placed on isolation precautions, without delay for waiting for diagnostic test results. The nurse needs to follow communicable disease reporting regulations and anticipate the administration of a multidrug regimen, such as isoniazid, rifampin, and pyrazinamide.

Essential Documentation

The nurse needs to:

- Document the results of the tuberculin skin test, interferon gamma release assay (IGRA),chest x-rays, and sputum cultures, if TB is a new diagnosis for the patient.
- Confirm and document that the case has been reported to local health authorities. Include the name of the person making the report and the name of the agency receiving it.
- Record the nursing assessment findings of TB, such as fatigue, weakness, anorexia, weight loss, night sweats, low-grade fever, cough, mucopurulent sputum, and chest pain.
- Chart precautions taken to prevent the transmission of the disease.
- Record all drugs given on the medication administration record, according to the facility's policy.
- Document nursing interventions, such as administering oxygen or suctioning, and the patient's response to them.
- Record the time that the health care provider was notified of any concerns and complications (include the name of the health care provider, orders given, the nurse's actions, and the patient's response).

- Document patient teaching given, including information on drugs, hygiene, preventing the spread of infection, the importance of proper nutrition, and the importance of proper follow-up and compliance with instructions for taking drugs. (See *Preventing tuberculosis*, below.)

Tuberculosis		
3/24/2019	1400	**NURSING INTERVENTION:** Pt. admitted to R/O TB. PPD injected subdermally in left forearm at 1340. CXR performed, IGRA test drawn, and sputum sent for culture. Pt. placed in private isolation room with negative-pressure ventilation. **NURSING ASSESSMENT:** Pt. reports recent weight loss of 10 lb, productive cough, night sweats, and low-grade fever. P 84, BP 142/78, RR 20, tympanic T 100.1°F. ______ **NURSING INTERVENTION:** Administering O_2 at 4 L/min via NC. Following standard and airborne precautions when interacting with pt. ______ **PATIENT TEACHING:** Explained isolation precautions to pt.'s family as well as the need for him to wear a mask when he leaves his room. Instructed pt. to throw all tissues in hazardous medical waste receptacle. **NURSING INTERVENTION:** Administered rifampin, isoniazid, and pyrazinamide, per orders. See MAR. All medications and procedures explained to pt. ______ ______ **Carla Marron, RN**

PREVENTING TUBERCULOSIS

The nurse needs to explain respiratory and standard precautions to the hospitalized patient with TB. The patient needs to inform pertinent health care providers, including the patient's dentist and ophthalmologist, that the patient has TB so that they can institute infection-control precautions.

Nurses and providers should wear a specific N95 respirator mask, which protects against inhalation of 0.3-micron particles when caring for the patient with TB. The patient should wear a surgical mask and be placed in isolation. Before discharge, the patient must be told to take precautions to prevent spreading the disease, such as wearing a mask around others, until the health care provider confirms that contagion is no longer possible.

The nurse needs to teach the patient other specific precautions to avoid spreading the infection—for instance, to cough and sneeze into tissues and to dispose of the tissues properly. It is important to stress the importance of thorough hand washing in hot, soapy water after handling tissues with secretions. Also, instruct the patient to wash eating utensils separately in hot, soapy water.

SELECTED READINGS

Anderson, L. (2018). Delivering artificial nutrition and hydration safely by feeding pumps. *British Journal of Nursing, 27*(18), 1032–1033.

Bird, S. (2014). Advance care planning. *Australian Family Physician, 43*(8), 526–528.

Booth, A. T., and Lehna, C. (2016). Advanced directives and advanced care planning for healthcare professionals. *Kentucky Nurse, 64*(2), 7–10.

Choi, F. H. (2015). Application of advanced directives. *CONNECT: The World of Critical Care Nursing, 9*(4), 134–134.

Coutaux, A. (2017). Non-pharmacological treatments for pain relief: TENS and acupuncture. *Joint Bone Spine, 84*(6), 657–661.

Everitt, E. (2016). Caring for patients with a tracheostomy. *Nursing Times, 112*(19), 16–20.

Felicilda-Reynaldo, R. F. (2013). Circulation savers: Thrombolytic therapy. *Medsurg Nursing, 22*(6), 393–397.

Lethaby, A., Temple, J., & Santy, J. (2013). Pin site care for preventing infections associated with external bone fixators and pins. *Cochrane Database of Systematic Reviews, 2004*(1), CD004551.

Lim, M., Yong, B. Y., Mar, M. Q., Ang, S. Y., Chan, M. Q. M., Lam, M., ... Lopez, V. (2018). Caring for patients on home enteral nutrition: Reported complications by home carers and perspectives of community nurses. *Journal of Clinical Nursing, 27*(13–14), 2825–2835.

Lowth, M. (2016). Tuberculosis: A clear and present danger. *Practice Nurse, 46*(10), 38–44.

McLeod-Sordjan, R. (2014). Death preparedness: A concept analysis. *Journal of Advanced Nursing, 70*(5), 1008–1019.

Miller, B. (2017). Nurses in the know: The history and future of advance directives. *Online Journal of Issues in Nursing, 22*(3), 1.

Miller, E. T., & Summers, D. (2014). Update on transient ischemic attack nursing care. *Stroke, 45*(5), e71–e73.

Rencuzogullari, I., Cağdaş, M., Karakoyun, S., Karabağ, Y., & Çınar, T. (2018). Successful treatment of massive thrombosis in different locations with prolonged thrombolytic therapy: A life-saving intervention. *American Journal of Emergency Medicine, 36*(9), 1722.e1–1722.e3.

Rogers, B., Kennedy, M., Wiselka, M., Morris, T., & Venkatraman, N. (2018). Current recommended management of tuberculosis. *Prescriber, 29*(10), 18–22

Russell, M. S., & Russell, M. D. (2015). Breathe easy: Safe tracheostomy management. *AHRQ WebM&M*. Retrieved from https://psnet.ahrq.gov/webmm/case/354/breathe-easy-safe-tracheostomy-management

Schellinger, P. D., & Köhrmann, M. (2018). Intravenous thrombolytic therapy remains the basis and mainstay of revascularizing therapy! *Stroke, 49*(10), 2285–2286.

Siddon, A. J., Kenney, B. C., Hendrickson, J. E., & Tormey, C. A. (2018). Delayed haemolytic and serologic transfusion reactions: Pathophysiology, treatment and prevention. *Current Opinion in Hematology, 25*(6), 459–467.

Watters, K. F. (2017) Tracheostomy in infants and children. *Respiratory Care, 62*(6), 799–825.

U

UNRESPONSIVENESS BY PATIENT

Assessment of unresponsiveness is a crucial link in activating early life-saving techniques. Unresponsiveness is checked by calling the patient's name and shaking the patient's shoulder. If the patient remains unresponsive, the nurse needs to call for help and take immediate measures to ensure airway, breathing, and circulation until the code team arrives.

Guidelines established by the American Heart Association require a written, chronological account of a patient's condition while cardiopulmonary resuscitation (CPR) is being performed. This is usually charted on the code record, which documents detailed observations and interventions as well as drugs administered to the patient. (See "The code record," page 62.) The nurse needs to remember to follow Advanced Cardiac Life Support guidelines when responding to a code.

Some facilities use a resuscitation critique documentation to identify actual or potential problems with the CPR process. This documentation tracks personnel responses and response times as well as the availability of appropriate drugs and functioning equipment.

Essential Documentation

The nurse should never rely on memory. All events should be recorded as they occur. Writing "recorder" after the nurse's name indicates that the nurse documented the code but did not participate. The nurse needs to:

- Document the date and time that the code was called.
- Record the patient's name, the location of the code, the name of the person who discovered that the patient was unresponsive,

the patient's condition, and whether the unresponsiveness was witnessed.

- Record the time that the health care provider or nurse practitioner was notified, his or her name, and the names of other members who participated in the code, as well as the time that the family was notified.
- Note the exact time for each code intervention and include vital signs, heart rhythm, laboratory test results (arterial blood gas or electrolyte values), type of treatment (CPR, defibrillation, or cardioversion), drugs (name, dosage, and route), procedures (intubation, temporary or transvenous pacemaker, or central venous line insertion), and the patient's response during these interventions.
- Indicate the time that the code ended and the patient's status. Some facilities require that the health care provider leading the code and the nurse recording the code review the code record and sign it.

The nurse's note should also include the fact that a code sheet was used to document the events of the code, the events leading up to the code, the assessment findings that prompted the code to be called, the name of the person who initiated CPR, and any other interventions performed before the code team arrived.

Unresponsive Patient

1/4/2019	1650	**NURSING ASSESSMENT:** Summoned to pt.'s room at 1557 by a shout from roommate. Found pt. unresponsive in bed without respirations or pulse. Roommate stated, "He was watching TV; then all of a sudden he started gasping and holding his chest." Code called at 1559. ______ **NURSING INTERVENTION:** Initiated CPR with Leslie Adams, RN. Code team arrived at 1600 and continued resuscitative efforts. (See code record). Pt. moaned and opened eyes at approx. 1610. Notified Dr. F. Brower at home at 1615 and explained situation – will be in immediately. Report called to Tom Kennedy, RN, and pt. transferred to ICU at 1638. Family notified of pt.'s condition and transfer. ______
		______ **Michelle Robbins, RN**

URINARY CATHETER INSERTION, INDWELLING

Also known as a Foley or retention catheter, an indwelling urinary catheter remains in the bladder to provide continuous urine drainage. A balloon inflated at the catheter's distal end prevents it from slipping out of the bladder after insertion.

An indwelling catheter is inserted using sterile technique and only when absolutely necessary. Insertion should be performed with extreme care to prevent injury to the patient and possible infection. Facility policy should be followed for sending laboratory specimens upon insertion to differentiate preexisting infections from catheter-related infections.

An indwelling catheter is most commonly used to relieve bladder distention caused by urine retention and to allow continuous urine drainage when the urinary meatus is swollen from childbirth, surgery, or local trauma. Other indications for an indwelling catheter include urinary tract obstruction caused by a tumor or enlarged prostate, urine retention or infection from neurogenic bladder paralysis caused by spinal cord injury or disease, protection of a wound from contamination by urine, and any illness in which the patient's urine output must be closely monitored.

Essential Documentation

The nurse should:

- Record the date and time that the indwelling urinary catheter was inserted.
- Note the size and type of catheter used.
- Describe the amount, color, and other characteristics of the urine emptied from the bladder.
- Record intake and output on the patient's intake and output record. (See "Intake and output," pages 210 to 212.)
- If large volumes of urine have been emptied, describe the patient's tolerance of the procedure.
- Note whether a urine specimen was sent for laboratory analysis.
- Document patient response and any patient teaching performed.

Indwelling Urinary Catheter Insertion		
5/12/2019	1115	**PATIENT TEACHING:** Explained reason for insertion of indwelling urinary catheter to pt. prior to hysterectomy. Pt. stated she understood the need but wasn't looking forward to its insertion. Reassured her that the insertion shouldn't be painful if she relaxes. Showed her how to do breathing exercises during insertion. ——— **NURSING INTERVENTION:** #16 Fr. Foley catheter inserted at 1045. Emptied 450 mL from bladder. ——— **NURSING ASSESSMENT:** Urine dark amber, no odor, or sediment. Specimen sent to lab for U/A and culture. Pt. states she has no discomfort and can't feel catheter in place. See I/O flow sheet. ——— **Molly Malone, RN**

SELECTED READING

Hinkle, J. L. & Cheever, K. H. (2017). *Brunner & Suddarth's Textbook of Medical Surgical Nursing.* 14th ed. Philadelphia, PA: Lippincott Williams & Wilkins/Wolters Kluwer Health.

V

VAGAL MANEUVERS

When a patient suffers sinus, atrial, or junctional tachyarrhythmias, vagal maneuvers—the Valsalva maneuver and carotid sinus massage—can slow the heart rate. These maneuvers work by stimulating parasympathetic nerve endings, which respond as they would to an increase in blood pressure. They send this message to the brainstem, which in turn stimulates the parasympathetic nervous system to increase vagal tone and decrease the heart rate. Usually performed by a health care provider, vagal maneuvers may also be performed by an advanced practice nurse under a health care provider's supervision.

In the Valsalva maneuver, the patient holds his or her breath and bears down, raising the intrathoracic pressure. When this pressure increase is transmitted to the heart and great vessels, venous return, stroke volume, and systolic blood pressure decrease. Within seconds, the baroreceptors respond to the changes by increasing the heart rate and causing peripheral vasoconstriction. When the patient exhales at the end of this maneuver, blood pressure rises to its previous level. This increase, combined with the peripheral vasoconstriction caused by bearing down, stimulates the vagus nerve, decreasing the heart rate.

There is also a modified Valsalva maneuver. Patients with supraventricular tachycardia (SVT) perform straining maneuver while in a semirecumbent position, then immediately lie supine with their legs raised to 45 degrees for 15 seconds before returning to the semirecumbent position. The purpose of this postural modification is to boost relaxation phase venous return and vagal stimulation.

In carotid sinus massage, manual pressure applied to the left or right carotid sinus slows the patient's heart rate. The patient's response to carotid sinus massage depends on the type of arrhythmia. If the patient has sinus tachycardia, the patient's heart rate will slow gradually during the procedure and speed up again after it. In atrial tachycardia, the arrhythmia may stop, and the heart rate may remain slow. With atrial fibrillation or flutter, the ventricular rate may not change; atrioventricular block may even worsen. Nonparoxysmal tachycardia and ventricular tachycardia will not respond to carotid sinus massage.

Essential Documentation

The nurse should record the date and time of the procedure, who performed it, and why it was necessary. Note the patient's response, any complications, and the interventions taken. If possible, obtain a rhythm strip before, during, and after the procedure.

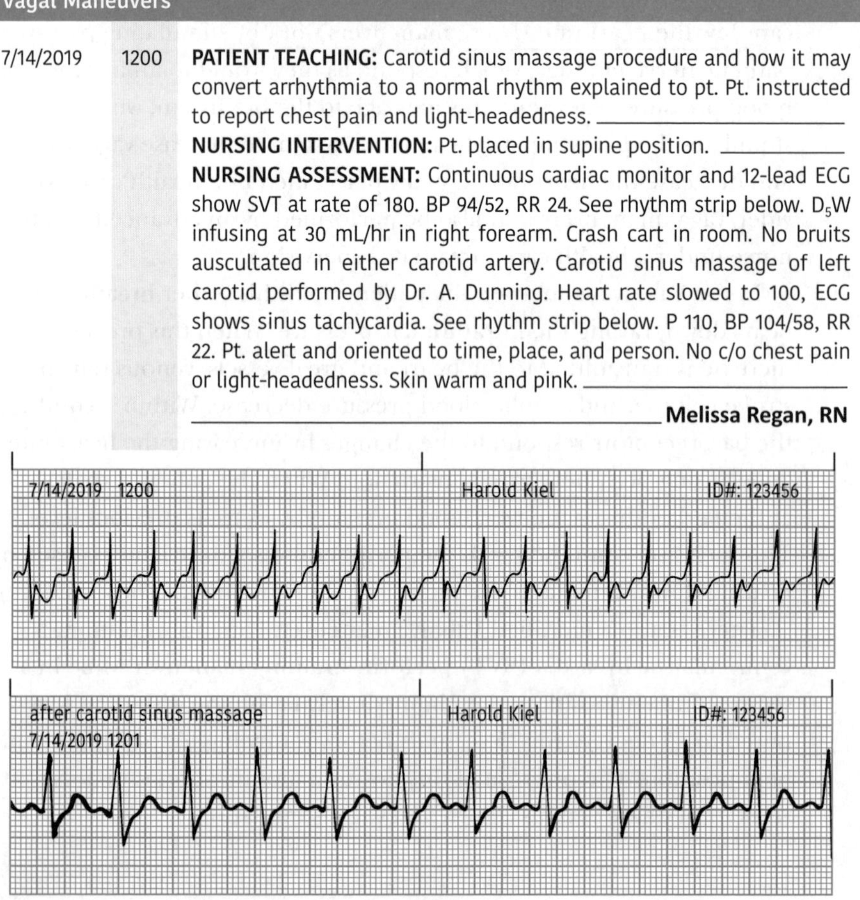

Vagal Maneuvers

7/14/2019	1200	**PATIENT TEACHING:** Carotid sinus massage procedure and how it may convert arrhythmia to a normal rhythm explained to pt. Pt. instructed to report chest pain and light-headedness. ______ **NURSING INTERVENTION:** Pt. placed in supine position. ______ **NURSING ASSESSMENT:** Continuous cardiac monitor and 12-lead ECG show SVT at rate of 180. BP 94/52, RR 24. See rhythm strip below. D_5W infusing at 30 mL/hr in right forearm. Crash cart in room. No bruits auscultated in either carotid artery. Carotid sinus massage of left carotid performed by Dr. A. Dunning. Heart rate slowed to 100, ECG shows sinus tachycardia. See rhythm strip below. P 110, BP 104/58, RR 22. Pt. alert and oriented to time, place, and person. No c/o chest pain or light-headedness. Skin warm and pink. ______ ______ **Melissa Regan, RN**

VENTRICULAR ASSIST DEVICE

A temporary life-sustaining treatment for the failing heart, the ventricular assist device (VAD) diverts systemic blood flow from a diseased ventricle into a centrifugal pump, thus temporarily reducing ventricular work, which allows the myocardium to rest and contractility to improve. The VAD functions somewhat like an artificial heart. The major difference is that the VAD assists the heart, whereas the artificial heart replaces it.

The permanent VAD is implanted in the patient's chest cavity, although it still provides only temporary support. The device receives power through the skin by a belt of electrical transformer coils (worn externally as a portable battery pack). It can also be operated by an implanted, rechargeable battery for short periods of time.

Candidates for the VAD include patients with massive myocardial infarction, end stage heart failure, irreversible cardiomyopathy, acute myocarditis, an inability to be weaned from cardiopulmonary bypass, valvular disease, bacterial endocarditis, or heart transplant rejection. The device may also be used in patients awaiting a heart transplant.

Essential Documentation

The nurse should record the date and time of the entry. Note the patient's condition after the insertion of the VAD. Record the results of the cardiopulmonary findings (including hemodynamic measurements) as well as neurologic and renal assessments. Document pump adjustments and the patient's response. Chart signs and symptoms of poor perfusion and ineffective pumping (e.g., arrhythmias, hypotension, slow capillary refill, cool skin, oliguria or anuria, or anxiety and restlessness), pulmonary embolism (such as dyspnea, chest pain, tachycardia, productive cough, or low-grade fever), and stroke or neurologic deficits.

Record the time that the health care provider was notified of complications, the provider's name, orders given, nursing interventions, and the patient's response. Document any drugs given (such as heparin); the dosage, frequency, and route; and the patient's response. Record the appearance of the cannula insertion site, site care, and dressing changes. Document all patient teaching and emotional support provided. Patient teaching may be recorded on a patient-teaching flow sheet. Use flow sheets to record frequent assessments, including vital signs, intake and output, intravenous therapy, hemodynamic parameters, and laboratory test values (e.g., complete blood count and coagulation studies).

Ventricular Assist Device (VAD)		
8/27/2019	1030	**NURSING ASSESSMENT:** VAD continues to function without problems. No pump adjustments made. Pt. states he feels much better since VAD insertion 3 days ago. Pt. is alert and oriented to time, place, and person. Moving all extremities, 5/5 hand grip bilaterally. Skin warm, pink, and dry. Breath sounds clear. Urine output remains greater than 60 mL/hr. Peripheral pulses 2/4 bilaterally upper extremity and lower extremity, capillary refill less than 3 sec bilaterally lower extremities. P 70 and regular, BP 110/68, RR 18, oral T 98.8°F. Cardiac monitor shows NSR, no arrhythmias noted. CO 5.6 L/min. PAP 25/16, PCWP 15 mm Hg, CVP 8 cm H_2O, MAP 36.6, and LAP 10 mm Hg. Cannula site without redness, warmth, drainage, or bleeding. ______
		NURSING INTERVENTION: Site cleaned and dressed according to policy. CBC w/diff, electrolytes, BUN, creatinine, PT-PTT drawn this a.m. Results pending. See flow sheets for documentation of frequent VS, I.V. therapy, I/O, hemodynamic parameters, and lab values. Transplant coordinator in to talk with pt. about transplant process. ______
		______ **Carol Allen, RN**

VIOLENT PATIENT

When a patient demonstrates violent behavior, quick action is needed to protect the patient, other patients, and the staff from harm. The nurse should follow the facility's policy for dealing with a violent patient. Call for help immediately and contact security. The health care provider, nursing supervisor, and risk manager should also be informed of the patient's violence. Stay with the patient, but do not crowd the patient.

If the nurse's own safety is threatened, the nurse should have another co-worker stay with the nurse and the patient. Remove dangerous objects from the area. Never block the nurse's exit or the patient's exit from a room. Use communication skills to try to calm the patient. Do not challenge the patient or argue with him or her. Use a calm and nonthreatening tone of voice and stance. Listen to the patient, and acknowledge the patient's anger.

Depending on their policies, some institutions prepare to handle violent individuals by mobilizing personnel. The nurse may be required to call a specific code through the paging operator, such as "code orange, room 462B." Specific staff members would respond to the call, such as security personnel, and individuals trained to handle volatile situations. The patient would then be approached and physically subdued and restrained enough to ensure safety without harming the patient, staff, or other patients. When the patient is restrained, he or she will need to be closely monitored and assessed, and the cause of the episode will need to be determined. A patient who is restrained should have a health care provider, such as a CNA, on one on one patient care 100% of the time. The patient may also require continued chemical or physical restraints if the violent behavior persists and no physical cause is determined.

Essential Documentation

The nurse should record the date and time of the note. Chart the location of the incident. Describe the patient's violent behaviors, and record exactly what the patient said in quotes. Record immediate nursing interventions and the patient's response. Chart the names of the people notified, such as the health care provider, the nursing supervisor, security, and the risk manager, when they were notified, and their responses. Note any injuries that occurred as a result of the violence. Complete an incident report, according to facility policy, repeating the exact information in the nurse's note. Include the names, addresses, and telephone numbers of witnesses.

Violent Patient		
3/9/2019	1715	**NURSING ASSESSMENT:** Heard shouts and a crash from pt.'s room at 1645. Upon entering room, saw dinner tray and broken dishes on floor. Pt. was standing, red-faced, with fist in air yelling, "My dog gets better food than this." ________
		NURSING INTERVENTION: Called for help and maintained a distance of approx. 5' from pt. When Ann Stilson, RN, and Jason Black, RN, arrived, I told them to wait in hall. Pt. was throwing books and other items from nightstand to floor. Firmly told pt. to stop throwing things and that I wanted to help him. I stated, "I can see you're angry. How can I help you?" Pt. responded, "Try getting me some decent food." Asked a nurse in the hall to call dietary office to see what other choices were on menu for tonight. Told pt. I would try to get him other food choices. Asked pt. to sit down with me to talk. Pt. sat on edge of his bed and I sat on chair approx. 4' from pt. Pt. started to cry and said, "I'm so scared. I don't want to die." Listened to pt. verbalize his fears for several minutes. When asked, pt. stated he would like to speak with chaplain and would agree to talk with a counselor. He apologized for his behavior and stated he was embarrassed. Contacted Dr. L. Hartwell at 1705 and told him of pt.'s behavior. Doctor approved of psych. consult and gave verbal order. On-call psychiatrist paged at 1708. Hasn't yet returned call. Nursing supervisor, Jack Fox, RN, also notified of incident. Pt. has no visible injuries. Will further assess pt. when calmer. ________
		________ **Kristen Burger, RN**

VISION IMPAIRMENT

A visual impairment in a patient may range from only a minor loss of vision to total blindness. If the patient has a visual impairment, determine what the patient can see and whether he or she uses any assistive devices to enhance vision. Perform a safety assessment, orient the patient to his or her room and the unit, and remove possible hazards (e.g., wastebaskets, electric cords, and other obstructions). Assess the patient's ability to maneuver around the environment. A patient with a recent loss of vision, such as the patient wearing an eye patch after eye surgery, may require more assistance than a patient who has had a gradual decline in vision or long-term visual loss.

Essential Documentation

The nurse should record the length of time that the patient has had a visual impairment. Describe the degree of vision loss—for example, whether the patient can see faces, shapes, and objects; read large print; or has a loss of peripheral vision or depth perception. Document whether assistive devices are being used, such as glasses, contact lenses, or a pocket magnifying glass. Describe the patient's ability to move around the environment safely. Record nursing interventions, such as obtaining a brighter light for the room and arranging personal objects within reach. Chart that the nurse notified other departments of the patient's visual impairment. Document patient teaching, such as orienting the patient to the room, the unit, and the use of the call bell. Include other instructions, such as calling for help when getting out of bed.

Vision Impairment		
4/16/2019	1900	**NURSING ASSESSMENT:** Pt. admitted for right hip replacement in a.m. Has had a gradual decline in vision over last 5 years due to macular degeneration. Pt. states she can see shapes and objects but has difficulty identifying faces from a distance. She uses a handheld magnifying glass to read large print books and also enjoys listening to books on tape. Pt. was able to safely maneuver around her room and unit; however, wastebasket and foot stool were moved against the wall. **NURSING INTERVENTION:** Showed pt. location of call bell attached to side rail of bed and emergency pull-cord in bathroom. Dietary office notified and will send an aide to read food choices to pt. Visual impairment marked in medical record, recorded on preop. checklist.
		________________ **Marcy Phillips, RN**

VITAL SIGNS, FREQUENT

A patient may require frequent monitoring of vital signs after surgery or certain procedures and diagnostic tests or during a critical illness. A frequent vital signs flow sheet or electronic health record allows the nurse to quickly document vital signs the moment they are taken without having to take the time to write a progress note. A flow sheet also allows the nurse to readily detect changes in the patient's condition.

Sometimes, recording only vital signs isn't sufficient to give a complete picture of the patient's status. In such a case, the nurse will also need to write a progress note. Make sure the data on the vital signs flow sheet are consistent with the data in the progress note.

Essential Documentation

The nurse should record the date on the flow sheet. Chart the specific time each set of vital signs is taken. If there is a significant change in vital signs, write a progress note documenting the change, the time the health care provider was notified, the provider's name, any orders given, nursing actions, and the patient's response. (See *Frequent vital signs flow sheet*, page 430.)

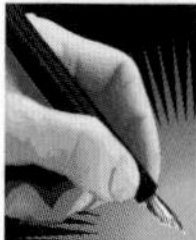

AccuChart

FREQUENT VITAL SIGNS FLOW SHEET

When the patient requires frequent vital sign assessments, a flow sheet such as this may help facilitate documentation by eliminating the need to continually make entries in the notation section of the chart. In this example, blood pressure is monitored every 15 minutes.

FREQUENT VITAL SIGNS FLOW SHEET

DATE	TIME	KEY	BP	P	RR	T	CVP	PAP			COMMENTS	TITRATED I.V.'S	MEDS STAT AND PRN	INITIALS
								S/D	M	W				
5/13/19	0900	S	122/84	98	18	98$_6$								MC
	0915	S	124/82	94	18									MC
	0930	S	122/78	92	20									MC
	0945	S	120/80	94	18									MC
	1000	S	128/78	94	20									MC

Key: S = Stethoscope D = Doppler P = Palpation T = Transducer

SELECTED READINGS

Appelboam, A., Reuben, A., Mann, C., Gagg, J., Ewings, P., Barton, A., Lobban, T., ... (2015). Postural modification to the standard Valsalva maneuver for emergency treatment of supraventricular tachycardias (REVERT): A randomized controlled trial. *Lancet, 386*(10005), 1747–1753.

Blair, A. (2018). The use of left ventricular assist devices in end-stage heart failure. *Critical Care Nursing Quarterly, 41*(4), 376–382.

Chan, T., Friedman, D. S., Bradley, C., & Massof, R. (2018). Estimates of incidence and prevalence of visual impairment, low vision, and blindness in the United States. *JAMA Ophthalmology, 136*(1), 12–19.

Cheng, K. S. (2018). How to prepare for and survive a violent patient encounter: When the unthinkable happens, having a plan that you have practiced regularly can make all the difference. *Family Practice Management, 25*(6), 5–10.

Çorbacıoğlu, Ş. K., Akıncı, E., Çevik, Y., Aytar, H., Öncül, M. V., Akkan, S., & Uzunosmanoğlu, H. (2017). Comparing the success rates of standard and modified Valsalva maneuvers to terminate PSVT: A randomized controlled trial. *The American Journal of Emergency Medicine, 35*(11), 1662–1665.

Dennis, J. L. (2018). Reporting violent patient incidents. *Journal of Healthcare Risk Management, 38*(2), 7.

Pasquier, M., Clair, M., Pruvot, E., Hugli, O., & Carron, P. N. (2017). Carotid sinus massage. *The New England Journal of Medicine, 377*(15), 1–4.

Scott, A. (2018). Spotlight on sight loss. *Community Practitioner, 91*(9), 31–33.

Taylor, C., Lynn, P., & Bartlett, J. L. (2019). *Fundamentals of nursing: The art and science of person-centered care.* Philadelphia, PA: Lippincott.

Twa, M. D. (2018). Assistive technology for vision impairment. *Optometry &* Vision *Science, 95*(9), 689–691.

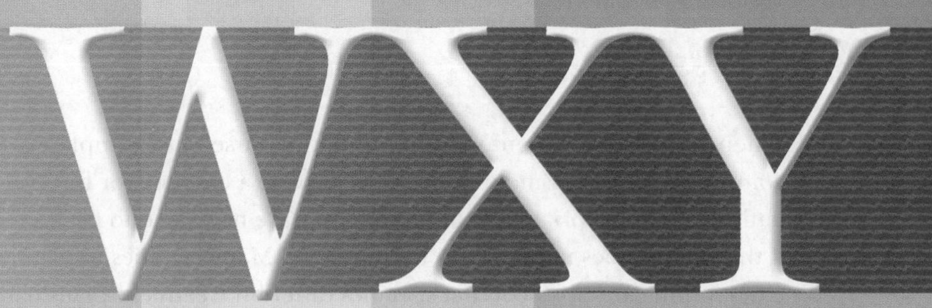

WALKER USE

A walker consists of a metal frame with handgrips and four legs buttressing the patient on three sides. One side remains open. Because this device provides greater stability and security than do other ambulatory aids, it is recommended that the patient with insufficient strength (especially upper body) and balance use a walker instead of crutches or a cane.

Essential Documentation

The nurse needs to:

- Record the date and time of each entry.
- Record the type of walker used, such as a standard, stair, or reciprocal walker.
- Note whether any attachments are used, including platform attachments or wheels.
- Describe the degree of guarding that the patient requires.
- Document the distance walked and the patient's tolerance.
- Document all education related to the use of the walker.

Walker Use		
8/20/2019	1200	**NURSING ASSESSMENT:** Pt. ambulated with reciprocal walker without assistance from own room to day room using 2-point gait, approx. 50'. Required only occasional verbal cues. Pt. was slightly SOB at end of walk. VS before walk P 82, BP 130/78, RR 18. After walk P 94, BP 138/82, RR 26. **PATIENT TEACHING:** Reinforced sitting and standing using the walker. Pt. gave proper demo. ______ **Carole Parker, RN**

WOUND ASSESSMENT

When caring for a patient with a wound, the nurse must complete a comprehensive assessment in order to provide a baseline for the evaluation and appropriateness of treatment. Care may need to be altered if the wound does not respond to treatment. Many facilities have a specific wound care protocol that specifies different treatment plans based on wound assessment. Wound dressings should be assessed routinely, noting any excessive or new drainage requiring a dressing change.

Essential Documentation

The nurse needs to:

- Document the date and time with each entry. Many facilities also have a special form or flow sheet on which to document wounds. (See *Wound and skin assessment tool,* pages 435 and 436.) Include the following for wound assessment:
  - wound size, including length, width, and depth in centimeters
  - wound appearance: color, edema, irregularities, surrounding tissue
  - wound shape
  - wound site, drawn on a body plan to document exact location
  - wound stage
  - characteristics of drainage, if any, including amount, color, and presence of odor
  - characteristics of the wound bed, including description of tissue type, such as granulation tissue, slough, or epithelial tissue
  - character of the surrounding tissue
  - presence or absence of eschar
  - presence or absence of pain
  - presence or absence of undermining or tunneling (in centimeters).

Wound Assessment		
9/14/2019	1330	**NURSING ASSESSMENT:** Pt. admitted to unit for fem-pop bypass tomorrow. Pt. has open wound at tip of 2nd left toe, approx. 0.5 cm × 1 cm × 0.5 cm deep. Wound is round with even edges. Wound bed is pale with little granulation tissue. No drainage, odor, eschar, or tunneling noted. Pt. reports pain at wound site, rates pain as 4 on scale of 0 to 10, w/10 being the worst pain imaginable. Surrounding skin cool to touch, pale, and intact. ______
		PATIENT TEACHING: Pt. understands not to cross legs or wear tight garments. ______
		______ **Mark Silver, RN**

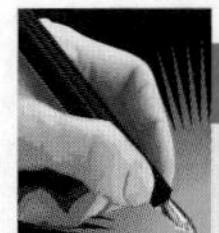

ACCUCHART

WOUND AND SKIN ASSESSMENT TOOL

A comprehensive wound and skin assessment may include a pictorial representation as a tool to identify a wound site. Using the wound and skin assessment tool below, the nurse identified the left second toe as a partial-thickness wound, vascular ulcer, that is blue in color using the classification of terms that follows.

PATIENT'S NAME (LAST, MIDDLE, FIRST)	ATTENDING PHYSICIAN	ROOM NUMBER	ID NUMBER
Brown, Ann	Dr. A. Dennis	123-2	01726

WOUND ASSESSMENT:

NUMBER	1	2	3	4	5	6
DATE	7/03/19					
TIME	12:15					
LOCATION	left second toe					
STAGE	II					
APPEARANCE	G					
SIZE-LENGTH	0.5 cm					
SIZE-WIDTH	1 cm					
COLOR/FLR.	RD					
DRAINAGE	0					
ODOR	0					
VOLUME	0					
INFLAMMATION	0					
SIZE INFLAM.	0					

KEY

Stage:
- I. Red or discolored
- II. Skin break/blister
- III. Sub 'Q' tissue
- IV. Muscle and/or bone

Appearance:
- D = Depth
- E = Eschar
- G = Granulation
- IN = Inflammation
- NEC = Necrotic
- PK = Pink
- SL = Slough
- TN = Tunneling
- UND = Undermining
- MX = Mixed (specify)

Color of Wound Floor:
- RD = Red
- Y = Yellow
- BLK = Black
- MX = Mixed (specify)

Drainage:
- 0 = None
- SR = Serous
- SS = Serosanguineous
- BL = Blood
- PR = Purulent

Odor:
- 0 = None
- MLD = Mild
- FL = Foul

Volume:
- 0 = None
- SC = Scant
- MOD = Moderate
- LG = Large

Inflammation:
- 0 = None
- PK = Pink
- RD = Red

(continued)

WOUND AND SKIN ASSESSMENT TOOL *(continued)*

WOUND ANATOMIC LOCATION:
(circle affected area)

Anterior Posterior Left lateral Right lateral

Left foot Right foot Left hand Right hand

Wound care: Cleaned wound with NSS; dry sterile dressing applied.

Signature: Mark Silver, RN Date 7/03/19

WOUND CARE

Preventing infection is an important intervention while caring for a surgical wound. Hand hygiene and wound covering will prevent pathogens from entering a wound. Protecting the skin around a wound decreases the chance for maceration and excoriation. The use of dressings and or pouches can maintain the integrity of the surrounding skin as well as aid in monitoring drainage, which may contribute to potential fluid and electrolyte imbalances.

Essential Documentation

The nurse needs to:

- Document the date and time of wound care as well as supplies used with dressing changes. Commonly, a flow sheet is used for continual monitoring of a wound.
- Record the amount of soiled dressing and packing removed.
- Describe wound appearance (size, condition of margins, wound bed, and presence of necrotic tissue) and odor (if present).
- Chart the type, color, consistency, and amount of drainage for each wound.
- Indicate the presence and location of drains.
- Note any additional procedures, such as irrigation, packing, or application of a topical medication.
- Record the type and amount of new dressing or pouch applied.
- Note the patient's tolerance of the procedure and any instructions given.
- Document special or detailed wound care instructions and pain management steps on the care plan or flow sheet.
- Document in the record any patient teaching completed about wound care.

Wound Care		
6/17/2019	1030	**NURSING ASSESSMENT:** Dressing removed from right mastectomy incision. 1.5 cm round area of serosanguineous drainage noted on dressing. No odor noted. 11-cm incision well-approximated, staples intact. Skin around incision intact, no redness. ______ **NURSING INTERVENTION:** Site cleaned with sterile NSS. Six sterile 4" × 4" gauze pads applied. Jackson Pratt drain at lateral edge of incision emptied for 10 mL serosanguineous fluid, no odor noted. See I/O flow sheet for shift totals. ______ **PATIENT TEACHING:** Explained dressing change and signs and symptoms of infection to report. Pt. verbalized understanding. Pt. states incision is tender but doesn't require pain medication. ______ ______ **Mark Silver, RN**

WOUND DEHISCENCE

Although surgical wounds typically heal without incident, occasionally the edges of a wound may fail to join or may separate even after they seem to be healing normally. This complication, called *dehiscence,* may be partial and superficial or complete, with disruption of all layers. It commonly occurs from 3 to 11 days after surgery.

Dehiscence occurs most commonly in abdominal wounds after a sudden strain, such as a sneeze or cough, vomiting, or sitting up in bed. Obese patients are at higher risk due to the constant strain placed on the wound and the slow healing of fatty tissue. Other factors that may contribute to dehiscence include poor nutrition (either from inadequate intake or diabetes mellitus), chronic pulmonary or cardiac disease, and localized wound infection.

If wound dehiscence occurs, the nurse should stay with the patient as a fellow health care provider contacts the surgeon. The patient is to be placed in a reclining position with the knees slightly flexed. The wound needs to be covered with sterile gauze pads soaked in sterile normal saline solution, then with dry sterile gauze pads, which are secured in place. The nurse will stay with the patient until the health care provider gives further instructions. Depending on the extent of the degree of dehiscence, the patient may need sutures or adhesive strips to close the wound.

Essential Documentation

The nurse should:

- Document the date and time the complication occurred and the patient's activity prior to the dehiscence.
- Document the appearance of the wound—that is, the amount, color, consistency, and odor of drainage.
- Document the patient assessment (including vital signs and pain level) as well as surgeon notification.

Wound Dehiscence		
8/24/2019	0945	**NURSING ASSESSMENT:** During dressing change at 0925, noted dehiscence of distal 2" of midline abdominal incision. Superficial layers of tissue observed, no evisceration noted. ________ **NURSING INTERVENTION:** Pt. placed in reclined position with knees flexed. Pt. states, "I felt something give when I coughed." Pt. denies

Wound Dehiscence (*continued*)

pain. Wound covered with sterile 4" × 4" gauze soaked in NSS, then covered with dry sterile dressing. ______
NURSING ASSESSMENT: P 100, BP 150/84, RR 18, T 98.6°F. ______
NURSING INTERVENTION: Dr. B. McBride notified at 0930. Adhesive strips ordered and applied to wound. Pt. to be kept on bed rest until. Dr. McBride visits pt. at 1030. ______
PATIENT TEACHING: Pt. instructed to stay in bed with knees flexed and to call nurse for assistance with moving in bed. Reviewed splinting incision with pillow if he has to cough or sneeze. Call bell placed within reach, and pt. demonstrated how to use it. ______
______ **Maureen Dunlop, RN**

WOUND EVISCERATION

A severe complication of wound dehiscence, evisceration occurs when a portion of the viscera (usually a bowel loop) protrudes through the incision. Evisceration can lead to peritonitis and septic shock, a potentially fatal condition.

Wound evisceration most commonly occurs 6 to 7 days after surgery and may be caused by poor nutrition, chronic pulmonary or cardiac disease, localized wound infection, or stress on the incision from coughing. A midline abdominal incision has a higher risk of wound evisceration.

If wound evisceration occurs, the nurse will stay with the patient as a fellow health care worker contacts the surgeon. The patient is to be placed in a reclining position with the knees slightly flexed if evisceration occurs with an abdominal incision. If the wound is in another region, the patient needs to be in a position that places decreased tension on the wound edges. The exposed viscera need to be covered with sterile gauze pads soaked in normal saline solution. Then, a sterile, waterproof drape should be placed over the dressings to keep the dressings moist. Preparing the patient for surgery should be anticipated.

Essential Documentation

The nurse needs to:

- Document the date and time the complication occurred and the patient's activity prior to the evisceration.
- Document the patient assessment (including vital signs and pain level) as well as surgeon notification.

- Include a description of the wound and the eviscerated organ as well as any drainage.
- Document that interventions were completed.
- Document that patient education and support were provided.

Wound Evisceration		
10/18/2019	1135	**NURSING ASSESSMENT:** Called to room by pt. who stated, "I think I felt something pulling when I coughed." Pt. lying curled on side splinting abdomen with arms, moaning. Eviscerated bowel pink and moist, no drainage. ________ **NURSING INTERVENTION:** Area covered with sterileNSS-soaked gauze. Sterile, waterproof drape placed over dressing. ________ **NURSING ASSESSMENT:** Skin color pale, diaphoretic. P 112, BP 92/58, RR 28, tympanic T 98.2°F. ________ **NURSING INTERVENTION:** Stayed with pt. while Karen Schultz, RN, called Dr. J. Brown who came by immediately, orders given. O_2 at 2 L/min by NC applied. IV line started in right antecubital with 18G catheter on first attempt. 1,000 mL lactated Ringer's solution infusing at 100 mL/hr. Being kept NPO for probable surgery. Pt. fearful and weeping. Offering reassurance and explaining all procedures. See flow sheet for VS. ________ ________ **Carla Molino, RN**

SELECTED READINGS

American Nurses Association. (2010). *Principles for nursing documentation.* Retrieved from https://www.nursingworld.org/~4af4f2/globalassets/docs/ana/ethics/principles-of-nursing-documentation.pdf

Annesley, S. H. (2019). Current thinking on caring for patients with a wound: A practical approach. *British Journal of Nursing, 28*(5), 290–294.

Chetter, I. C., Oswald, A. V., McGinnis, E., Stubbs, N., Arundel, C., Buckley, H., Bell, K., ... Saramago, P. (2019). Patients with surgical wounds healing by secondary intention: A prospective, cohort study. *International Journal of Nursing Studies, 89*, 62–71.

Duclos-Miller, P. (2016). *Improving nursing documentation and reducing risk.* Retrieved from https://hcmarketplace.com/aitdownloadablefiles/download/aitfile/aitfile_id/1806.pdf

Edwards, J. (2018). Assessment and management of chronic wounds. *Independent Nurse, 7*, 17–19.

Nazarko, L. (2018). Choosing the correct wound care dressing: an overview. *Journal of Community Nursing, 32*(5), 42–52.

Stout, K. (Ed.). (2018). *Nursing documentation made incredibly easy.* Philadelphia, PA: Wolters Kluwer.

Taylor, C., Lillis, C., Lynn, P., & LeMone, P. (2015). *Fundamentals of nursing.* Philadelphia, PA: Wolters Kluwer.

Z

Z-TRACK INJECTION

The Z-track method of intramuscular injection prevents leakage, or tracking, into the subcutaneous tissue. It is typically used to administer drugs that irritate and discolor subcutaneous tissue, primarily iron preparations such as iron dextran. It may also be used in an elderly patient who has a decreased muscle mass. Lateral displacement of the skin during the injection helps to seal the drug in the muscle.

Discomfort and tissue irritation may result from drug leakage into subcutaneous tissue. Failure to rotate sites in patients who require repeated injections could interfere with the absorption of medication. Unabsorbed medications may build up in deposits that can reduce the desired pharmacologic effect and may lead to abscess formation or tissue fibrosis.

Essential Documentation

The nurse needs to:

- Record the date and time of the entry, the medication and dosage given, and the site of injection on the patient's medication administration record (MAR).
- Include the patient's response to the injected drug, if appropriate. (See *Z-track injection* page 442.)

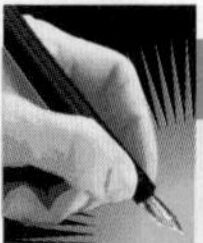

AccuChart

Z-TRACK INJECTION

A medication chart may be used to document medication administration by Z-track injection. An example of a record of dosage and administration is provided below.

Patient Name: David Stein   Medical record number: 97531

NURSE'S FULL SIGNATURE, STATUS AND INITIALS	INIT.		INIT.		INIT.
Roy Charles, RN	RC				
Theresa Hopkins, RN	TH				

DIAGNOSIS: Heart failure, atrial flutter, COPD

ALLERGIES: ASA   DIET: Cardiac

ROUTINE/DAILY ORDERS FINGERSTICKS/INSULIN COVERAGE			DATE: 1/10		DATE: 1/11		DATE: 1/12		DATE: 1/13		DATE: 1/14		DATE: 1/15		DATE: 1/16		DATE: 1/17		DATE: 1/18		DATE: 1/19	
ORDER DATE	MEDICATIONS DOSAGE, ROUTE, FREQUENCY	TIME	SITE	INT.	SITE	INT.	SITE	INT.	SITE	INT.	SITE	INT.	SITE	INT.	SITE	INT.	SITE	INT.	SITE	INT.	SITE	INT.
1/10/19	Iron dextran 50 mg I.M. daily by Z-track × 3 doses	0900	right GM	RC	left GM	TH	right GM	TH														

SELECTED READING

Yilmaz, D., Khorshid, L., & Dedeoğlu, Y. (2016). The effect of the Z-track technique on pain and drug leakage in intramuscular injections. *Clinical Nurse Specialist, 30*(6), E7–E12.

Standardized Systems

NURSING MINIMUM DATA SET

The Nursing Minimum Data Set (NMDS) is a means of standardizing nursing information. It contains three categories of data: nursing care, patient demographics, and service elements. Nursing care includes nursing diagnoses, interventions, outcomes, and nursing intensity. Patient demographics include the patient's personal information, date of birth, sex, race or ethnicity, and place of residence. Service includes any service agency number, health record number, date of episode of admission or encounter, date of discharge or termination, disposition of the patient and expected payer of medical bills.

Nursing Benefits

The NMDS allows the nurse to collect nursing diagnoses and intervention data and identify the nursing needs of various patient populations. It also lets the nurse track patient outcomes and describe nursing care in various settings, including the patient's home. This system helps establish accurate estimates for nursing service costs and provides data about nursing care that may influence health care policy and decision making.

With the NMDS, the nurse can compare nursing trends locally, regionally, and nationally, which allows for a comparison of nursing data from various clinical settings, patient populations, and geographic areas. However, the NMDS does more than provide valuable information for research and policy making. It also helps the nurse to provide better patient care. For instance, examining the outcomes of patient populations will help the nurse set realistic outcomes for an individual patient, formulate accurate nursing diagnoses, and plan interventions.

The standardized format of the NMDS also encourages more consistent nursing documentation. All data are coded, making documentation and information retrieval faster and easier. Currently, NANDA International assigns numerical codes to all nursing diagnoses so that they can be used with the NMDS.

VOICE-ACTIVATED SYSTEMS

Some hospitals have instituted voice-activated nursing documentation systems, which are most useful in hospital departments that have a high volume of structured reports, such as the operating room. The software program uses a specialized knowledge base of nursing words, phrases, and report forms, combined with automated speech recognition (ASR) technology. This system allows the user to record prompt and complete nursing notes by voice. The ASR system requires little or no keyboard use; the nurse simply speaks into a telephone handset, and the text appears on the computer screen.

The software program includes information on the nursing process, nursing theory, nursing standards of practice, report forms, and a logical format. The system uses trigger phrases that cue the system to display passages of report text. The nurse can use the text displayed to design an individualized care plan or to fill in standard facility forms.

Although voice-activated systems are designed to work most efficiently with these trigger phrases, they also allow word-for-word dictation and editing. The system increases the speed of reporting and frees the nurse from paperwork so that the nurse can spend more time at the bedside.

ADDITIONAL ELECTRONIC SYSTEM FEATURES

Depending on the system type, an electronic documentation system may provide the ability to print out patient schedules. The system may also be equipped with barcode technology.

Patient Schedules

Most systems have the ability to print out schedule lists for patients. For example, the nurse can print out a schedule of patients who require fingerstick glucose level tests. If the situation requires the nurse to delegate the task, the list may be given to ancillary staff members. The list lets them know exactly when they are supposed to obtain the fingerstick glucose level for each patient.

MAINTAINING PATIENT CONFIDENTIALITY

The American Nurses Association and the American Records Association offer these guidelines for maintaining the confidentiality of computerized medical records.

Never Share

The nurse should never give his or her password or computer code to anyone—including another nurse in the unit, a nurse serving temporarily in the unit, or a health care provider. The health care facility can issue a short-term password that allows infrequent users to access certain records.

Log Off

After logging into a computer terminal, the nurse should not leave the terminal unattended. Although some computer systems have a timing device that automatically logs off the user after an idle period, the nurse should get into the habit of logging off the system before leaving the terminal.

Don't Display

The nurse should not leave information about a patient displayed on a monitor where others can see it. Also, the nurse should not leave print versions or excerpts of the medical record unattended.

The Joint Commission Abbreviations to Avoid

OFFICIAL "DO NOT USE" LIST

To reduce the risk of medical errors, The Joint Commission has created an official "Do Not Use" list of abbreviations.[1] In addition, The Joint Commission offers suggestions for other abbreviations and symbols to avoid.

Abbreviation	Potential problem	Use instead
U (unit)	Mistaken for "0" (zero), the number "4" (four), or "cc"	Write "unit"
IU (International Unit)	Mistaken for IV (intravenous) or the number 10 (ten)	Write "International Unit"
Q.D., QD, q.d., qd (daily)	Mistaken for each other	Write "daily"
Q.O.D., QOD, q.o.d., qod (every other day)	Period after the Q mistaken for "I" and the "O" mistaken for "I"	Write "every other day"
Trailing zero (X.0 mg)* Lack of leading zero (.X mg)	Decimal point is missed	Write X mg Write 0.X mg
MS	Can mean morphine sulfate or magnesium sulfate	Write "morphine sulfate"
MSO_4 and $MgSO_4$	Confused for one another	Write "magnesium sulfate"

[1]Applies to all orders and all medication-related documentation that is handwritten (including free-text computer entry) or on preprinted forms.

*Exception: A "trailing zero" may be used only where required to demonstrate the level of precision of the value being reported, such as for laboratory results, imaging studies that report the size of lesions, or catheter/tube sizes. It may not be used in medication orders or other medication-related documentation.

ADDITIONAL ABBREVIATIONS, ACRONYMS, AND SYMBOLS

(For possible future inclusion in the official "Do Not Use" list)

Abbreviation	Potential problem	Use instead
> (greater than) < (less than)	Misinterpreted as the number "7" (seven) or the letter "L" Confused for one another	Write "greater than" Write "less than"
Abbreviations for drug names	Misinterpreted due to similar abbreviations for multiple drugs	Write drug names in full
Apothecary units	Unfamiliar to many practitioners Confused with metric units	Use metric units
@	Mistaken for the number "2" (two)	Write "at"
cc	Mistaken for U (units) when poorly written	Write "mL" or "milliliters"
µg	Mistaken for mg (milligrams), resulting in 1,000-fold overdose	Write "mcg" or "micrograms"

Institute for Safe Medication Practices (ISMP) Drug Sound-Alike/ Look-Alike Names

TABLE 1. U.S. FOOD AND DRUG ADMINISTRATION–APPROVED LIST OF COMMONLY CONFUSED GENERIC DRUG NAMES	
Drug Name with Tall Man Letters	Confused with
aceta**ZOLAMIDE**	aceto**HEXAMIDE**
aceto**HEXAMIDE**	aceta**ZOLAMIDE**
bu**PROP**ion	bus**PIR**one
bus**PIR**one	bu**PROP**ion
chlorpro**MAZINE**	chlorpro**PAMIDE**
chlorpro**PAMIDE**	chlorpro**MAZINE**
clomi**PHENE**	clomi**PRAMINE**
clomi**PRAMINE**	clomi**PHENE**
cyclo**SERINE**	cyclo**SPORINE**
cyclo**SPORINE**	cyclo**SERINE**
DAUNOrubicin	**DOXO**rubicin
dimenhy**DRINATE**	diphenhydr**AMINE**
diphenhydr**AMINE**	dimenhy**DRINATE**
DOBUTamine	**DOP**amine
DOPamine	**DOBUT**amine
DOXOrubicin	**DAUNO**rubicin
glipi**ZIDE**	gly**BURIDE**
gly**BURIDE**	glipi**ZIDE**
hydr**ALAZINE**	hydr**OXY**zine—**HYDRO**morphone
HYDROmorphone	hydr**OXY**zine—hydr**ALAZINE**
hydr**OXY**zine	hydr**ALAZINE**—**HYDRO**morphone
medroxy**PROGESTER**one	methyl**PREDNIS**olone—methyl**TESTOSTER**one
methyl**PREDNIS**olone	medroxy**PROGESTER**one—methyl**TESTOSTER**one
methyl**TESTOSTER**one	medroxy**PROGESTER**one—methyl**PREDNIS**olone

(continued)

TABLE 1. U.S. FOOD AND DRUG ADMINISTRATION–APPROVED LIST OF COMMONLY CONFUSED GENERIC DRUG NAMES (*continued*)

Drug Name with Tall Man Letters	Confused with
mito**XANTRONE**	Not specified
ni**CAR**dipine	**NIFE**dipine
NIFEdipine	ni**CAR**dipine
predniso**LONE**	predni**SONE**
predni**SONE**	predniso**LONE**
risperi**DONE**	r**OPINIR**ole
r**OPINIR**ole	risperi**DONE**
sulf**ADIAZINE**	sulfi**SOXAZOLE**
sulfi**SOXAZOLE**	sulf**ADIAZINE**
TOLAZamide	**TOLBUT**amide
TOLBUTamide	**TOLAZ**amide
vin**BLAS**tine	vin**CRIS**tine
vin**CRIS**tine	vin**BLAS**tine

From Institute for Safe Medication Practices. (2016). *Look-alike drug names with recommended tall man letters*. Retrieved from https://www.ismp.org/recommendations/tall-man-letters-list

TABLE 2. INSTITUTE FOR SAFE MEDICATION PRACTICES (ISMP) LIST OF COMMONLY CONFUSED DRUG NAMES***

Drug Name with Tall Man Letters	Confused with
ALPRAZolam	**LOR**azepam—clonaze**PAM**
a**MIL**oride	am**LODIP**ine
am**LODIP**ine	a**MIL**oride
ARIPiprazole	**RABE**prazole
AVINza	**INV**anz*
aza**CITID**ine	aza**THIO**prine
aza**THIO**prine	aza**CITID**ine
car**BAM**azepine	**OX**carbazepine
CARBOplatin	**CIS**platin
ce**FAZ**olin	cefo**TE**tan—cef**OX**itin—cef**TAZ**idime—cef**TRIAX**one
cefo**TE**tan	ce**FAZ**olin—cef**OX**itin—cef**TAZ**idime—cef**TRIAX**one
cef**OX**itin	ce**FAZ**olin—cefo**TE**tan—cef**TAZ**idime—cef**TRIAX**one
cef**TAZ**idime	ce**FAZ**olin—cefo**TE**tan—cef**OX**itin—cef**TRIAX**one
cef**TRIAX**one	ce**FAZ**olin—cefo**TE**tan—cef**OX**itin—cef**TAZ**idime
Cele**BREX**	Cele**XA***
Cele**XA**	Cele**BREX***

TABLE 2. INSTITUTE FOR SAFE MEDICATION PRACTICES (ISMP) LIST OF COMMONLY CONFUSED DRUG NAMES (*continued*)

Drug Name with Tall Man Letters	Confused with
chlordiaze**POXIDE**	chlorpro**MAZINE****
chlorpro**MAZINE****	chlordiaze**POXIDE**
CISplatin	**CARBO**platin
clo**BAZ**am	clonaze**PAM**
clonaze**PAM**	clo**NID**ine—clo**ZAP**ine—clo**BAZ**am—**LOR**azepam
clo**NID**ine	clonazepam—clo**ZAP**ine—Klono**PIN***
clo**ZAP**ine	clonaze**PAM**—clo**NID**ine
DACTINomycin	**DAPTO**mycin
DAPTOmycin	**DACTIN**omycin
DEPO-Medrol*	**SOLU**-Medrol*
diaze**PAM**	dil**TIAZ**em
dil**TIAZ**em	diaze**PAM**
DOCEtaxel	**PACL**itaxel
DOXOrubicin**	**IDA**rubicin
DULoxetine	**FLU**oxetine—**PAR**oxetine
e**PHED**rine	**EPINEPH**rine
EPINEPHrine	e**PHED**rine
epi**RUB**icin	eri**BUL**in
eri**BUL**in	epi**RUB**icin
fenta**NYL**	**SUF**entanil
flavox**ATE**	fluvoxa**MINE**
FLUoxetine	**DUL**oxetine—**PAR**oxetine
flu**PHENAZ**ine	fluvoxa**MINE**
fluvoxa**MINE**	flu**PHENAZ**ine-flavox**ATE**
guai**FEN**esin	guan**FACINE**
guan**FACINE**	guai**FEN**esin
Huma**LOG***	Humu**LIN***
Humu**LIN***	Huma**LOG***
hydr**ALAZINE****	hydro**CHLORO**thiazide—hydr**OXY**zine**
hydro**CHLORO**thiazide	hydr**OXY**zine**—hydr**ALAZINE****
HYDROcodone	oxy**CODONE**
HYDROmorphone**	morphine—oxy**MOR**phone
HYDROXYprogesterone	medroxy**PROGESTER**one**

(continued)

TABLE 2. INSTITUTE FOR SAFE MEDICATION PRACTICES (ISMP) LIST OF COMMONLY CONFUSED DRUG NAMES *(continued)*	
Drug Name with Tall Man Letters	Confused with
hydr**OXY**zine**	hydr**ALAZINE****—hydro**CHLORO**thiazide
IDArubicin	**DOXO**rubicin****—idaru**CIZU**mab
idaru**CIZU**mab	**IDA**rubicin
in**FLIX**imab	ri**TUX**imab
INVanz*	**AVIN**za*
ISOtretinoin	tretinoin
Klono**PIN***	clo**NID**ine
La**MIC**tal*	Lam**ISIL***
Lam**ISIL***	La**MIC**tal*
lami**VUD**ine	lamo**TRI**gine
lamo**TRI**gine	lami**VUD**ine
lev**ETIRA**cetam	lev**OCARN**itine—levo**FLOX**acin
lev**OCARN**itine	lev**ETIRA**cetam
levo**FLOX**acin	lev**ETIRA**cetam
LEVOleucovorin	leucovorin
LORazepam	**ALPRAZ**olam—clonaze**PAM**
medroxy**PROGESTER**one**	**HYDROXY**progesterone
met**FORMIN**	metro**NIDAZOLE**
methazol**AMIDE**	meth**IMA**zole—met**OL**azone
meth**IMA**zole	met**OL**azone—methazol**AMIDE**
met**OL**azone	meth**IMA**zole—methazol**AMIDE**
metro**NIDAZOLE**	met**FORMIN**
metyra**PONE**	metyro**SINE**
metyro**SINE**	metyra**PONE**
mi**FEPRIS**tone	mi**SOPROS**tol
mi**SOPROS**tol	mi**FEPRIS**tone
mito**MY**cin	mito**XANTRONE****
mito**XANTRONE****	mito**MY**cin
Nex**AVAR***	Nex**IUM***
Nex**IUM***	Nex**AVAR***
ni**CAR**dipine**	ni**MOD**ipine—**NIFE**dipine**
NIFEdipine**	ni**MOD**ipine—ni**CAR**dipine**
ni**MOD**ipine	**NIFE**dipine**—ni**CAR**dipine**
Novo**LIN***	Novo**LOG***
Novo**LOG***	Novo**LIN***

TABLE 2. INSTITUTE FOR SAFE MEDICATION PRACTICES (ISMP) LIST OF COMMONLY CONFUSED DRUG NAMES (*continued*)	
Drug Name with Tall Man Letters	**Confused with**
OLANZapine	**QUE**tiapine
OXcarbazepine	car**BAM**azepine
oxy**CODONE**	**HYDRO**codone—Oxy**CONTIN***—oxy**MOR**phone
Oxy**CONTIN***	oxycodone—oxy**MOR**phone
oxy**MOR**phone	**HYDRO**morphone**—oxy**CODONE**—Oxy**CONTIN***
PACLitaxel	**DOCE**taxel
PARoxetine	**FLU**oxetine—**DUL**oxetine
PAZOPanib	**PONAT**inib
PEMEtrexed	**PRALA**trexate
penicill**AMINE**	penicillin
PENTobarbital	**PHEN**obarbital
PHENobarbital	**PENT**obarbital
PONATinib	**PAZO**Panib
PRALAtrexate	**PEME**trexed
Pri**LOSEC***	**PRO**zac*
PROzac*	Pri**LOSEC***
QUEtiapine	**OLANZ**apine
qui**NID**ine	qui**NINE**
qui**NINE**	qui**NID**ine
RABEprazole	**ARIP**iprazole
ra**NITI**dine	ri**MANTA**dine
rif**AMP**in	rif**AXIM**in
rif**AXIM**in	rif**AMP**in
ri**MANTA**dine	ra**NITI**dine
Risper**DAL***	r**OPINIR**ole**
risperi**DONE****	r**OPINIR**ole**
ri**TUX**imab	in**FLIX**imab
romi**DEP**sin	romi**PLOS**tim
romi**PLOS**tim	romi**DEP**sin
r**OPINIR**ole**	Risper**DAL***—risperi**DONE****
Sand**IMMUNE***	Sando**STATIN***
Sando**STATIN***	Sand**IMMUNE***
s**AX**agliptin	**SIT**agliptin

(continued)

TABLE 2. INSTITUTE FOR SAFE MEDICATION PRACTICES (ISMP) LIST OF COMMONLY CONFUSED DRUG NAMES (*continued*)

Drug Name with Tall Man Letters	Confused with
SEROquel*	**SINE**quan*
SINEquan*	**SERO**quel*
SITagliptin	s**AX**agliptin—**SUMA**triptan
Solu-**CORTEF***	**SOLU**-Medrol*
SOLU-Medrol*	Solu-**CORTEF***—**DEPO**-Medrol*
SORAfenib	**SUNI**tinib
SUFentanil	fenta**NYL**
sulf**ADIAZINE****	sulfa**SALA**zine
sulfa**SALA**zine	sulf**ADIAZINE****
SUMAtriptan	**SIT**agliptin—**ZOLM**itriptan
SUNItinib	**SORA**fenib
TEGretol*	**TREN**tal*
tia**GAB**ine	ti**ZAN**idine
ti**ZAN**idine	tia**GAB**ine
tra**MAD**ol	tra**ZOD**one
tra**ZOD**one	tra**MAD**ol
TRENtal*	**TEG**retol*
val**ACY**clovir	val**GAN**ciclovir
val**GAN**ciclovir	val**ACY**clovir
ZOLMitriptan	**SUMA**triptan
Zy**PREXA***	Zyr**TEC***
Zyr**TEC***	Zy**PREXA***

* Brand names always start with an uppercase letter. Some brand names incorporate tall man letters in initial characters and may not be readily recognized as brand names. An asterisk follows all brand names on the ISMP list.

** These drug names are also on the FDA list.

*** The ISMP list is not an official list approved by FDA. It is intended for voluntary use by health care practitioners and drug information and technology vendors. Any manufacturers' product label changes require FDA approval.

From Institute for Safe Medication Practices. (2016). *Look-alike drug names with recommended tall man letters*. Retrieved from https://www.ismp.org/recommendations/tall-man-letters-list

Common Charting Mistakes to Avoid

Recording information in the patient's chart is an important part of the nurse's job. There are many ways that charting mistakes can be made. When the nurse is aware of the following eight common pitfalls, the nurse can not only avoid making these mistakes but can also avoid being involved in litigation.

Failing to Record Pertinent Health or Drug Information

Suppose the patient has a food or drug allergy or a disease such as diabetes or hemophilia. The patient's caregivers need to know this information, but the nurse inadvertently forgets to chart it. This will not only endanger the patient, but can lead to litigation.

Failing to Record Nursing Actions

The nurse should record everything that is done for a patient as soon as possible. Chart what is observed and the actions taken as a result of the observation. Not charting something will affect the next shift. The nurses on the next shift will not know if the same observation is new or a change if the prior nurse does not chart the observation. Also, timing is everything. Waiting too long to chart nursing actions means the nurse has to rely on memory, which can cause inaccurate or incomplete information.

Failing to Record That Medications Have Been Given

The nurse should record every medication given when it is given and include the dose, route, and time. Failing to do so could result in a patient being overmedicated, which could be terminal in some cases. If the nurse is the one who observes that a medication has been ordered and not charted as having been administered, the nurse should question it. Make sure that the medication has not already been given rather than making the mistake of doubling the dose.

Electronic health records and electronic medication records have made the administration of medication more efficient and safer for patients. Medications and patient hospital bracelets often have specific barcodes that will ensure patients do not mistakenly receive double doses of medications. The nurse should always double-check medication orders with another nurse or nurse supervisor if there is any doubt or ambiguity in the medication order. The nurse should be sure to observe the 12 rights of medication administration:

1. Right patient
2. Right medication
3. Right dosage of medication
4. Right route of medication
5. Right time for medication
6. Right assessment of patient prior to administration of medication
7. Right medication preparation
8. Right expiration date on medication
9. Right of patient to refuse medication
10. Right of patient to understand reason for medication
11. Right documentation of medication administration
12. Right evaluation of medication effect

(continued)

Recording on the Wrong Chart

The nurse cannot be too careful in any situation that might lead to confusion between two patients, who could have the same last name, same room, same condition, or even the same health care provider. Always match the chart with the wristband of the patient before any nursing action.

Failing to Document a Discontinued Medication

If a patient is taken off a medication for any reason, the nurse needs to document that order promptly. Not doing so could result in serious complications for the patient. Commonly, the health care provider will make a computerized physician order entry that discontinues the drug.

Failing to Record Drug Reactions or Changes in the Patient's Condition

Monitoring the patient's response to treatment is not enough. The nurse should recognize an adverse reaction or a worsening of the patient's condition, then intervene before the patient is seriously harmed.

Writing Incomplete Records

In most instances, the mistake of writing incomplete records rarely causes a lawsuit, but in the midst of proceedings, it can help add to the argument of inadequate care. Thus, the nurse should give all charting careful attention. Make sure to include everything needed and to accompany all documentation with the nurse's initials and the time and date.

Adapted from Special Report: *How to Properly Document to Reduce Your Liability Risk*.

Charting Checkup: When the Nurse Is on Trial—How to Protect Oneself

If the nurse is named in a malpractice suit that goes to court, the nurse's documentation could be the best defense . . . if the nurse's charting offers a full record of the patient care provided. How and what the nurse documented—and what the nurse did not document—will greatly influence the trial.

Believable Evidence

The outcome of a malpractice trial usually comes down to one simple question: Whom does the jury believe? The patient presents evidence that he or she was injured because the nurse's care did not meet accepted standards of care. In turn, the nurse presents evidence that the standard of care was provided. But if for some reason the nurse's evidence is not believable—and there can be many reasons why it is not—the jury will accept the patient's evidence. The patient's attorney may then convince the jury that the nurse was negligent.

Was It Negligence?

If the nurse did act negligently and the nurse's charting truthfully reflects the care he or she gave, the patient record will be the attorney's best evidence against the nurse—as it should be. These cases are often settled out of court. But if the nurse was not negligent, a carefully and accurately charted patient record is the nurse's best defense.

The problem is that sloppy charting practices can make a nurse appear negligent even when he or she is not. That is an important point to remember: If the nurse's charting is unclear, is incomplete, or conveys a negative attitude toward the patient, the jury may perceive the nurse as negligent, even if the nurse gave the patient excellent care.

The nurse can help to protect him- or herself by knowing how to chart, what to chart, when to chart, and even who should chart. The nurse should also know how to handle sensitive issues, such as difficult or uncooperative patients, and how to avoid misinterpreting medical records. Remember, it is not only what the nurse charts but also how the nurse charts that is important.

Keep It Objective

The nurse's documentation should contain only objective, verifiable information, not opinion. If the nurse charts information that is subjective, the nurse should be sure to back it up with documented facts. For example, the nurse should not record that a patient fell out of bed unless the nurse actually saw the patient fall. If the nurse finds the patient lying on the floor, that is what the nurse should record. If the patient tells the nurse that he fell out of bed, that is what the nurse should record. If the nurse heard a thud, went to the room, and found the patient on the floor, that is what the nurse should record.

Describe events and behaviors clearly, without putting labels on them. For example, the nurse should not say that the patient was "saying strange things" or "acting weird" because this could mean something different to every member of the jury. Instead, the nurse should record exactly what the patient said or did; the nurse should not comment on what he or she thought about it.

(continued)

Be Specific

The nurse should use only approved abbreviations and should document in quantifiable terms. If the patient is in pain, for example, the nurse should not just record that the patient appears to be in pain. The nurse should record why the patient is in pain: "Pt. requested pain medication after stating that she felt lower back pain radiating to her right leg, 6 on a scale of 0 to 10. No numbness or tingling, no edema. Color of extremity pink, temperature warm."

Remain Neutral

The nurse should not use negative words to describe the patient or patient actions. If the nurse uses unflattering words like *obnoxious*, *bizarre*, or *drunk*, it is only too easy for the patient's attorney to convince a jury that the nurse did not like the patient and, therefore, did not take good care of the patient. If the patient is uncooperative, for example, the nurse should not chart "Pt. is uncooperative"; instead, the nurse should record what the patient says or does and let the facts tell the story: "I attempted to give the patient his medication, but he said, 'I have had enough pills. Leave me alone.' I attempted to find out why he wouldn't take his medication, but he wouldn't answer me. Patient's health care provider notified that he would not take medication." Likewise, the nurse should not simply record that the patient was drunk; instead, the nurse should record the results of a blood-alcohol test or that the patient refused to consent to one. Nor should the nurse say that a patient was violent or abusive without describing exactly what the patient said or did.

Keep the Record Intact

The nurse must be careful to keep patient charts complete and intact. A jury will be suspicious if pages from a medical record are discarded, even if the nurse did it for innocent reasons, such as spilled coffee or a torn page.

If an original page must be replaced with a copy, the nurse should cross-reference it with a note like "Recopied from page 4" or "Recopied on page 6." Make sure to attach the original page. If a page is damaged, note "Reconstructed charting," and attach the damaged page.

Avoiding Assumptions

The nurse should always record the facts about patients, not his or her own thoughts or conclusions. In the following example, the nurse did not document the facts. Instead the nurse documented opinion and assumption.

Attorney: Would you please read your fifth entry from January 6?
Nurse: Patient fell out of bed...
Attorney: Thank you. Did you see the patient fall out of his bed?
Nurse: No.
Attorney: Did anyone see the patient fall out of his bed?
Nurse: Not that I know of.
Attorney: So these notes reflect only what you assume happened to the patient. Is that correct?
Nurse: I guess so.
Attorney: Is it fair to say, then, that you charted something as fact even though you didn't know that it was?
Nurse: I suppose so.
Attorney: Thank you.

Adapted from Special Report: *How to Properly Document to Reduce Your Liability Risk.*

The NANDA International Nursing Diagnoses

This is a list of Nursing Diagnoses and Domains according to NANDA-International 2018-2020.

DOMAIN 1. HEALTH PROMOTION

Class 1. Health awareness

- Decreased diversional activity engagement
- Readiness for enhanced health literacy
- Sedentary lifestyle

Class 2. Health management

- Frail elderly syndrome
- Risk for frail elderly syndrome
- Deficient community health
- Risk-prone health behavior
- Ineffective health maintenance
- Ineffective health management
- Readiness for enhanced health management
- Ineffective family health management
- Ineffective protection

DOMAIN 2. NUTRITION

Class 1. Ingestion

- Imbalanced nutrition: less than body requirements
- Readiness for enhanced nutrition
- Insufficient breast milk production
- Ineffective breastfeeding
- Interrupted breastfeeding
- Readiness for enhanced breastfeeding
- Ineffective adolescent eating dynamics
- Ineffective child eating dynamics
- Ineffective infant feeding dynamics

- Ineffective infant feeding pattern
- Obesity
- Overweight
- Risk for overweight
- Impaired swallowing

Class 2. Digestion

This class does not currently contain any diagnoses

Class 3. Absorption

This class does not currently contain any diagnoses

Class 4. Metabolism

- Risk for unstable blood glucose level
- Neonatal hyperbilirubinemia
- Risk for neonatal hyperbilirubinemia
- Risk for impaired liver function
- Risk for metabolic imbalance syndrome

Class 5. Hydration

- Risk for electrolyte imbalance
- Risk for imbalanced fluid volume
- Risk for deficient fluid volume
- Excess fluid volume

DOMAIN 3. ELIMINATION AND EXCHANGE

Class 1. Urinary function

- Impaired urinary elimination
- Functional urinary incontinence
- Overflow urinary incontinence
- Reflex urinary incontinence
- Stress urinary incontinence
- Urge urinary incontinence
- Risk for urge urinary incontinence
- Urinary retention

Class 2. Gastrointestinal function

- Constipation
- Risk for constipation

- Perceived constipation
- Chronic functional constipation
- Risk for chronic functional constipation
- Diarrhea
- Dysfunctional gastrointestinal motility
- Risk for dysfunctional gastrointestinal motility
- Bowel incontinence

Class 3. Integumentary system

This class does not currently contain any diagnoses

Class 4. Respiratory function

- Impaired gas exchange

DOMAIN 4. ACTIVITY/REST

Class 1. Sleep/rest

- Insomnia
- Sleep deprivation
- Readiness for enhanced sleep
- Disturbed sleep pattern

Class 2. Activity/exercise

- Risk for disuse syndrome
- Impaired bed mobility
- Impaired physical mobility
- Impaired sitting
- Impaired standing
- Impaired transfer ability
- Impaired walking

Class 3. Energy balance

- Impaired energy field
- Fatigue
- Wandering

Class 4. Cardiovascular/pulmonary responses

- Activity intolerance
- Risk for activity intolerance
- Ineffective breathing pattern

- Decreased cardiac output
- Risk for decreased cardiac output
- Impaired spontaneous ventilation
- Risk for unstable blood pressure
- Risk for decreased cardiac tissue perfusion
- Risk for ineffective cerebral tissue perfusion
- Ineffective peripheral tissue perfusion
- Risk for ineffective peripheral tissue perfusion
- Dysfunctional ventilatory weaning response

Class 5. Self-care

- Impaired home maintenance
- Bathing self-care deficit
- Dressing self-care deficit
- Feeding self-care deficit
- Toileting self-care deficit
- Readiness for enhanced self-care
- Self-neglect

DOMAIN 5. PERCEPTION/COGNITION

Class 1. Attention

- Unilateral neglect

Class 2. Orientation

This class currently does not contain any diagnoses

Class 3. Sensation/Perception

This class currently does not contain any diagnoses

Class 4. Cognition

- Acute confusion
- Risk for acute confusion
- Chronic confusion
- Labile emotional control
- Ineffective impulse control
- Deficient knowledge
- Readiness for enhanced knowledge
- Impaired memory

Class 5. Communication

- Readiness for enhanced communication
- Impaired verbal communication

DOMAIN 6. SELF-PERCEPTION

Class 1. Self-concept

- Hopelessness
- Readiness for enhanced hope
- Risk for compromised human dignity
- Disturbed personal identity
- Risk for disturbed personal identity
- Readiness for enhanced self-concept

Class 2. Self-esteem

- Chronic low self-esteem
- Risk for chronic low self-esteem
- Situational low self-esteem
- Risk for situational low self-esteem

Class 3. Body image

- Disturbed body image

DOMAIN 7: ROLE RELATIONSHIP

Class 1. Caregiving roles

- Caregiver role strain
- Risk for caregiver role strain
- Impaired parenting
- Risk for impaired parenting
- Readiness for enhanced parenting

Class 2. Family relationships

- Risk for impaired attachment
- Dysfunctional family processes
- Interrupted family processes
- Readiness for enhanced family processes

Class 3. Role performance

- Ineffective relationship
- Risk for ineffective relationship
- Readiness for enhanced relationship
- Parental role conflict
- Ineffective role performance
- Impaired social interaction

DOMAIN 8. SEXUALITY

Class 1. Sexual Identity

This class currently does not contain any diagnoses

Class 2. Sexual function

- Sexual dysfunction
- Ineffective sexuality pattern

Class 3. Reproduction

- Ineffective childbearing process
- Risk for ineffective childbearing process
- Readiness for enhanced childbearing process
- Risk for disturbed maternal-fetal dyad

DOMAIN 9. COPING/STRESS TOLERANCE

Class 1. Post-trauma responses

- Risk for complicated immigration transition
- Post-trauma syndrome
- Risk for post-trauma syndrome
- Rape trauma syndrome
- Relocation stress syndrome
- Risk for relocation stress syndrome

Class 2. Coping responses

- Ineffective activity planning
- Risk for ineffective activity planning
- Anxiety
- Defensive coping

- Ineffective coping
- Readiness for enhanced coping
- Compromised family coping
- Disabled family coping
- Readiness for enhanced family coping
- Death anxiety
- Ineffective denial
- Fear
- Grieving
- Complicated grieving
- Risk for complicated grieving
- Impaired mood regulation
- Powerlessness
- Risk for powerlessness
- Readiness for enhanced power
- Impaired resilience
- Risk for impaired resilience
- Readiness of enhanced resilience
- Chronic sorrow
- Stress overload

Class 3. Neurobehavioral Stress

- Acute substance withdrawal syndrome
- Risk for acute substance withdrawal syndrome
- Autonomic dysreflexia
- Risk for autonomic dysreflexia
- Decreased intracranial adaptive capacity
- Neonatal abstinence syndrome
- Disorganized infant behavior
- Risk for disorganized infant behavior
- Readiness for enhanced organized infant behavior

DOMAIN 10. LIFE PRINCIPLES

Class 1. Values

This class currently does not contain any diagnoses

Class 2. Beliefs

- Readiness for enhanced spiritual well-being

Class 3. Value/belief/action congruence

- Readiness for enhanced decision-making
- Decisional conflict
- Impaired emancipated decision-making
- Risk for impaired emancipated decision-making
- Readiness for enhanced emancipated decision-making
- Moral distress
- Impaired religiosity
- Risk for impaired religiosity
- Readiness for enhanced religiosity
- Spiritual distress
- Risk for spiritual distress

DOMAIN 11. SAFETY/PROTECTION

Class 1. Infection

- Risk for infection
- Risk for surgical infection

Class 2. Physical injury

- Ineffective airway clearance
- Risk for aspiration
- Risk for bleeding
- Impaired dentition
- Risk for dry eye
- Risk for dry mouth
- Risk for falls
- Risk for corneal injury
- Risk for injury
- Risk for urinary tract injury
- Risk for perioperative positioning injury
- Risk for thermal injury
- Impaired oral mucous membrane integrity
- Risk for impaired oral mucous membrane integrity
- Risk for peripheral neurovascular dysfunction
- Risk for physical trauma
- Risk for vascular trauma
- Risk for pressure ulcer

- Risk for shock
- Impaired skin integrity
- Risk for impaired skin integrity
- Risk for sudden infant death
- Risk for suffocation
- Delayed surgical recovery
- Risk for delayed surgical recovery
- Impaired tissue integrity
- Risk for impaired tissue integrity
- Risk for venous thromboembolism

Class 3. Violence

- Risk for female genital mutilation
- Risk for other-directed violence
- Risk for self-directed violence
- Self-mutilation
- Risk for self-mutilation
- Risk for suicide

Class 4. Environmental hazards

- Contamination
- Risk for contamination
- Risk for occupational injury
- Risk for poisoning

Class 5. Defensive processes

- Risk for adverse reaction to iodinated contrast media
- Risk for allergic reaction
- Latex allergic reaction
- Risk for latex allergic reaction

Class 6. Thermoregulation

- Hyperthermia
- Hypothermia
- Risk for hypothermia
- Risk for perioperative hypothermia
- Ineffective thermoregulation
- Risk for ineffective thermoregulation

DOMAIN 12. COMFORT

Class 1. Physical comfort

- Impaired comfort
- Readiness for enhanced comfort
- Nausea
- Acute pain
- Chronic pain
- Chronic pain syndrome
- Labor pain

Class 2. Environmental comfort

- Impaired comfort
- Readiness for enhanced comfort

Class 3. Social comfort

- Impaired comfort
- Readiness for enhanced comfort
- Risk for loneliness
- Social isolation

DOMAIN 13. GROWTH/DEVELOPMENT

Class 1. Growth

This class currently does not contain diagnoses

Class 2. Development

- Risk for delayed development

Index

Note: Locators followed by 'i' refers to an illustration and 't' refers to a table